Kennedy's PAEDIATRIC OPERATIVE DE

Kennedy's PAEDIATRIC OPERATIVE DENTISTRY

Fourth Edition

M. E. J. CURZON BDS (Lon), MS(Rochester), PhD (Lon), FRCD (Canada), FDSRCS (England)

Professor of Child Dental Health, University of Leeds.
Consultant in Paediatric Dentistry,
Leeds General Infirmary, Leeds, England.
Formerly Senior Clinical Instructor in Pediatric Dentistry,
Eastman Dental Center, Rochester, New York.

J. F. ROBERTS BDS (Bristol), Cert Pediatric Dentistry, Eastman Dental Center, Rochester, New York

Private Practitioner in Paediatric Dentistry, London.
Visiting Lecturer in Paediatric Dentistry, University of Leeds.
Clinical Senior Lecturer in Paediatric Dentistry,
Guy's Hospital, London, England.

D. B. KENNEDY BDS (Lon), LDSRCS (England), MSD (Indiana), MSD (Washington), FRCD (Canada), FACD

Private Practitioner in Paediatric Dentistry and Orthodontics,
Vancouver and Richmond, British Columbia, Canada.
Guest Lecturer, Department of Restorative Dentistry,
Faculty of Dentistry, University of British Columbia, Vancouver.
Formerly Chief Examiner in Paediatric Dentistry,
Royal College of Dentists of Canada.
Formerly Lecturer in Paediatric Dentistry, Guy's Hospital, London.
Visiting Lecturer in Orthodontics, University of Washington, Seattle, Washington.

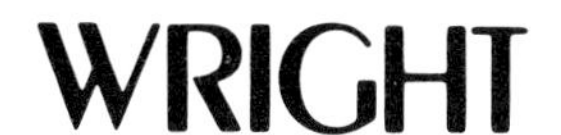

Wright
An imprint of Butterworth-Heinemann
Linacre House, Jordan Hill, Oxford OX2 8DP
A division of Reed Educational & Professional Publishing Ltd

A member of the Reed Elsevier plc group

OXFORD LONDON BOSTON

NEW DELHI SINGAPORE SYDNEY

TOKYO TORONTO WELLINGTON

First published by John Wright & Sons Ltd 1976
Second edition 1979
Third edition 1986
Reprinted 1992
Fourth edition 1996

British Library Cataloguing in Publication Data
A catalogue record for this book is
available from the British Library

Library of Congress Cataloguing in Publication Data
A catalogue record for this book is
available from the Library of Congress

ISBN 0 7236 1016 9

Typeset by Bath Typesetting Ltd
Printed and bound in Great Britain at the Bath Press, Avon

Contents

Preface to the fourth edition

The opportunity to prepare a fourth edition of this book has enabled a number of changes to be made, taking into account the many improvements in operative dentistry for children that have come about during the last 10 years. The addition of two more authors has brought to the text enhanced expertise and experience in clinical paediatric dentistry. The information and advice given here is based upon extensive, day-to-day clinical practice by all three authors within their respective practices. The book has also been expanded up to 20 chapters, principally in the area of pulp therapy for primary teeth, now so important in the preservation of such teeth. All other chapters have been rewritten and the opportunity taken to update the material and provide new illustrations where needed.

Our aim throughout has been to give guidance on quality restorative care for children. We firmly believe that each and every child, should they develop dental caries, deserves the best care that dentistry can give. We hope that this book will aid undergraduate dental students to develop the skills to carry out quality dentistry. Postgraduate dentists and general dental practitioners, we also hope, will benefit from this text in understanding the principles and standards to be achieved in paediatric dentistry.

We are very grateful to the publishers for giving us the opportunity to prepare this new edition. The support and patience of our wives and staff during the preparation of this book has been very much appreciated.

M.E.J.C.
J.F.R.
D.B.K.

Preface to the first edition

Many parents do not recognize the importance of restoring the primary dentition. Yet malocclusions can sometimes be attributed to the premature loss of primary teeth, or aggravated by that loss. Paediatric dentistry can play a vital role in the dental development of the young patient by providing natural space maintainers for the permanent teeth and by instilling in the child positive attitudes towards oral health.

Operative dentistry is just one aspect of overall dental health care for the child. However, it requires the utmost in technical skill and attention to detail. It cannot be divorced from epidemiology, diagnosis, treatment planning, behaviour management and preventive care. This book in no way attempts to cover all aspects of paediatric dentistry, rather it is limited to all facets of operative dentistry concerning the primary and young permanent dentition. Cavity preparations are described in detail and variations from previously accepted norms justified. An attempt has been made to justify each particular procedure by identifying the indications, contraindications, and reasons for success or failure.

The book is subdivided into chapters dealing with specific topics so that the practitioner can quickly refer to a particular area to find assistance for his problem. The glossary may help remind or update him regarding terminology which may be hazy in his memory. This subdivision may also be of value to the dental student, either during his review or as supplementary reading for a technique course on paediatric operative dentistry. Because of the organization of material by topic, there will be repetition in areas which overlap; perhaps the reader will consider this as reinforcement of important information.

The philosophy of providing the highest standard of care is presented, together with practical hints which help attain this goal. Whilst references to scientific studies support the text, every effort has been made to make the book of practical value by providing solutions to everyday problems. These practical hints can be readily incorporated into a busy practice.

D. B. K.

Acknowledgements

This book has involved the time and support of a number of colleagues and associates during its preparation and revision. Firstly, we wish to thank Mary Seager of Butterworth-Heinemann for encourgaing us to undertake the preparation of the fourth edition and her patience during its gestation. Secondly, as each chapter completed its revision by us it has been reviewed by a colleague and we wish to acknowledge the effort and dedication of Monty Duggal, Stephen Fayle, Elizabeth O'Sullivan, Maxine Pollard, Jack Toumba and Callum Youngson. Peter Hirschmann has contributed advice on radiographic techniques and Gavin Fairpo has been most helpful in sorting out the problems of computer transfer of the texts. Their comments and suggestions have been invaluable.

Many of the line drawings and photographs have been redrawn or replaced. The drawings have been expertly done by Anna Durban of the University of Leeds Audio-Visual Department and the photographs by Angus Robertson and Simon Charters of the Leeds Dental Institute Photographic and Illustration Department. We are indebted to them for their patience and willingness to achieve what we wanted.

PART I

Principles of restorative care for children

CHAPTER 1

The basis for paediatric operative dentistry

A rationale for the preservation of primary teeth

The preservation of the primary dentition until its normal, anticipated exfoliation can be justified on the following grounds:

- maintenance of arch length;
- maintenance and improvement of appearance;
- maintenance of a healthy oral environment;
- psychology of keeping teeth;
- prevention and relief of pain;
- function of chewing and speech.

Maintenance of arch length

Premature loss of primary molars is a local aetiological factor in the development of a malocclusion. Usually orthodontists recommend the preservation of primary teeth since the best space maintainer is the retained healthy primary tooth. While the preservation of the primary dentition will not always prevent a malocclusion, it will usually make it less severe. In addition, the permanent molar relationship will be symmetrically maintained, an important consideration when assessing the difficulty of active orthodontic treatment. On the other hand, the premature loss of primary molars often aggravates a developing malocclusion. The effect of the premature loss is to reveal and localize any crowding that is present (Houston et al., 1992). This can be used to the patient's advantage in the planned extraction of primary teeth, such as the extraction of primary canines so that permanent incisors erupt into better alignment. It is to be hoped that much space closure and concurrent correction of crowding will occur spontaneously to reduce the need for subsequent appliance therapy.

Early loss of primary molars causes more severe effects than the early loss of primary incisors. Usually, the greater the degree of initial crowding present, the greater the likelihood of space loss when a primary tooth is lost. As a rule, the earlier the tooth is lost, the more severe the effects. Conversely, the older the child, the less serious the effects. It is more harmful to lose a second primary molar at age 3 than at age 8 years. The location of the lost primary tooth is also significant. In the mixed dentition, the loss of those primary teeth adjacent to permanent teeth produces a more serious problem. At the distal aspect of the primary dentition the first permanent molar is prevented from mesial migration by the presence of the primary molars. Therefore the premature loss of the second primary molar can have drastic consequences if it occurs before or during the eruption of the first permanent molar. The mesial migration of the first permanent molar, if not prevented, will result in the second premolar (which erupts later) being blocked out lingually from the arch.

Adjacent to the permanent incisors in the mixed dentition is the primary canine. Its premature loss can, under conditions of crowding and adverse musculature, encourage deviation of the centre line in the maxillary arch and deepening of the overbite by tipping of the permanent incisors distally and lingually in the mandibular arch. Although this discussion has been mainly directed towards the effects of extraction, it should be recognized that mesial migration of posterior teeth can occur as a result of interproximal caries.

The effects of premature loss of primary incisors on the developing occlusion are usually negligible. Once the primary canines are fully erupted (at about age 3 years), no space loss is likely to follow removal of primary incisors. This does not apply to the period of infancy (under 3 years of age) when the retention of primary incisors prior to the eruption of primary canines is justified. This is because their early removal would encourage the primary canines to assume a more mesial position and thus impinge upon space for the permanent incisors. Their maintenance is also justified on the basis of appearance.

Maintenance of a healthy oral environment

Two groups of micro-organisms, lactobacilli and mutans streptococci, have been closely linked with the carious process as based on Miller's chemicoparasitic theory (Marsh, 1993). Their presence in the oral cavity in excessive numbers is not considered beneficial. It has been proven that restoration of carious lesions reduces the count of these bacteria in the oral flora (Alalusuua et al., 1987). Children with a low prevalence of decay usually have low counts. Thus, reducing oral micro-organisms by restorative dentistry to the primary dentition may indirectly reduce the incidence of decay in the permanent dentition. Nikiforuk and Pulver (1969), in a review article, reported that there was an infective, transmissible factor in dental caries; it may be that the organisms present in untreated lesions of primary teeth are partially responsible for the caries in adjacent permanent teeth. Irrespective of this, there is generally a proportional relationship between caries in the primary dentition and the caries that occurs later in the same child's permanent dentition, although in individual children this may not always be so. In children from certain immigrant groups in the UK, high levels of caries in primary teeth are often not followed by corresponding levels in the permanent teeth.

Restoring carious primary teeth will certainly improve the health of the oral environment and a sound, healthy dentition may be far reaching in its good effects. For example, parents frequently complain that their child has a poor appetite. A child does not want to eat if teeth hurt every time he or she chews. While many children manage to eat without a full complement of teeth, few can function properly when their teeth are ravaged by caries. A restoration to correct occlusion and contour, and the alleviation of pain and discomfort, can allow the child to enjoy proper function during mastication. Once function has been restored and pain and infection eliminated, these children will be able to enjoy eating harder, more detergent food. In our experience parents sometimes comment that growth improves once the dentition has been restored to full function.

Psychology of tooth extraction

The extraction of teeth implies that they are unimportant. For far too long the philosophy that primary teeth are of no importance and if decayed should be left or extracted has conditioned some people to think that teeth are not necessary and even an encumbrance to be 'got rid of' at the earliest opportunity. Indeed within the last generation in parts of the North of England, Scotland, in New England (USA) and in the maritime provinces of Canada, total tooth extraction was considered the best twenty-first birthday present. The rationale was that once they had all been removed, there would be no further trouble with teeth. Undoubtedly this attitude has not been helped by the over-willingness of some dentists to resort to extraction of the primary teeth, thus engendering a lifelong poor attitude to dental health.

By making all efforts to restore and preserve the primary dentition the psychological message imparted is 'teeth are important'. The authors have noted time and time again, within their practices, that the restoration of the primary teeth brings about a complete change of attitude to dental health care. It cannot be emphasized too strongly the need to keep the primary dentition intact no matter how carious it is.

It has also been our experience that mothers of children with nursing-bottle caries can become much more positive in their attitudes towards the problem if the teeth are restored.

Restoration of broken-down maxillary incisors not only restores the appearance but emphasizes prevention.

Prevention and relief of pain

From the viewpoint of both the child and the dentist, the prevention of pain is more desirable and easier to handle than its relief. One of the most difficult problems that the dentist faces daily is the need to provide emergency treatment for patients in pain. Management of the child presents a great problem since the child's awareness of dental problems is significantly correlated with a negative behavioural response (Wright et al., 1983). The lack of sleep, restlessness and distress from toothache unfavourably influence the child's behaviour. The dentist must then attempt to relieve the pain of a child who is not receptive to treatment. Furthermore, the emergency patient often has to be accommodated into an already busy daily schedule, often at the expense of other patients presenting for routine care. Depending on the ability of the child, the dentist, and the parent to cope with the situation, a traumatic early dental experience may occur which can unfavourably condition the child against dentistry for a lifetime.

Prevention of pain is the key to success. Treatment can then be performed on a more cooperative child; furthermore, when lesions are diagnosed early, the operative dentistry is less extensive, easier to do and less time-consuming.

Maintenance and improvement of appearance

No one can be sure of the real value of the dentition to an individual since different people have different attitudes towards their teeth, both in terms of appearance and function. Parents are certainly aware of the cosmetic value of orthodontic treatment and of the aesthetic restoration of anterior teeth. Children, too, are becoming more aware of their appearance, perhaps because they live in an era of acute peer evaluation. Children want to be like everyone else; they want to avoid ridicule and criticism from their peers. Much criticism may be directed towards unsightly teeth and may be psychologically traumatic. Older children can certainly express their desires for an aesthetic smile to be like their peers. However, the younger preschool child seldom has that ability because of a limited vocabulary and the strong parental influences exerted at this age. Our personal experience in the aesthetic restoration of primary incisors with strip crowns (Chapter 11) has been most favourable.

Function of the primary dentition and speech

Parents often associate the premature loss of primary incisors with the development of speech problems such as lisping. They should be reassured that usually no permanent habits result from such loss. Any lisping that might follow primary incisor removal will often be reversible when the permanent incisors erupt. All children go through the transition from primary to mixed dentition during which they are temporarily without incisors, but most do not develop permanent speech anomalies, demonstrating the adaptability of the tongue. It should be remembered that the child's speech is developed between 18 and 36 months of age.

The extent of the problem

Paediatric operative dentistry cannot be divorced from epidemiology, diagnosis, behaviour guidance, treatment planning and preventive care. Population groups most susceptible to dental caries should be identified from epidemiological data. The clinician then targets susceptible areas for each age group and tooth type during the clinical examination.

Epidemiology

The prevalence and incidence of a disease refer to the number of individuals showing evidence of that disease either at one point in time (prevalence) or the change in the extent over a period of time (incidence).

The experience of dental decay in a community is measured by evaluating the total effects of the carious process (past and present) up to the time of the examination. It is measured in terms of Decayed, Missing, or Filled Teeth or Surfaces (DMFT or DMFS) for permanent teeth, using capital letters. For primary teeth, the index of decayed, extracted (or indicated for extraction) or filled teeth and surfaces using lower case letters (deft or defs) is usual. These definitions serve as references for the following material.

Epidemiological surveys from many parts of the Western world indicate that dental caries experience among children and young adults has declined since the 1970s. For the majority of children in Western countries the level of dental caries is now low. Nevertheless, when decay does occur, even if in only one tooth in a mouth, it is essential to preserve that tooth. However, in some subpopulations the dental needs of young children are high, and may have started to increase again. These are generally inner-city, low socioeconomic or immigrant groups (Grindefjord et al., 1993). Their restorative dental needs remain high.

In other countries of the world, dental decay is either very prevalent or, if low, may be showing signs of increasing (Marthaler, 1990). In either case there is still a need for high-quality restorative care coupled with the necessary preventive programmes. Therefore, there remains a need for good paediatric dental care in every country. Patterns of treatment will vary by age groups and these are discussed next.

Primary dentition (age 0–2 years, infancy)

About 8% of 2-year-olds exhibit dental caries and 5% will have one or more obvious carious lesions (Wendt et al., 1991). Nursing caries remains a problem affecting between 5% and 10% of children even in Western societies (Curzon and Pollard, 1994). It is therefore essential to carry out a full examination of the primary dentition as soon as the teeth have started to erupt, usually by the end of the first year of life. The use of a mirror and blunt explorer (so as not to damage the enamel on probing) is essential in the diagnostic process. When posterior contacts are closed, bitewing radiographs are essential for the detection of interproximal caries (*Fig.* 1.1). In the absence of bitewing radiographs, as many as 75% of interproximal lesions may be undetected (Kidd and Pitts, 1990). It has also been shown that bitewing radiographs identify, with clinical examination, 82% of occlusal caries in first permanent molars (Ketley and Holt, 1993).

Nursing-bottle mouth syndrome or nursing caries

Two interesting facts arise from the review by Ripa (1988). First, a greater caries prevalence has been noted in the lower social groups; this has been confirmed by others (Dilley et al., 1980; Johnsen et al., 1984). Second, the aetiological role of certain feeding habits was identified. In cases of nursing-bottle caries, the mean age for discontinuation of the bottle was 23±2 months, compared with the recommended discontinuation at age 12 months (Dilley et al., 1980). These feeding habits may produce a condition in infants and young children known as nursing-bottle mouth syndrome. The cause is traced to prolonged use of natural or artificial drinks and juices containing sugars (sucrose, fructose, glucose or lactose) that are often syrupy in texture, taken from a nursing bottle. Milk with sugar added is also a problem. Such drinks are given in a reservoir feeder, pacifier, or 'dinky cup' (Winter et al., 1971). Although sweetened syrups and juices are the most common culprits, unsweetened milk has the potential to produce dental caries if left stagnant over the tooth surfaces for a sufficient time. Indeed, Dilley et al. (1980) found that milk was the predominantly used liquid in their study of 75 patients with nursing-bottle decay. In fact, prolonged nursing with human milk from 'at will' breast-feeding can

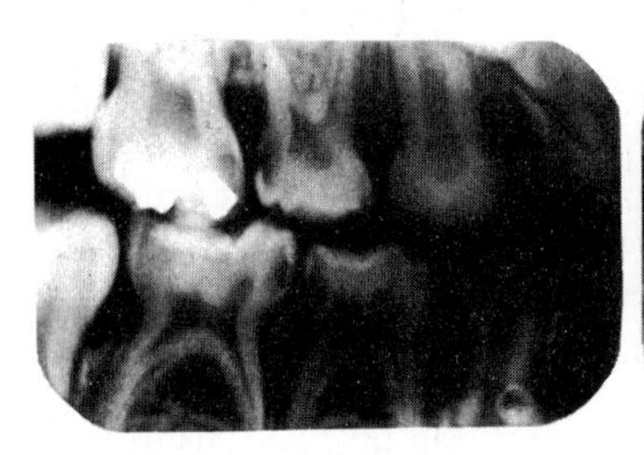
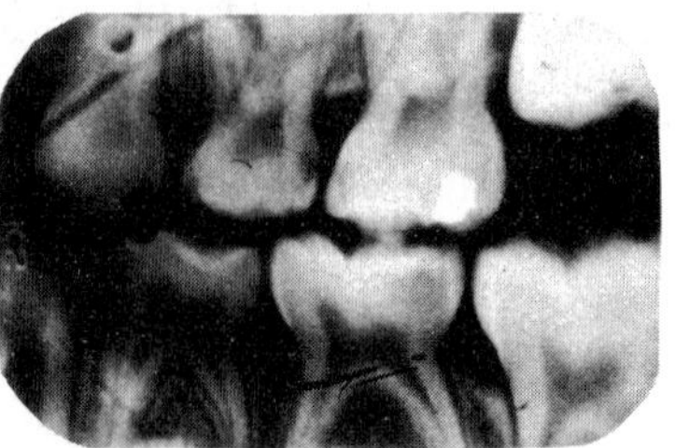

Fig. 1.1. Bitewings of 5-year-old demonstrating interproximal lesions in all four quadrants.

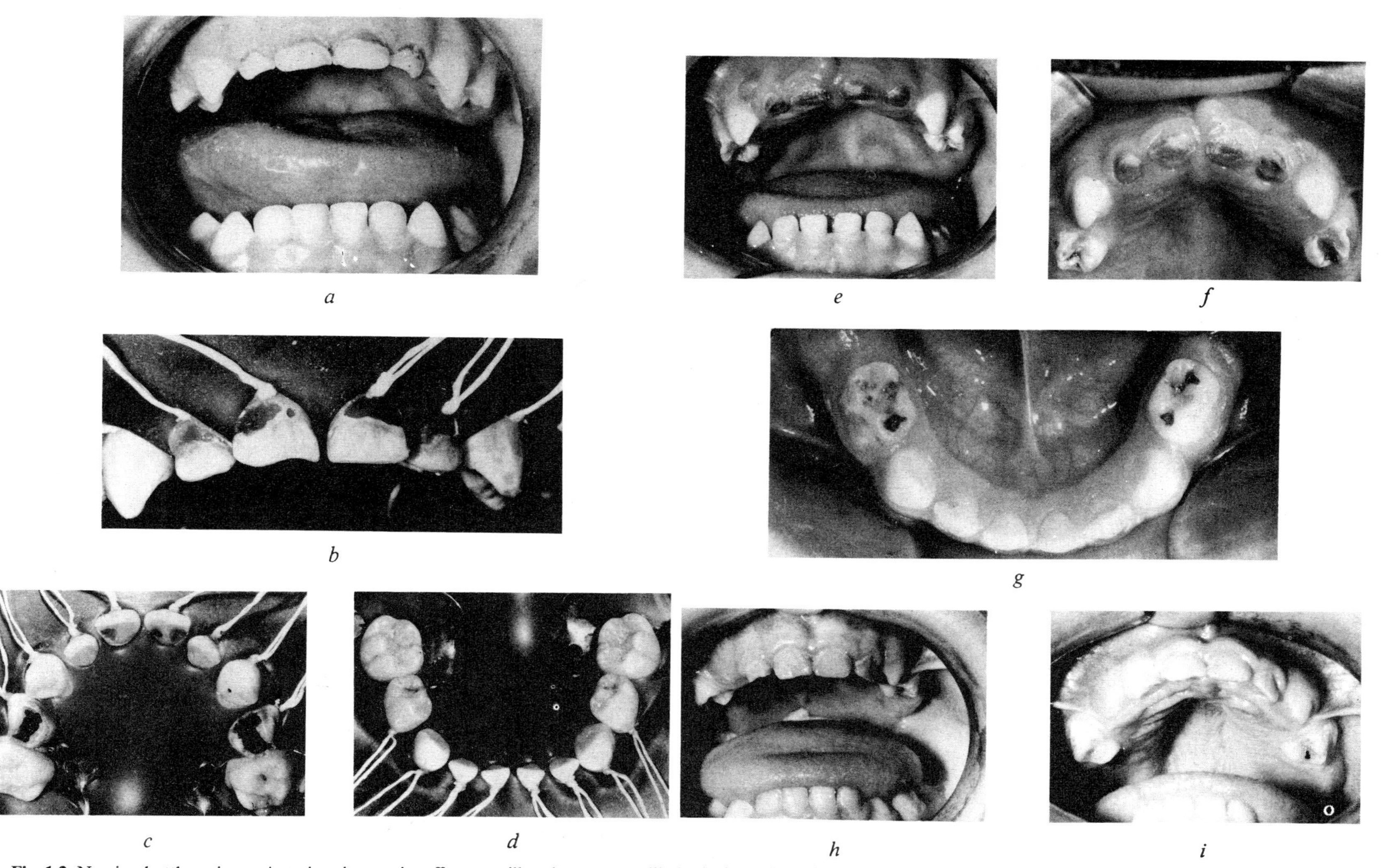

Fig. 1.2. Nursing-bottle caries. *a*, Anterior view: caries affects maxillary but not mandibular incisors. Age 20 months with apple juice in a bottle when going to bed. *b*, *c*, *d*. More extensive case. Age 26 months with apple juice in bottle when going to bed. *b*, Anterior view: class 5 lesions. *c*, Maxillary view: caries affects first primary molar more than primary canine or second primary molar. *d*, Mandibular view. Incisors are not affected. Occlusal surfaces of first primary molars carious. *e*, *f*, *g*, Severe case. Age 18 months with juice in bottle when going to bed and honey on dummy/pacifier. *e*, Anterior view. Crowns destroyed to gingival margin. *f*, Maxillary view. Note destruction of primary molars also. *g*, Mandibular view. *h*, *i*, Nursing caries in a case of 'at-will' breast feeding. Age 19 months. *h*, Anterior view. *i*, Maxillary view.

also produce decay in infants (Roberts, 1982; Curzon and Drummond, 1987). The pattern of carious attack is identical to nursing-bottle caries (*Fig.* 1.2). Indeed, parents may require exhaustive questioning to reveal the true aetiology of the condition. Nursing caries affects primarily the labial surfaces of the maxillary primary incisors and the occlusal surfaces of the first primary molars (Curzon and Pollard, 1994) (*Fig.* 1.2). The anterior lesions, if untreated, will encompass the lingual and interproximal areas of the maxillary incisors in a circumferential manner. By nature of the suckling habit, the lower lip protects the mandibular incisors. The primary canines and second primary molars are rarely affected, owing to the eruption sequence combined with the cessation of the feeding habit. Decreased salivary flow during sleep aggravates the condition by reducing the diluting and buffering effects of the saliva.

The description above refers to the initial clinical appearance of nursing-bottle mouth. If the lesions are left untreated, tooth destruction continues so that eventually the maxillary primary incisors may be flush with the gingiva (*Fig.* 1.2*e,g*). The parents may present their child for treatment at this stage reporting that 'the teeth came in soft and brown and just broke off'. Such a history may lead to the inaccurate diagnosis of a developmental anomaly of the primary dentition.

Nursing caries differs in aetiology from the extensive carious lesions seen in the primary molars of preschool and school-age children (*Figs* 1.3 and 1.4). In this instance, the extensive tooth destruction may not necessarily be traced to infant feeding habits if the second primary molars are decayed. Rather, a detailed account of the child's dietary habits may reveal a craving for foods high in refined carbohydrates, often as snacks. Frequent use of these foods has been shown to be responsible for a higher incidence of decay (Gustafsson et al., 1954).

When the parents are unaware or apathetic about the need to seek dental care at an early age, the tooth destruction will continue unimpeded. This condition may be inaccurately labelled as rampant caries while it is actually a result of neglect in seeking care. By contrast, rampant caries is a suddenly appearing, widespread, rapidly burrowing type of caries resulting in early involvement of the pulp and affecting those teeth usually regarded as immune to ordinary decay. This often affects the teenager and young adolescent (McDonald and Avery, 1974).

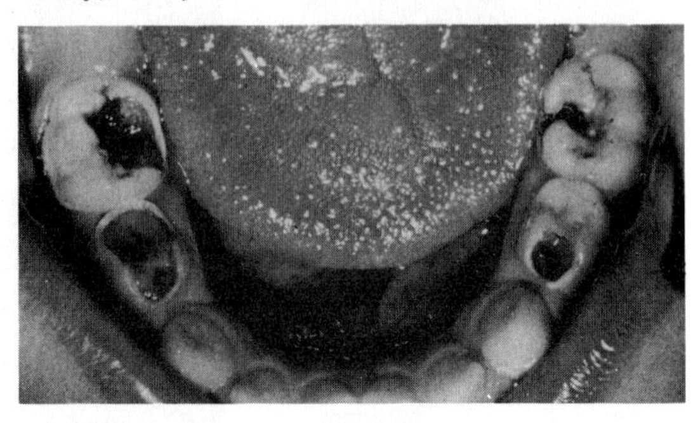

Fig. 1.3. Gross destruction of mandibular primary molars in a 3-year-old child.

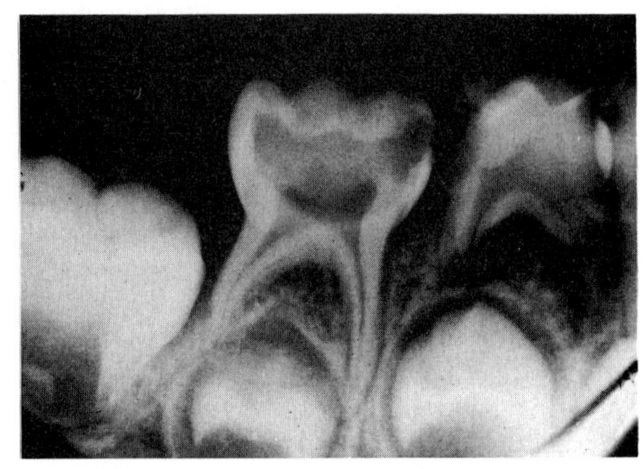

Fig. 1.4. Mandibular periapical radiograph demonstrating large lesions in primary molars of a 3-year-old.

Primary dentition (age 3 years)

For those children who do not have nursing-bottle caries, the prevalence of decay in the primary dentition in the UK has significantly fallen in recent years (OPCS, 1994). In 5-year-olds, the proportion of children with known decay (either decayed or restored teeth) decreased from 71% in 1973 to 48% in 1983 to 47% in 1993, indicating the slowing down of the decline. It should be remembered that epidemiological data taken with the absence of bitewing radiographs may under-report the presence of decay when posterior contacts are closed.

Location of caries – primary dentition (age 3–6 years)

The location and diagnosis of individual lesions are discussed in subsequent chapters, and an

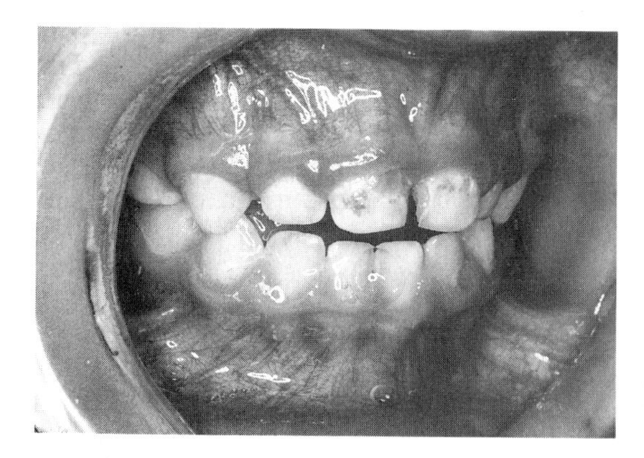

a

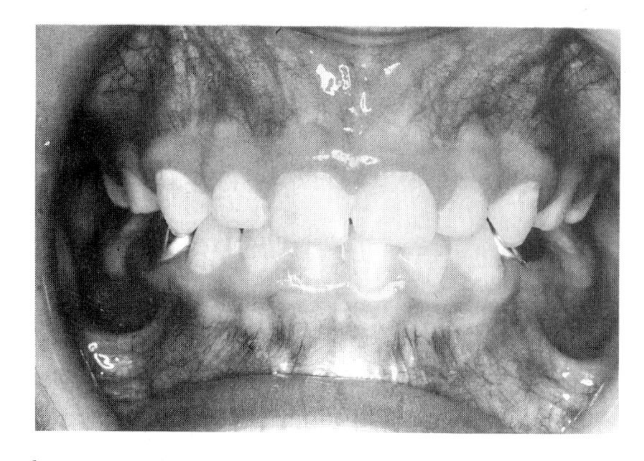

b

Fig. 1.5. *a*, Nursing caries presenting as decay on labial and mesial surfaces of maxillary incisors. *b*, Teeth shown in (*a*) restored with strip crowns (see Chapter 11).

outline only will be given here. Occlusal lesions in primary molars are more common than interproximal lesions in preschool children. In these young children, posterior contacts may not close until age 3 years, which may explain this observation; however, once posterior contacts close, the prevalence of interproximal lesions will increase. Second primary molars have more occlusal lesions than first primary molars, likewise the mandibular molars have more than the maxillary because of the depth and anatomy of the occlusal fissures. The labial and lingual surfaces of primary teeth seldom decay, except in the case of nursing caries (*Fig.* 1.5). Mandibular primary incisors seldom decay, probably because of the spacing that occurs in the area and their close proximity to the ducts of the submandibular salivary gland, which means that they benefit from the diluting and buffering properties of saliva.

Hennon et al. (1969) found the following areas of primary teeth to be most commonly affected by caries:

	Maxillary	*Mandibular*
Second molar	occlusal–lingual	occlusal–buccal
First molar	occlusal	occlusal–buccal
Canine	buccal	buccal
Lateral incisor	mesial	mesial
Central incisor	mesial	mesial

The mixed dentition (age 12 years)

A comparison of studies performed in recent years with those of previous decades reveals a significant decrease of approx. 30–50% in dental decay in children. Similarly, there is a marked increase in the number of decay-free children (Bohanan and Bader, 1984). This reduction in decay is subject to regional variation, e.g. children in Scotland have more decay than those living in the South of England (OPCS, 1994). While the overall decay rate has reduced in prosperous Western countries it appears that certain children are more susceptible than others to developing dental decay. Specifically at age 6 years the US Rand Study (1982) demonstrated that 80% of the dental decay occurred in 20% of children. This should force the clinician to target these children for more stringent diagnostic and preventive procedures. The proportion of 7-year-olds in the UK with decayed or filled permanent teeth continued to decline between 1983 and 1993 (OPCS, 1994). These reductions in decay should not lead to complacency, particularly as they appear to be slowing down and tapering off. Prevention must still remain the main emphasis in the dental care of children, coupled with high-quality restorations when needed.

Location of caries in the mixed dentition

The newly erupted first permanent molars and permanent incisors have areas that are susceptible to plaque retention and subsequent development of caries. These are the occlusal surfaces in permanent molars, the lingual developmental pit and groove in maxillary permanent molars, the buccal developmental pit and groove in mandibular permanent molars and lingual pits in maxillary permanent incisors, notably the lateral incisor. Probably because of the depth and inclination of the occlusal fissures, the mandibular permanent molars decay more frequently than maxillary molars. It has been shown that the best predictor of caries in the permanent molars is the level of caries in the primary dentition (Gray et al., 1991).

In addition to these susceptible areas, the closing of posterior contacts may result in the development of Class 2 lesions. In the mixed dentition the mesial surface of the first permanent molar is placed at risk if caries affects the second primary molar. Also, the interproximal surfaces of maxillary incisors may be at risk in those children with closed anterior contacts and a high caries incidence. Only 16% of the decay experience in 5–11-year-old children occurred interproximally, with 84% of the disease occurring in pit and fissures in North American children in 1981 (Bohanan and Bader, 1984). The effect of fluoride has brought about a marked decline in the number of interproximal lesions in the mixed and young permanent dentition. This has occurred in both fluoridated and non-fluoridated communities, and confirms the belief that occlusal pit and fissure caries is least influenced by fluoride.

The early permanent dentition (age 12–15 years)

There is an unnecessarily high incidence of caries in the young permanent dentition (age 12–15 years) among British schoolchildren. The most recent survey (OPCS, 1994) showed that among 12-year-olds the proportion with active decay fell from 39% in 1983 to 24% in 1993, while among 15-year-olds the same proportions were 42% to 30%, respectively. The proportions for those 14-year-olds with any past or present decay experience fell from 81% to 53% and for 15-year-olds from 93% to 63% between 1983 and 1993. This still means that approximately half of young teenagers have dental decay. The young permanent dentition is thus potentially a time of high caries activity (*Fig.* 1.6), unless measures can be implemented to prevent the disease.

There appears to be a difference in decay rates between North American and UK children in the early permanent dentition. Bohanan and Bader (1984) reported that by age 13 years, 20% of North American children had 60% of the dental decay. This should encourage the clinician to target both diagnostic and preventive procedures for those children at risk. Despite marked reductions in decay in younger children over the past decade, the number of 15-year-olds in the UK with some decay in 1983 was 93%, compared with 97% in 1973 (OPCS, 1984).

Location of caries in the early permanent dentition

In this age group the order of susceptibility of teeth to caries attack is:

(1) first permanent molar (most susceptible);
(2) second permanent molar;
(3) premolars;
(4) maxillary anterior teeth;
(5) canine and mandibular incisors (least susceptible).

There is often a bilateral symmetry of caries attack in these children.

The occlusal surfaces of recently erupted second molars and premolars are susceptible to caries

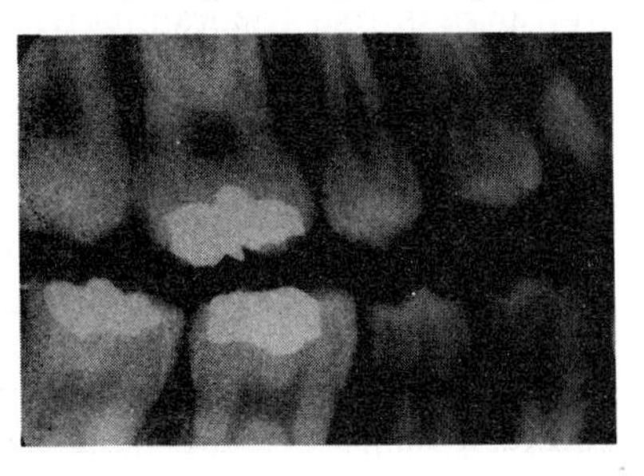

a

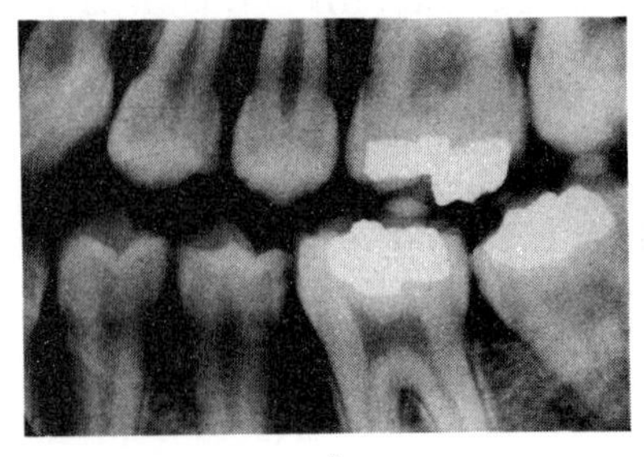

b

Fig. 1.6. Bitewings of a 13-year-old demonstrating developing interproximal lesions between several posterior teeth.

by virtue of their morphology. By comparison, buccal and lingual surfaces of these teeth, together with permanent canines and mandibular incisors, are seldom attacked by caries. The exception to this is the lingual pit of maxillary lateral incisors, which has been reported to be carious in 11% of the 12–15-year-old age group.

There are more occlusal than interproximal lesions in the 12- and 13-year-olds due to the recent eruption of, and early occlusal attack on, second molars and premolars. Certainly the occlusal surface of second permanent molars appears to become carious very quickly after eruption; it is also a clinical impression that the spread of occlusal decay in mandibular second permanent molars is very fast. However, after age 13 years, there is an increased percentage of interproximal compared with occlusal lesions (Berman and Slack, 1973) (*Fig.* 1.6).

Diagnosis

Before any treatment, a thorough examination including appropriate radiographs is necessary to obtain diagnostic records. Also included should be a medical, familial and dental history, and an assessment of the child's co-operative ability, the occlusion and the oral home care.

From the epidemiological surveys the clinician should direct particular attention to those areas that are commonly decayed in the various age groups. The need for bitewing radiographs to diagnose interproximal lesions cannot be overemphasized. When considering interproximal lesions in primary molars, the clinician must remember that the distance between the external enamel surface and pulp is less in primary than permanent teeth (Chapter 2). A Class 2 lesion into dentine on one primary molar surface is often accompanied by enamel decalcification on the interproximal surface of the adjacent primary tooth; such decalcifications, or radiographic etches of enamel, indicate the need for a preventive programme to remineralize these lesions. This may well be possible by the application of fluoride (varnish or gel) to the demineralized surface when the cavity has been cut in the adjacent tooth, but prior to placing the restoration.

Treatment planning

Reference has already been made to diagnostic records and treatment planning (see also Chapter 4). Apart from orthodontic extractions, it is assumed that the dentist will strive to restore the primary dentition to normal contour and function, thus allowing the primary teeth to be the natural space maintainers. Restorable teeth should be saved unless they do not meet the criteria outlined in Chapter 16 for teeth that cannot be saved because of a poor prognosis of pulp pathology.

Dental appointments for the child are inconvenient to the parents because of difficulty with transport, baby-sitting responsibilities for other children, lost time from school for the child and from work for some parents. Therefore, treatment should be planned effectively to minimize the number of visits. Contrary to common opinion in Great Britain, Lenchner's study (1966) does not support the hypothesis that the length of the appointment affects a child's behaviour and attitude towards dentistry. He found that children can tolerate appointments of 48–175 min without significant deterioration in behaviour patterns. His experiences have been routinely replicated in our practices. The operator should therefore be encouraged to make full use of local anaesthetic by performing quadrant dentistry. Full-arch dentistry can also be accomplished for many children, particularly recall patients who may require two Class 1 restorations in first permanent molars.

The prevalence of dental caries will often determine that more than one restoration must be placed in a quadrant, as interproximal caries commonly affects adjacent primary molars simultaneously. When planning treatment, dentists must also take into account the child's past decay experience and the prognosis for co-operation in the preventive recommendations. Incipient lesions should be restored in those caries-active children who require other operative work in that quadrant.

Sequencing of appointments can help in favourably conditioning a child's response to treatment. Unless emergency care is required, the treatment sequencing outlined below is recommended, since it gradually introduces the child to dentistry (see Chapter 4). In some children, the examination and preventive visits can be condensed into one appointment. This is compatible also with the reduced prevalence of dental caries, and addresses the problem of a working parent's busy schedule.

When possible, maxillary teeth should be

treated first since the maxillary infiltration is easier to administer than the mandibular block (see Chapter 6). Also, infiltrations should be less painful for the child, although the experienced dentist should be able to administer a painless block providing topical anaesthesia is used first. The first and also the last appointment of the sequence should be short to give the child confidence initially and to leave a favourable memory of dental treatment finally.

Unfortunately, such sequencing cannot always be arranged when there are extensive lesions or when emergency treatment is required. Emergency treatment should be limited to relief of pain because of the limited tolerance of the child who is distressed by pain and lack of sleep. When possible, extraction should be delayed until pain has been relieved by placement of a temporary dressing or a first-stage pulp treatment (Chapter 16).

Conservative treatment at the emergency visit has substantial advantages. Firstly, pain is relieved and yet the child and parents do not form an association between pain and extraction; secondly, the busy practitioner can schedule a further appointment for complete examination and diagnostic records. Children who present for emergency treatment frequently have many large lesions, although only one of these may cause the pain. Also, many of the large open lesions have probably been present for several months. One extra week without care, until diagnostic records are made, is probably of no consequence, provided pain from the offending tooth is relieved.

Dental practitioners should not be tempted to perform pulp therapy at an emergency visit. Some may be horrified by the accumulated effects of dental neglect and recommend wholesale extractions at the emergency visit. Neither approach takes into account other potential dental problems, such as space loss and crowding.

Preventive care

However high the standard of operative dentistry may be, its success lies partially in the ability of the patient and parents to maintain a favourable oral environment for the restorations. Thus preventive dentistry must go hand in hand with any operative work. (The preventive aspects of operative dentistry are discussed in greater detail in Chapter 8.) By making projections of the future in treatment planning, the dentist can prevent unnecessary repetition of work. For example, the astute diagnostician who sees a 4-year-old with interproximal caries in the primary molars and decalcification along the gingival margin may be wise to consider placing steel crowns on these teeth, partially as a preventive measure. This is especially true if the prognosis for home care is poor and the restorations are larger than the 'textbook ideal' since they have a long life ahead of them. Preformed, or stainless-steel crowns, once placed, seldom require further treatment (Roberts and Sherriff, 1992), and that cannot always be said of Class 2 alloys in primary molars in 4-year-olds. Thus the crown may be a more economical restoration, despite the sense of false economy given by the alloy, which may require replacement.

References

Alalusuua S. et al. (1987) Caries in the primary dentition and salivary *Streptococcus mutans* and lactobacillus levels as indicators of caries in permanent teeth. *Pediatr. Dent.* **9**, 126.

Berman D. S. and Slack G. L. (1973) Susceptibility of tooth surfaces to carious attack. *Br. Dent. J.* **134**, 135.

Bohanan H. M. and Bader J. D. (1984) Future impact of public health and preventive methods on the incidence of dental caries. *J. Can. Dent. Assoc.* **50**, 229.

Curzon M. E. J. and Drummond B. K. (1987) Case report – rampant caries in an infant related to prolonged on-demand breast feeding and a lacto-vegetarian diet. *J Paediatr. Dent.* **3**, 25.

Curzon M. E. J. and Pollard M. A. (1994) Nursing caries: its extent and prevalence. In: *Proceedings of Conference on Carbohydrates in Infant Nutrition and Dental Caries.* Ed. Graf. R. Darmstadt, Milupa Scientific.

Dilley G. I., Dilley D. M. and Machen J. B. (1980) Prolonged nursing habit: a profile of patients and their families. *J. Dent. Child.* **47**, 102–7.

Gray M. M., Marchmont M. D. and Anderson R. J. (1991) The relationship between caries experience in the deciduous molars at 5 years and in the first permanent molars of the same child at 7 years. *Community Dent. Health.* **8**, 3.

Grindefjord M., et al, (1993) Caries prevalence in 2.5 year old children. *Caries Res.* **27**, 505.

Gustafsson B. E. et al. (1954) Vipeholm dental caries study. *Acta Odont. Scand.* **11**, 232.

Hennon D. K., Stookey G. K. and Muhler J. C. (1969) Prevalence and distribution of dental caries in preschool children. *J. Am. Dent. Assoc.* **79**, 1405.

Houston W. J. B., Stephen C. D and Tulley W. J. (1992) *A Textbook of Orthodontics*, 2nd edn. London, Wright.

Johnsen D. C. et al. (1984) Background comparisons of pre-$3\frac{1}{2}$-year-old children with nursing caries in four practice settings. *Pediatr. Dent.* **6**, 50.

Ketley C. E. and Holt R. D. (1993) Visual and radiographic diagnosis of occlusal caries in first permanent molars and in second primary molars. *Br. Dent. J.* **174**, 364.

Kidd E. A. M. and Pitts N. B. (1990) A reappraisal of the value of the bitewing radiograph in the diagnosis of posterior proximal caries. *Br. Dent. J.* **169**, 195.

Lenchner V. (1966) The effect of appointment length on behaviour of the pedodontic patient and his attitude towards dentistry. *J. Dent. Child.* **33**, 61.

McDonald R. E. and Avery D. R. (1974) *Dentistry for the Child and Adolescent*. 4th edn. St Louis, Mosby.

Marsh P. D. (1993) Antimicrobial strategies in the prevention of dental caries. *Caries Res.* (suppl 1) **27**, 72.

Marthaler T. M. (1990) Changes in the prevalence of dental caries: How much can be attributed to changes in the diet? *Caries Res.* (suppl 1) **24**, 3.

Nikiforuk G. and Pulver F. (1969) Practical aspects of current caries research and epidemiological data. *J. Dent. Child.* **36**, 249.

Office of Population Censuses and Surveys (1984) *Children's Dental Health.* (1984) London, HM Government Statistical Service.

Office of Population Censuses and Surveys (1994) *Children's Dental Health: Dental Caries among Children in the United Kingdom in 1993.* SS 94/1 London, HM Government Statistical Service.

Rand Corporation (1982), Bell R. M., Klein S. P., Bohanan H. M., Graves R. E. and Disney J. A. (R-2862-RWJ).

Ripa L. W. (1988) Nursing bottle caries: a comprehensive review. *Pediatr. Dent.* **10**, 268.

Roberts G. J. (1982) Is breast feeding a possible cause of dental caries? *J. Dent.* **45**, 274.

Roberts J. F. and Sherriff M. (1992) The fate and survival of amalgam and preformed crown molar restorations placed in a specialist dental practice. *Br. Dent. J.* **169**, 237.

Wendt L-K., Hallonsten A-L. and Koch G. (1991) Dental caries in one- and two-year old children living in Sweden. *Swed. Dent. J.* **15**, 1.

Winter G. B. et al. (1971) The prevalence of dental caries in pre-school children aged 1 to 4 years. *Br. Dent. J.* **130**, 271.

Wright G. Z., Starkey P. E. and Gardiner D, E. (1983) *Child Management in Dentistry*. 2nd edn. Butterworth-Heinemann.

Chapter 2

Anatomy of primary and permanent teeth

Anatomical variations between primary and permanent teeth dictate different approaches to both cavity design and pulp therapy. The essential differences are depicted in *Figs* 2.1 and 2.2 and will be discussed in relation to their clinical significance (see also McDonald and Avery, 1994).

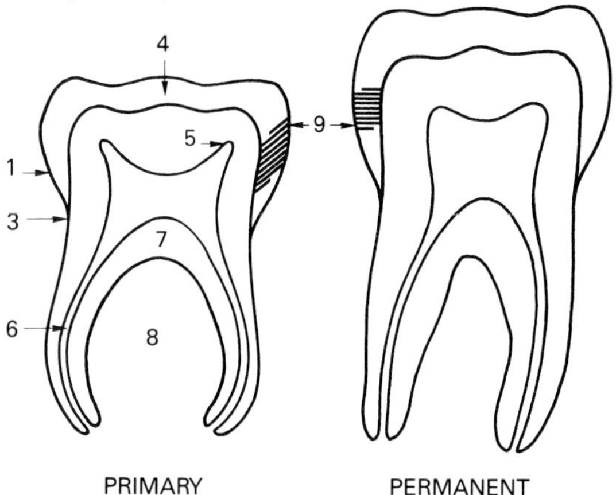

Fig. 2.1. Differences between primary and permanent teeth: cross-sectional view in buccolingual plane. 1. Bulbous crown and cervical prominence. 2. Narrow occlusal table. 3. Cervical constriction (apical to cervical enamel prominence). 4. Thin enamel. 5. Pulp horns. 6. Fine canals. 7. Thin pulpal floor. 8. Position of follicle of developing permanent tooth. 9. Enamel rod inclination.

Crown morphology

The crowns of the primary teeth are more bulbous than their permanent successors. The molar crowns are wider mesiodistally than

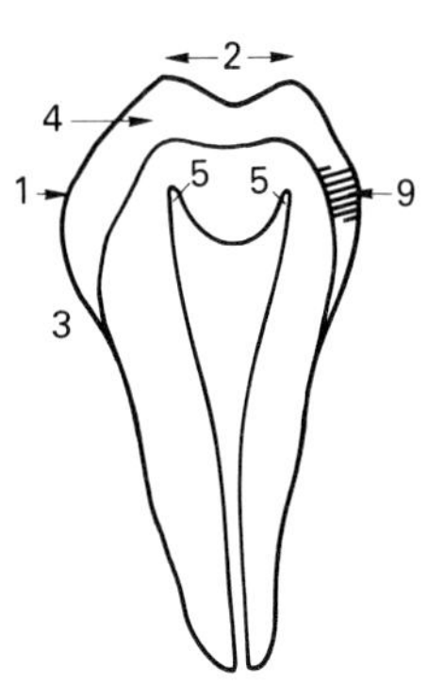

Fig. 2.2. Mesiodistal view of mandibular primary molar, labelled as in *Fig*. 2.1.

they are occlusogingivally. The mesiodistal and incisogingival dimensions of the primary incisors and canines are similar.

The primary molars exhibit a very narrow occlusal table in a buccolingual plane because of the occlusal convergence of the buccal and lingual walls. This narrow table is more pronounced in the first than in the second primary molar. This should automatically reduce the buccolingual dimensions of the design of the occlusal part of any Class 1 or 2 cavity to prevent weakening of cusps. Because of the broad, gingivally located contact areas, there will be gingival divergence of buccal and lingual walls. As a result, the interproximal margins of a Class 2 cavity must extend widely at the gingival aspect of the embrasures so as to be available for cleansing. The isthmus area, where the interproximal box and the occlusal lock meet, is narrow exactly at a point where strength is needed to withstand the forces of occlusion and the trauma of opposing cusps. Furthermore, the occlusal aspects of the interproximal box leave little margin for error since overextension will leave unsupported enamel or alloy. These are major causes of the high failure rate of Class 2 alloys from ditched interproximal margins and fractured isthmuses. This is more noticeable in mandibular first primary molars because of their very narrow occlusal table (Berkovitz et al., 1992)

The relation of the small occlusal table of the primary molar to the bulbous crown is important when deciding when to restore with a plastic restoration (amalgam, composite resin etc.) or with a stainless steel preformed crown. As described above, it is very easy to undermine the walls of a primary tooth and weaken the crown to the point of fracture. The loss of the marginal ridge also indicates probable pulpal pathology (Stoner, 1967) and the need for pulp therapy. Experience shows that, certainly for the first primary molar, mesial and distal caries means a weakened tooth which when restored with amalgam or other plastic material will inevitably lead to failure. The anatomy of the primary molar dictates that the stainless steel crown should be the restoration of choice where there has been breakage of the marginal ridge or where mesial and distal caries occurs, especially in first primary molars.

There is a marked cervical prominence of enamel in primary molars gingival to which is an equally marked cervical constriction. The placement of the floor of the interproximal box in a Class 2 cavity is dictated by these anatomical differences. When the gingival floor of the interproximal box is placed too far cervically it becomes too narrow. The operator may then be tempted to re-establish the gingival floor by moving the axial wall farther pulpally, unfortunately at the risk of exposing the pulp. The lingual and buccal aspects of the cervical prominence of enamel can be used to retain a stainless-steel crown, whose margins fit apical to this in the gingival sulcus.

Enamel of primary teeth is thinner than that of permanent teeth. The thin enamel, together with the relatively large pulp horns, means that there may be only a very small distance between the outer enamel surface and the pulp. The clinical significance of this is threefold. Firstly, it is imperative that lesions be diagnosed at an early stage, as failure to do so may result in the undetected caries penetrating to the pulp between recall visits. This is especially true with Class 2 lesions, since the distance between the mesial surface of the mandibular first primary molar and the pulp may be as little as 1.6 mm (Wheeler, 1965). Bitewing radiographs are thus very important when posterior contacts are closed. Secondly, the operator must re-evaluate the size of the burs used and adapt them to the size of the primary molar. Overextension of a cavity either buccally or lingually at the embrasures, or pulpally, is to be avoided. The diameter of the pear-shaped No. 330 bur, which is ideal for primary teeth, is about 1.0 mm. Burs of this dimension are recommended. Thirdly, care must be taken to provide restorative material in sufficient bulk for retention without exposing the pulp.

Contact areas

The contact areas between primary molars are broader, flatter and situated farther gingivally than those between permanent molars (Berkovitz et al., 1992). The clinical significance of this is threefold. Firstly, interproximal lesions need to be extensive before they are clinically observable as a grey shadow undermining the marginal ridge. This, together with the larger pulp horns, thin enamel, and Stoner's observation (1967) that broken down marginal ridges are often associated with pulp exposure, makes early diagnosis of Class 2 lesions even more imperative. Because the contact areas are broad and flat, interproximal exploration may be fruitless, leaving the bitewing radiograph as the best diagnostic aid of primary molar Class 2 lesions. Secondly, the buccal and lingual margins of the interproximal box must extend far enough towards the embrasure at the gingival margin to make them accessible for cleansing. Again, to discourage marginal failure, care must be taken to ensure that occiusal enamel is not left unsupported. Thirdly, as caries starts at or below the contact area, so the gingival seat must be taken below the contact. This also allows the correct placement of a matrix band, and makes the cavosurface margin accessible for cleaning. However, when caries extends subgingivally it is impossible to establish optimal gingival-floor depth.

Enamel structure

The enamel rods of permanent teeth incline horizontally or apically in the gingival one-third. This requires the use of a gingival-margin trimmer in permanent teeth to ensure that there will be no unsupported enamel rods. The inclination of enamel rods in the gingival one-third of primary molars is towards the occlusal (*Fig.* 2.1). Thus, there is no need for cavo-surface bevelling since all enamel rods of the gingival wall will accordingly be supported.

Pulp and root morphology

1. Relative to placement of restorations

The pulp horns of primary teeth are more prominent than those of permanent teeth and are relatively closer to the surface when the thinner primary enamel is considered. Cavity design must allow for these horns, which are situated below the appropriate cusps. Therefore, in a Class 2 cavity with a narrow isthmus, tunnelling, grooving or rounding of the axio-pulpal line angle can be carried out without fear of pulp exposure. This will provide a greater bulk of alloy at the weak isthmus area.

The first primary mandibular molar has an occlusal ridge of enamel below which is a pulp horn (Hibbard and Ireland, 1957). This horn can be very fine and extend well up into the enamel ridge. If a mesial–occlusal–distal (MOD) restoration is attempted, there is a considerable risk of exposing this pulp horn, frequently without knowing. On innumerable occasions the authors have been referred children with abscessed mandibular first primary molars containing an MOD amalgam. A dentist will have placed the restoration and in so doing inadvertently exposed the pulp, which has then died and abscessed. MOD restorations are contraindicated in these circumstances and a stainless-steel crown should be used. Pre-operative bitewing radiographs will give the operator an idea of the superficially placed pulp horns and allow the cavity preparation to be planned accordingly.

2. Relative to pulp therapy

The pulp horns are extensions of the bulky coronal pulp that accounts for most of the young primary tooth's pulp tissue; this is particularly true of primary molars. Maxillary molars have three pulp horns, which correspond to the three roots (mesiobuccal, distobuccal and palatal). Mandibular molars have four pulp horns located under the respective cusps: mesiobuccally, mesiolingually, distobuccally, and distolingually. There are two roots and usually two or three root canals; the mesial root may have one or two canals. Access to the coronal pulp chamber is best achieved through the occlusal surface by locating all the pulp horns and joining them with bur cuts. The roof of the pulp chamber can then be lifted off. The depth of the coronal pulp varies markedly; the preoperative radiograph gives the operator a good idea not only of its depth, but also of the thickness of the pulpal floor and the mesiodistal location of the entrance of the root canals. The thin pulpal floor may have accessory canals (Winter, 1962), though these are seldom visible radiographically. Accessory canals, together with the porous pulpal floor seen in non-vital primary molars (Moss et al., 1965), may account for the leakage of inflammatory products from the pulp chamber to the inter-radicular area. This may explain the high incidence of inter-radicular bone loss in non-vital primary molars compared with the peri-apical bone loss seen in non-vital permanent teeth. It is for this reason that a pulpectomy technique is advocated for non-vital primary teeth.

Where a primary tooth has become non-vital or partially non-vital and abscessed, the presence of the accessory canals means that a pulpectomy is indicated. In vital teeth the pulpotomy technique is appropriate because vital tissue will be maintained in the accessory canals. The structure of the pulp canal in the primary teeth therefore dictates which pulp therapy technique may or may not be used.

The primary pulp ages as does the permanent pulp, but at a faster rate. Thus the root canals of a primary molar in a 3-year-old may appear radiographically very wide while they may appear very fine or obliterated in the same child at age 8. Similarly, the primary pulp is capable of physiological and pathological changes such as secondary dentine formation, internal resorption, pulp stones and calcifications. Thorough radiographic preoperative assessment is mandatory to help establish the diagnosis of pulp pathology (Chapter 17).

The roots of primary teeth are longer and thinner mesiodistally than those of permanent successors, and are flared to allow for the development of the underlying premolars. The retention of primary molar roots after physiological resorption or extraction is due to their curvature and narrowness. The radicular pulp of the primary molars follows a thin, tortuous and branching path, as shown by Hibbard and Ireland (1957). In the past the multiple branching of the primary pulp was felt to make conventional endodontic procedures considerably more difficult than in permanent teeth. However, following the report by Starkey (1973), there has been a reapprasial of this and now pulpectomies in primary molars and incisors are recommended for non-vital or abcessed teeth (Duggal and Curzon, 1992). The treatment of pulpally involved primary teeth usually consists of removing part, or all, of the pulp and then applying some medicament to fix any remaining pulp tissue or to fill the root canal. The fact that a permanent successor is lying close to the primary molar roots means that burs, broaches and files must also be handled with extreme care. At the same time, any medicament placed in the pulp chamber and/or canals must be entirely resorbable, and not cause damage to succedaneous tooth.

References

Berkovitz B. K. B., Holland G. R. and Moxham B. J. (1992) *A Colour Atlas and Textbook of Oral Anatomy, Histology and Embryology*. London, Wolfe.

Duggal M. S. and Curzon M. E. J. (1989) Restoration of the broken down primary molar: I. pulpectomy technique. *Dental Update* **16**, 26.

Hibbard E. D. and Ireland R. L. (1957) Morphology of the root canals of the primary molar teeth. *J. Dent. Child.* **24**, 250.

McDonald R. E. and Avery D. R. (1994) Development and morphology of the primary teeth. In: *Dentistry for the Child and Adolescent*, 6th edn. St Louis, Mosby.

Moss S. J., Addelston H. and Goldsmith E. D. (1965) Histologic study of pulpal floor of deciduous molars. *J. Am. Dent. Assoc.* **70**, 372.

Starkey P. (1973) Pulpectomy and root canal filling in a primary molar. Report of a case. *J. Dent. Child.* **40**, 213.

Stoner J. E. (1967) Dental caries in deciduous molars. *Br. Dent. J.* **123**, 130

Wheeler R. C. (1965) *A Textbook of Dental Anatomy and Physiology*. Philadelphia, Saunders.

Winter G. B. (1962) Abscess formation in connection with deciduous molar teeth. *Archs Oral Biol.* **7**, 373.

Chapter 3

Principles and preventive aspects of paediatric operative dentistry

Preventive aspects of operative dentistry fall into the following categories:

- preservation of tooth structure;
- protection of interproximal surfaces
- protection of the occlusal surface (Chapter 8).

Before some of these individual aspects are discussed, it should be stated that a high standard of operative dentistry is essential to effective plaque control. Well-placed and properly contoured restorations whose margins are easily available for cleansing should provide longer service than those placed less meticulously.

Operative dentistry should be an adjunct to the practitioner's philosophy of preventive care for the child patient. Preventive measures, specifically applicable to the individual patient, must be instituted at the earliest possible time to alter the aetiological factors in caries formation.

Preservation of tooth structure

This section will outline many examples described in detail elsewhere in the text. However, it serves to bring together some important concepts in paediatric operative dentistry.

One aim should always be to place a restoration which will last as long as the tooth is in the mouth. This may not be possible in either primary or permanent teeth, since new lesions may develop on a different surface of the tooth and marginal deterioration of a restoration may result in subsequent replacement. However, every time a restoration is replaced there is a danger of increasing cavity size and weakening remaining tooth structure.

For example, the mandibular first permanent molar often requires an occlusal restoration within 2 years of its eruption. This same tooth may subsequently require a mesio-occlusal cavity when the second primary molar is present before the second premolar erupts. This restoration may then need to be replaced when the premolar erupts, if the interproximal margins are no longer cleanable. When the second permanent molar erupts, the mesio-occlusal restoration may have to be removed for the second time to include any distal lesion. And how many mesial–occlusal–distal restorations in teenagers are of the classic textbook dimensions?

This exaggerated example demonstrates that one tooth, in this case a first permanent molar, may be subjected to as many as four operative procedures in as little as 7 years, between ages 7 and 14. Cavity preparation in primary and young permanent teeth should therefore conserve sound tooth structure. Although all cavity margins must be extended into areas that can be adequately cleaned and decay must be removed, the preparations should have minimal intercuspal dimensions. As noted in Chapter 8, the intercuspal width of a Class 1 cavity determines the isthmus width of any Class 2 restoration subsequently placed in that tooth. Such minimal cavity preparations leave interproximal margins which are better supported and less likely to fail.

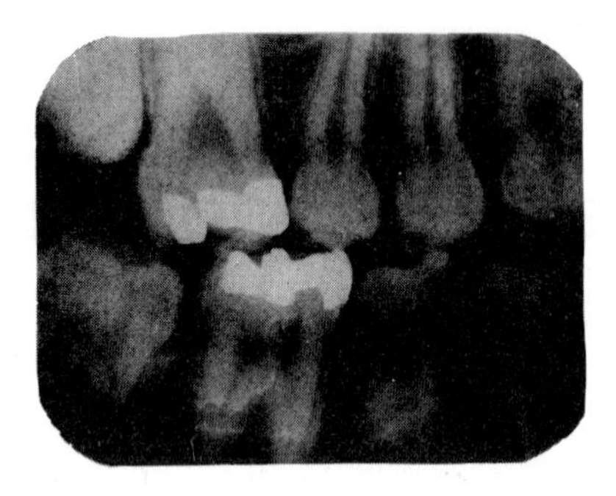
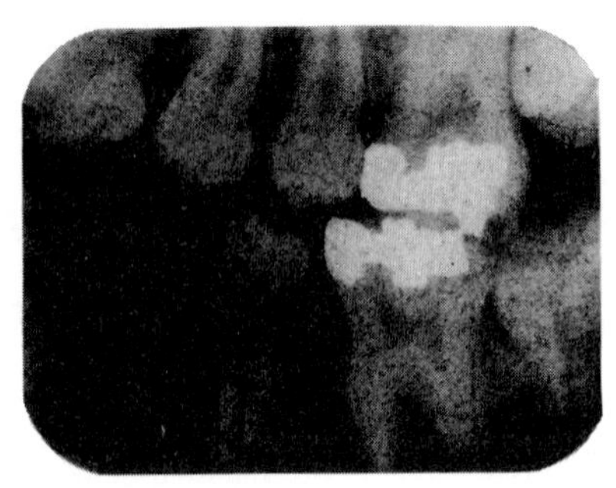

Fig. 3.1. Correctly placed mesio-occlusal restorations in first permanent molars. Note the depth of the proximal box.

One specific modification to this concept must be made for the mesio-occlusal cavity in a first permanent molar, adjacent to the second primary molar. The interproximal margins of the Class 2 cavity must be made so as to be easily cleaned with respect to both the adjacent second primary molar and the anticipated contact with the second premolar. Usually the contact area between first permanent and second primary molar is more occlusally located than the one between permanent molar and second premolar. Therefore the gingival seat of the interproximal box should be placed deliberately subgingival in anticipation of the premolar's eruption.

Failure to do this means that the floor of the box will not be easily cleaned with respect to the second premolar (*Fig.* 3.1). The buccal and lingual walls of the interproximal box should be easily cleaned with respect to the primary molar. Because of the subgingival preparation, additional care must be exercised in placing the matrix band and finishing the restoration.

These examples underline the fact that the dimension of time as it relates to paediatric operative dentistry is most important. The need for restorations in adults, and the types of restorations which are placed, may be directly related to the dentistry that patients received when they were children. It cannot be overemphasized that early diagnosis of the lesion enables the practitioner to perform minimal cavity preparations.

Protection of interproximal surfaces (adjacent to Class 2 restorations)

The proximal surface adjacent to a Class 2 cavity is put at risk during operative dentistry. Cardwell (1974) found that in more than 90% of cases, dental students traumatically damaged this surface when preparing a Class 2 cavity on the adjacent tooth; statistics are not available for dental practitioners. This traumatic damage is of minimal significance in the primary dentition since adjacent primary molars often require simultaneous restoration of Class 2 lesions (i.e. disto-occlusal on the first primary molar and mesio-occlusal on the second primary molar). The situation is different when a distal lesion in a second primary molar is being restored and the first permanent molar has erupted. It should be realized that the aetiological factors responsible for the distal lesion in the second primary molar will invariably cause some demineralization on the adjacent mesial surface of the first permanent molar. This demineralization may not be apparent radiographically but can be observed directly when the distal proximal box of the second primary molar has been prepared (McDonald, 1974).

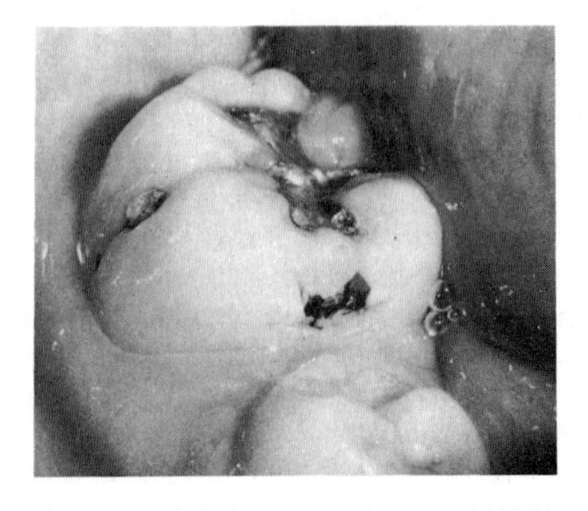

Fig. 3.2. Stannous fluoride staining on the mesial surface of the first permanent molar. An incipient lesion has been arrested.

Two methods can be used to protect interproximal surfaces adjacent to Class 2 cavities. First, precautions must be taken to prevent unnecessary mechanical damage and second, fluoride (in some form) should be applied to the proximal surface. This serves to aid in the remineralization of the enamel and can arrest the lesion (*Fig.* 3.2).

Prevention of mechanical damage

Unnecessary mechanical damage to proximal surfaces adjacent to Class 2 cavities is prevented by a combination of interproximal wedging, matrix protection, a correct sequence of cavity preparation, and patient control.

Interproximal wedges, in addition to protecting the interdental papillae, together with the rubber dam spring the teeth slightly apart to facilitate cavity preparation. A metal matrix band placed before the interproximal box is prepared and protects the adjacent surface. The occlusal surface should be prepared before the proximal box, as described in Chapter 9. The gingival, buccal and lingual extensions of the proximal box should be made before the contact is broken with hand instruments. Sudden movement by the child, together with poor finger rests while using rotary instruments, can result in trauma to the adjacent surface and the floor of the proximal base.

Fluoride – topical

McDonald (1974) compared the ability of directly applied 8% stannous fluoride and silver nitrate to prevent the progression of superficial lesions on the mesial surface of first permanent molars. The solutions were applied to the exposed mesial surface following cavity preparation of distal lesions in second primary molars with the rubber dam in place. Although stannous fluoride was more effective than silver nitrate at 1 year, it seemed to lose its effect after this time, as both solutions were equally effective in preventing the progression of the lesion at the 2-year evaluation. It is interesting that in approximately 75% of the untreated (control) teeth, the lesion progressed from an enamel radiolucency to radiographic involvement of the dentine in 2 years. By comparison, a single application of 8% stannous fluoride (or silver nitrate) prevented the progression of the lesion in 43% of teeth after 2 years (*Fig.* 3.2). Either stannous fluoride solution, acidulated phosphate fluoride (APF) gel or a fluoride varnish could be used.

A similar study comparing direct application of APF, stannous fluoride and silver nitrate to the exposed mesial surface of recently erupted first permanent molars was reported by Hyde (1973). All solutions were effective after 1 year, although the APF solution was superior to the others at the 2-year evaluation. This tends to confirm that stannous fluoride loses its effectiveness after a year and also that silver nitrate is least effective. The protection afforded by fluoride, though beneficial, may be insufficient over the long term since the opportunity to apply it directly occurs only once, namely when the adjacent Class 2 cavity is prepared.

However, this should not discourage the routine application of topical fluoride to quadrants isolated during operative dentistry; certainly any exposed surface will benefit from its application. In addition, 10% stannous fluoride is of benefit in indirect pulp treatment (Nordstrom et al., 1974). It is difficult to assess whether fluoride applied to isolated cavity preparations will reduce recurrent caries. The many variables in cavity preparation and amalgam manipulation make such a study very difficult to structure, although it has been attempted (Alexander, 1968). It seems more likely that recurrent caries is due to marginal failure resulting from faulty operative dentistry rather than lack of fluoride. However, the extent to which fluoride alters the rate of recurrent decay, or even prevents it, remains unknown.

Fluoride-impregnated cements

Since the second primary molar and first permanent molar may be in contact for as many as 5–6 years (between ages 6 and 12), other means of protecting the mesial surface of the permanent tooth must be considered. The difficulty of placing a Class 2 restoration in a partially erupted first permanent molar makes this preventive approach even more desirable. Placement of a material which continually releases fluoride would be of benefit. It has long been recognized that surfaces adjacent to silicate restorations seldom decay. This was explained by the fluoride flux in the silicate powder being continually released from the set restoration. However, the concept still applies to surfaces adjacent to fluoride-leaching glass-ionomer cements. Despite any shortcomings that glass-ionomer may have as a Class 2 cavity restorative material (Papanathasiou et al., 1994), its potential to protect adjacent proximal surfaces must be recognized (Hatibovic-Kofman and Koch, 1991).

Preventive aspects of cavity preparation

One object of cavity preparation is to remove carious material. The cavity is designed with possible future sites of attack in mind, and the completed cavity is then restored to correct contour with a suitable material. Black (1924) outlined an approach to cavity preparation and identified certain principles that should be followed. His recommendations have withstood the test of time but have been modified in the light of current concepts of conservation of tooth tissue and the preparation of cavities with prevention of further decay in mind. Both primary and permanent teeth lend themselves to these principles. It is recommended that during cavity preparation the following sequence be followed (Kidd and Smith, 1994):

(1) gain access to the caries;
(2) remove all caries;
(3) consider – design of cavity in relation to
- (i) final choice of materials,
- (ii) retention of restoration,
- (iii) protection of remaining tooth structure,
- (iv) optimal strength of restoration,
- (v) shape and protection of the cavity margins;

(4) refine and debride cavity;
(5) placement of restoration.

The above steps blend together and therefore cannot really be considered as separate activities, particularly with the use of high-speed cutting instruments. However, operators who keep these steps in mind will be well equipped to evaluate their own cavity preparations and find ways of improving their technique.

Access

Operator preference and, to a certain extent, patient behaviour will determine the extent of usage of high- and low-speed cutting and hand instrumentation. A bur commensurate with the tooth's size and projected cavity dimensions is recommended for use in the high-speed handpiece for cutting the majority of the preparations; the No. 330 pear-shaped bur is ideal for primary teeth.

For the child's comfort, as much of the cavity preparation as possible should be completed with the high-speed instruments. Cutting should commence at the occlusal pits and fissures. The chance of inadvertent pulp exposure is reduced by limiting the cavity to 0.5 mm pulpal to the amelodentinal junction. Axially, with only 0.5 mm of dentine, the cutting bur can come perilously close to pulp horns (particularly in first primary molars). However, the tooth needs to be prepared beyond the amelodentinal junction to allow retention grooves to be placed within the dentine and yet avoiding unsupported enamel. Slow-speed and hand instrumentation can then be used to finish the cavity.

Inadvertent pulp exposure tends to be avoided when the occlusal part of a Class 2 cavity is prepared before the interproximal box, since visibility of the box is improved. This also minimizes the risk of damaging the adjacent tooth. If this does occur it is of minimal clinical significance when there are adjacent interproximal areas on primary molars in need of simultaneous restoration. However, the situation becomes more serious when no lesion is present on the adjacent tooth, such as the mesial surface of the first permanent molar when a distal cavity is prepared in the second primary molar. Great care needs to be taken to prevent an iatrogenic area of plaque retention and subsequent cavity formation.

The small size of the Class 3 lesion makes it desirable to use slow-speed instrumentation from the outset. Often this is the best way to keep the cavity small enough to be aesthetically acceptable. This recommendation applies to both primary and permanent teeth. Bur size must be commensurate with tooth size, the projected cavity dimensions and the relatively superficial position of the pulp horns in primary teeth. The diameter of the pear-shaped No. 330 bur is approximately 1.00 mm. This, or similarly sized burs, are thus recommended for Class 1 and 2 cavity preparations. The same bur, No. 330, can be used for Class 3 and Class

5 cavities, indeed all intracoronal preparations in primary teeth.

Outline form

Black (1924) identified pits and fissures and interproximal contact surfaces as areas that were particularly susceptible to caries. He recommended that cavity preparations should include these danger areas so that the margins of the cavity and restorative material would be located in a so-called immune area; at least they would be in a self-cleansing or readily cleansed area. In effect, he was recommending extension for prevention. This means that the Class 1 amalgam cavity should not be confined to the carious defect. Rather the outline form should include pits and fissures throughout the occlusal surface. Failure to place the margins in an area amenable to cleansing increases the likelihood that new decay will develop later. Since Black's recommendations, advances in pit-and-fissure sealants and composite resins demand reassessment of the extension for prevention concept in the Class 1 restoration. Results on preventive resin restorations (Simonsen, 1991) suggest that extension for prevention may be unnecessarily destructive to tooth structure. The concept of the preventive resin restoration is to remove carious material only, followed by restoration; the remaining occlusal surface is sealed for prevention. With the present decline in dental decay, the preventive resin restoration is a viable and appropriate alternative to the routine Class 1 amalgam restoration (Chapter 8).

The interproximal box of a Class 2 cavity must allow the passage of an explorer tip between its margins and the adjacent tooth in three directions, buccally, lingually and gingivally. The extension of cavities is dictated by where it will be possible for the patient to clean with a toothbrush. The results of overextension have already been mentioned; underextension may result in the incomplete removal of caries, predisposition to the onset of new caries, and difficulty in matrix application.

Class 3 and 5 cavities differ from Class 1 and 2 cavities because the outline form need include only the carious lesion. Maintaining the principles of Class 1 and 2 cavity preparation would result in unnecessary tooth destruction when restoring an incipient Class 3 lesion. Unless there are indications of a remineralization potential, enamel decalcification adjacent to a Class 5 lesion would necessitate extending the Class 5 cavity to include that area in order to prevent recurrent caries (Chapter 12).

Elimination of decay

Unless indirect pulp treatment is being performed, all cavities must be rendered caries-free before any restorative material is inserted, including bases. The recommended outline form and depth may result in a caries-free cavity if the initial lesion is small. Should any caries remain, it may be removed with round burs run at slow speed and with spoon excavators. High-speed burs are less efficient than slow-speed burs for removing caries.

Particular emphasis should be placed on removing all softened and stained material at the amelodentinal junction; frequently such material persists under the cusps. If it is left, it will continue to proceed pulpally, in addition to undermining the enamel until a cusp may eventually fracture. Round burs run at a very slow speed with a light touch are preferred to spoon excavators since the hand instruments, when properly sharpened, often remove more material than is clinically necessary. This may be unfortunate if indirect pulp treatment was planned and an unwanted exposure is encountered. In asymptomatic teeth, it is acceptable to leave stained hard dentine at the base of the cavity if its removal would, in the operator's opinion, result in pulp exposure (as explained in Chapter 16).

Resistance and retention form

The ease of manipulation, low cost, and time-proven results of amalgam alloy make it the material of choice for all posterior cavity preparations in children. The restoration will be subjected to displacing forces either occlusally or interproximally and cavity design must contend with this problem. A cavity depth of 1.5 mm will usually provide sufficient bulk of restorative material for strength. As primary enamel is 1.0 mm thick the use of the No. 330 bur to the full length of the cutting head (1.5 mm) will prepare a cavity approximately 0.5 mm into dentine. An exception is the axiopulpal line angle of Class 2 cavities which may be rounded, tunnelled or grooved to provide additional bulk of restorative material at this point of weakness. The weakness may be aggravated by the trauma of opposing cusps and the placement of excessively deep anatomical grooves in the restoration.

The strength at the isthmus area of a Class 2 cavity is three times greater when the bulk of amalgam alloy is provided in depth rather than in width. Provided that a narrow outline form is made, the cavity can be deepened at the isthmus without fear of pulp exposure. Thus, just as with permanent teeth, there should be a tendency towards narrower and deeper preparations (Kidd and Smith, 1994).

Rounded internal line angles as produced by the No. 330 bur are recommended for both primary and permanent teeth. The advantages are threefold. First, they reduce the stress within the tooth that results from masticatory forces. Second, the rounded angles permit easier condensation of amalgam. Third, there is less chance of pulp horn exposure when a round rather than an inverted-cone bur is used.

The 90° angle at the cavosurface margin results in adequate support of alloy and enamel rods by dentine; the more acute angles are responsible for marginal deterioration (Jorgensen and Palbol, 1965). This is because the enamel rod/prism structure runs at 90° from the amelodentinal junction to enamel surface. It also facilitates carving of the alloy. The finishing of the cavity should be done with this in mind, irrespective of the marked variation from tooth to tooth in cuspal inclines.

Refinement and debridement of the cavity

The final stage of the preparation is the establishment of well-supported and finished margins and a cavity that is free of debris. Hatchets and chisels may be used to refine the proximal box to test the support of the enamel and break off weakened margins. Gingival margin trimmers may be used with care on the floor of the interproximal boxes in primary molars (Chapter 9) to remove weak enamel fragments; they are recommended for routine use in finishing Class 2 cavities in permanent molars.

Grieve (1968) examined the smoothness of interproximal margins produced by various finishing techniques, using tracings from photomicrographs as a measuring tool. The cavity prepared by a diamond instrument in the air-turbine had a very rough margin which required finishing before the restoration was inserted. The tungsten-carbide bur run at 20 000 rev/min produced the best results at the embrasure margins. This has been confirmed by the electron microscopic evaluation of Class 2 proximal margins (Boyde and Knight, 1970). However, the direction of bur rotation and the routine use of a chisel are also responsible for the production of smooth margins. Grieve also recommended the use of chisels on the gingival floor of the interproximal box of Class 2 preparations in permanent teeth. The chisels remove unsupported enamel and can also be used to refine the buccogingival and linguogingival line angles.

Pulp protection

It is important that the clinician recognizes the potential insult to the pulp from cavity preparation. On the one hand, it has been documented that the most apparently atraumatic cavity preparation causes histological pulp damage; of course, the greater the use of burs during the preparation, the more severe the pulp pathology. On the other hand, patients rarely complain of pain following the placement of restorations. However, this does not necessarily mean that pulp damage has not occurred, but rather that any damage is subclinical and, generally, reversible. The pulp can respond unfavourably to the following irritants:

- thermal change,
- dehydration,
- bacterial contamination.

Thermal change

It is currently accepted in Great Britain that all burs run at high speed (in the air-turbine) should be cooled with water or an air/water combination. The aim of this is to reduce the production of heat in the dentine, which will then be transferred to the pulp. However, high-speed burs probably remove tooth structure so fast that the heat is never allowed to penetrate close to the pulp. Furthermore, an air/water-spray coolant reduces visibility when working in the maxillary arch by indirect vision. In North America, the need for an air/water spray as a coolant is not uniformly accepted. In many dental schools and practices, air coolant is used as an alternative. Thus, it seems pertinent to review the evidence in support of each method.

When low speeds (500 rev/min) are used without any coolant, some transient disruption of the odontoblastic layer will be seen by microscopy. As bur speeds increase (still without any coolant), further damage takes the form of vacuolization of odontoblasts and aspiration of their nuclei. When the uncooled bur speed exceeds 3000 rev/min (still in the range of slow speed), the damage is no longer confined to that pulp immediately adjacent to the cavity preparation. Further clinical and histological evidence is provided from studies in which young permanent teeth with Class 5 cavities were cut with a bur in the air-turbine using either an air or an air/water spray coolant. These studies are particularly relevant since most cavity preparation is done with burs run in the air-turbine. Pulpal damage in the initial postoperative period (up to 6 weeks) was more severe in the air-cooled than in the air/water-cooled groups (Dachi and Stigers, 1968; Marsland and Shovelton, 1970). However, recovery from initial damage was complete in both cases.

Contrary to what might be supposed, the intrapulpal temperature is not raised with either method of cooling; rather it is lowered slightly (Bhaskar and Lilly, 1965). In support of air coolant, a 4-year clinical study of teeth prepared either with air or with air/water coolant revealed no clinical differences between each group; no one method caused clinically evident pulp damage (Bouschour and Matthews, 1966). Thus, there seems to be adequate evidence to support the use of air-cooled high-speed instrumentation on the basis of clinical rather than microscopic results.

The practitioner has to rely very much on the pulp's healing potential. Fortunately, in young teeth the highly cellular pulp and incompletely formed apices lend themselves freely to repair. However, the pulp may be insulted prior to operative dentistry by the size of the carious lesion. To avoid adding insult to injury, and thus to minimize pulp damage, an air/water-spray coolant is recommended for all rotary instrumentation at both high and low speeds. Also, this will wash debris from the cavity preparation, help prevent dehydration, and avoid the unpleasant odour that occurs with air-cooled burs. It is assumed that all burs, particularly those run at high speed, will be used with a light touch and an intermittent, gentle, paintbrush motion.

Dehydration

Excessive use of air coolant during the cavity preparation or debridement can cause pulp damage (Brannstrom, 1960). While the cavity must be dry to obtain maximum visibility and ideal conditions for inserting restorative materials, the dentist should be alert to potential pulpal damage caused by excessive dehydration.

Bacterial contamination

Laboratory studies (Beagrie, 1979) have indicated that bacteria left in cavity preparations prior to placement of the restorative material are a greater cause of pulpal inflammation than the material itself. It is, therefore, critical to ensure that cavity preparations are thoroughly washed and dried to eliminate all bacterial debris.

References

Alexander W. E. (1968) Effect of a stable 30% stannous fluoride solution on recurrent caries around amalgam restorations. Unpublished MSD thesis, Indiana University.

Beagrie G. S. (1979) Pulp irritation and silicate cement. *J. Can. Dent. Assoc.* **45**, 67.

Bhaskar S. N. and Lilly G. E. (1965) Intrapulpal temperature during cavity preparation. *J. Dent. Res.* **44**, 644.

Black G. V. (1924) *A Work on Operative Dentistry*, 5th edn, Vol. 2. Chicago, Chicago Medico-Dental.

Bouschour C. F. and Matthews J. L. (1966) A four-year clinical study of teeth restored after preparation with an air turbine handpiece with an air coolant. *J. Prosthet. Dent.* **16**, 306.

Boyde A. and Knight P. J. (1970) Scanning electron microscope studies of the preparation on the embrasure walls of Class II cavities. *Br. Dent. J.* **129**, 557

Brannstrom M. (1960) Dentinal and pulpal response. II. Application of an air stream to exposed dentin. Short observation period. *Acta Odont. Scand.* **18**, 17.

Cardwell J. A. (1974) Personal communication from study reported in 1972 as *J. Dent. Res.* **51**, 1269.

Dachi S. F. and Stigers R. W. (1968) Pulpal effects of water and air coolants used in high-speed cavity preparations. *J. Am. Dent. Assoc.* **76**, 95.

Grieve A. R. (1968) Finishing cavity margins. *Br. Dent. J.* **125**, 12.

Hatibovic-Kofman D. and Koch G. (1991) Fluoride release from glass ionomer cements *in vivo* and *in vitro*. *Swed. Dent. J.* **15**, 253.

Hyde E. J. (1973) Caries-inhibiting action of three different topically-applied agents on incipient lesions in newly erupted teeth: results after 24 months. *J. Can. Dent. Assoc.* **39**, 189.

Jorgensen K. D. and Palbol O. P. (1965) Experiments on the relationship between the strength and the angle of amalgam margins. *Acta Odont. Scand.* **23**, 513

Kidd E. and Smith B. G. N. (1994) *Pickard's Operative Dentistry*, 6th edn. Oxford University Press.

McDonald R. E. (1974) *Dentistry for the Child and Adolescent*, 2nd edn, p. 132. St Louis, Mosby.

Marsland E. A. and Shovelton D. S. (1970) Repair in the human dental pulp following cavity preparation. *Archs Oral Biol.* **15**, 411.

Nordstrom D. et al. (1974) The use of stannous fluoride for indirect pulp capping. *J. Am. Dent. Assoc.* **88**, 97.

Simonsen R. J. (1991) Retention and effectiveness of dental sealants after 15 years. *J. Am. Dent. Assoc.* **122**, 34.

Papanathasiou A. G., Curzon M. E. J. and Fairpo C. G. (1994) The influence of restorative material on the survival rate of restorations in primary molars. *Pediatr. Dent.* **16**, 282.

PART II

Diagnosis and patient management

Chapter 4

Treatment planning

A key issue in the restorative care of children is treatment planning. It cannot be too strongly emphasized that a treatment plan, written in some degree of detail, is essential in the management of the dental care of children. It is instrumental in providing high-quality care but is also a major part of the behavioural management of a child (Curzon and Duggal, 1994).

Because a child who has experienced dental caries will need preventive care as well as restoration of the diseased teeth, so a properly drawn up treatment plan must encompass both the preventive and restorative aspects of care. The two entities must be carried out together and indeed should overlap, for a high-quality restoration will help to prevent further dental caries. In another sense the placement of a stainless-steel crown on a tooth, in a mouth prone to decay, 'prevents' further decay by its full coverage of the tooth crown. It is a preventive restoration.

The philosphy of focusing entirely on prevention and delaying the restoration of the teeth until an adequate level of prevention is attained is, in our opinion, ill-founded. Put simply, prevention is not accepted by parents or child when there is pain. Treating children with diseased teeth solely with topical fluoride, diet anlaysis and oral hygiene does little good when broken-down teeth and abscesses are present. In our opinion the failure to restore decayed teeth with cavitation is negligent on the part of the dentist and borders on malpractice. In our experience the simultaneous restoration of the teeth encourages acceptance and implementation of the preventive programme.

Introductory procedures

Children who have not experienced restorative dentistry in the past but who now need treatment will need an introduction to clinical dentistry. This entails a sequenced approach gradually introducing the methods to be used: topical and local analgesia, rubber-dam placement, rotary intruments and completion of a restoration. The time taken for such an introduction is, of course, unknown and so a treatment plan must take account of this. Simple restorative procedures, often of a preventive nature, such as fissure sealants and preventive resin restorations, are ideal in these situations. These may be accomplished in one introductory visit or may need two or three short appointments.

Other children who have experienced restoration of their teeth before, or attempted restoration, present a different set of conditions and may require a different treatment planning approach. Some will quite adequately cope with advanced restoration of their teeth to include pulpectomies and preformed crowns. Others may have been put off by their previous experiences and require a reintroduction to dentistry, also with the use of preventive procedures to achieve this. In the following chapters, where the focus is on the restoration of teeth in children, it is assumed that the

Likes to be called '..............................'

DENTAL HISTORY

Name .... Date of birth ....

Address .... Siblings: 1. .... Age ....

.... 2. .... Age ....

3. .... Age ....

Medical history: ....

....

....

Past dental history:

Check-ups	Yes____No____		Extractions	Yes____No____
Fillings	Yes____No____		LA	Yes____No____
Fissure sealants	Yes____No____		GA	Yes____No____

Liked ....

Disliked ....

Parents' assessment of previous behaviour:	Excellent	Good	Fair	Poor	Bad
Parents' assessment of expected behaviour:	Good	Co-operative		Resistant	

Parent'(s) experience of dental treatment ....

....

EXTRAORAL EXAMINATION ....

....

INTRAORAL EXAMINATION ....

....

DENTAL CHARTING

R	17	16	5	4	3	2	1	1	2	3	4	5	26	27	L
	47	46	5	4	3	2	1	1	2	3	4	5	36	37	

DIAGNOSIS

....

....

....

Fig. 4.1. Example of a record form for the paediatric dental history. Note the recording of the child's usual manner of address, or nickname, for future reference.

overall behaviour of the child is co-operative or that steps have or will be taken to ensure co-operation. Similarly, in this chapter we have to assume that the dentist has, or will have, taken steps to manage the behaviour of the child. As discussed later in Chapter 6, pain control and behaviour management (Fayle and Pollard, 1994) are an integral part of paediatric dentistry but behavioural management techniques are covered extensively in other textbooks to which the reader is referred (for example, Wright et al., 1987).

History taking

Treament planning requires the obtaining of all the necessary information on the past and present dental status of the child. A plan of action by dental visits is then drawn up so that the child's teeth can be restored in the shortest possible time. An ideal approach involves the practice of quadrant dentistry.

Quadrant dentistry

This approach reduces the number of times local analgesia is used, makes maximum use of the time available and is economically beneficial to the parents as well as the dentist. Preferably under rubber dam, a whole quadrant of the dentition is isolated, together with local analgesia, and all the work needed in that quadrant is completed in one visit. This might include pulp treatment on two primary molars with stainless-steel crowns as well as single- or two-surface restorations of the first permanent molar and/or the distal surface of the primary canine. An experienced paediatric dentist should be able to complete the above treatment in an appointment lasting 45 min.

Diagnosis of the child's dental problems

Treatment planning starts with the first observations of the child. As the child enters the dental surgery or office with their parent or other carer the dentist should be observing their behaviour. The child's relationship to the parent or carer is noted, as it will affect the sequence of restorative procedures and hence the treatment plan. The history should include questions as to previous restorations carried out, or attempted. The previous use, or lack of use, of local analgesia is important. A question should also be asked about any previous experience with rubber dam. It is useful to know how successful previous restorations have been (did they 'fall out'?). A previous history of extractions only, whether with local analgesia or general anaesthesia, is important. All details should be recorded on a suitable dental history form, an example of which is shown in *Fig*. 4.1.

At the first examination visit no restorative work should be carried out other than the placement of dressings or temporary fillings. Temporaries should be placed, if the child is co-operative enough, in order to seal open cavities and prevent further food impaction.

Dental treatment needs' assessment

The present situation should be recorded, with all existing restorations charted, together with an indication of their quality. Some existing restorations may need replacing as soon as possible. Others might be left for a further course of treatment. The clinical examination should be carried out under good lighting conditions and transillumination (Pitts, 1993) may be useful. The following should be looked for, in particular in the primary teeth, and noted:

- staining of pits and fissures,
- discoloration of enamel,
- the condition of marginal ridges on teeth as to whether intact or broken.

The loss of a marginal ridge, as illustrated in *Fig*. 4.2, is important because a broken ridge is a good indicator that pulp therapy will be needed (Stoner, 1967). Recurrent caries around existing restorations and the integrity of the margins should be recorded. At the same time, the presence of sinuses and/or chronic or acute abscesses indicates pulp pathology, which may require pulpectomies or extractions (Duggal and Curzon, 1989).

The primary incisors should be looked at carefully as decay in these teeth may be an indicator of nursing caries and an appropriate aspect of the preventive programme implemented. If the teeth are still restorable, then strip crowns will need to be planned for (see Chapter

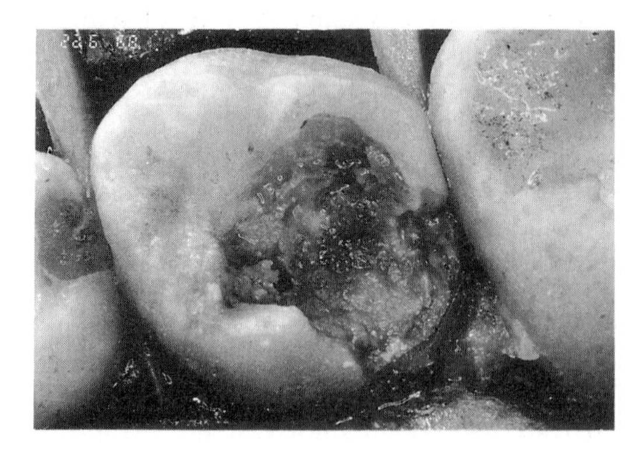

Fig. 4.2. Photograph of primary molar with broken marginal ridge. A pulp treatment, either a pulpotomy or pulpectomy, is needed here.

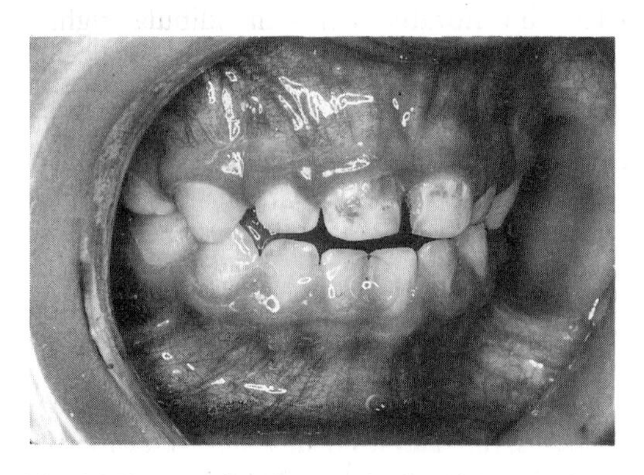

Fig. 4.3. Preoperative photograph of a child presenting with extensive caries of the primary dentition.

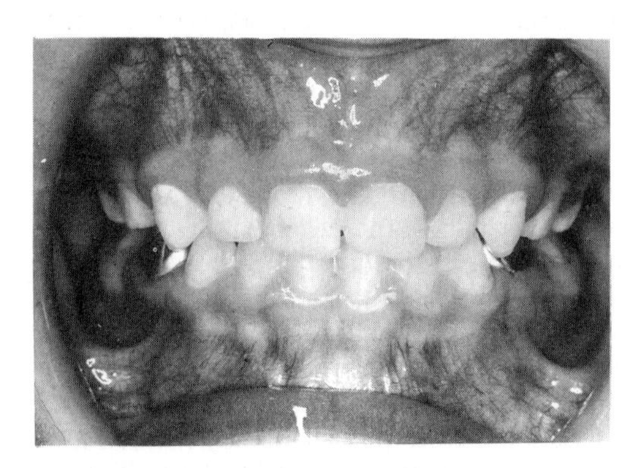

Fig. 4.4. Postoperative photograph of the child shown in *Fig.* 4.3 illustrating completed restorations preserving the primary dentition. Note the restoration of the maxillary incisors.

11). Even quite broken-down incisors should be restored (*Figs* 4.3 and 4.4). A complete charting of all dental conditions, caries, restorations, fractured teeth (not dealt with in this book) are needed prior to drawing up the treatment plan and also for medicolegal reasons. A new charting is needed for each recall course of treatment as well.

Radiographs

These are required before the drawing up of a treatment plan. For restorative dentistry, bitewings will be needed; if there is evidence of periapical pathology, then periapical radiographs of affected teeth will also be required. The types and sequence of taking radiographs are discussed in Chapter 5.

Planning by visits

A treatment plan should be written out by visits. The first visit will include the recording of the examination, dental charting, assessment of oral hygiene and the drawing up of the treatment plan. All subsequent visits should be laid out with specific notations as to which teeth are to be restored, with what material, whether local analgesia is required and which segment of the preventive programme is to be carried out.

A typical approach to the first dental visits for a new child patient might be:

- *Visit 1* An initial examination visit includes history-taking and radiographs. Open cavities might be dressed with zinc oxide.
- *Visit 2* Next comes a preventive visit which can include discussion of treatment, plaque scoring, review of oral hygiene, diet counselling, prophylaxis and topical fluoride application. The prophylaxis and fluoride treatment give both child and dentist the opportunity to establish further rapport in an essentially atraumatic setting; it also emphasizes the preventive philosophy of the practice to the parent and child.
- *Visit 3* Not until the third visit is any operative dentistry performed; by this time rapport should have been established (if it has not been, the need to use other means

for behaviour guidance, such as premedication, should have been determined at the second visit).

Subsequent visits will involve the restoration of the teeth, along with a continuing programme of preventive care, but all detailed in a treatment plan.

As each visit arrives the dental assistant is able, from a detailed treatment plan, to prepare all instruments and materials beforehand. This will include the punching of the required number of holes in a rubber dam, local analgesia needles, topical and cartridge. In other words, everything that will be needed so that the dentist can concentrate on the management of the child without having to waste time wondering which tooth to restore next.

Parental discussion

It is important that the full details of which teeth are to be restored be discussed with the parent(s), including the materials to be used, as well as an indication as to how many visits this will entail and over what period of time. Where local analgesia is required this should be discussed in case the parent is averse to its use. Similarly, the use of stainless-steel crowns, with implications for aesthetics, needs approval (Roberts, 1983). The success of the treatment will be in large measure dependent on the enthusiasm and support of the parent(s). In this book we assume that all treatment will be carried out and can be completed with the co-operation of parent and child. Where there are severe management problems then this will need to be discussed with the parent(s) and indeed the treatment plan may need to be modified with an open-ended number of visits in order to allow for behaviour management to be carried out first.

Order of restorations

When treating a child who has not previously experienced restorative care, a small restoration, or even a preventive restoration or fissure sealant, should be completed first. Using the simple behavioural technique of 'tell, show, do' and positive reinforcement, the child becomes acquainted with the sensations associated with rotary instruments. A small amount of topical anaesthetic ointment can also be used to introduce the child to the sensation of numbness of the mucosa. This is then followed up at the next visit, the first main restorative visit, with the use of local analgesia.

Because local analgesia is important for successful restoration of primary and young permanent teeth, and essential to behaviour management, it is advised that a maxillary infiltration be used, as far as possible, as a first choice. A right-handed dentist would therefore choose the upper left quadrant to start with. The sequence of quadrants for a right-handed dentist is then:

- first restorative visit – maxillary left,
- second restorative visit – maxillary right,
- third restorative visit – mandibular left,
- fourth restorative visit – mandibular right.

This treatment-planning approach, based upon the ease of giving local analgesia, would start with the maxillary right quadrant for a left-handed dentist.

However, nothing in paediatric dentistry is entirely rigidly laid down. While we earnestly recommend beginning restorative care in the maxillary left quadrant, if there is only one small preventive resin restoration or Class 1 lesion in the maxillary right quadrant, then obviously this is where one would start. The common-sense approach is always to start the introduction to dentistry with the simplest restoration and the easiest local analgesia.

Within each quadrant, all the work needed can be done under a single injection. When primary incisors need restoring then these should be left to last and completed at a fifth restorative visit. Should primary mandibular incisors be cariously involved, then in our experience the decay rate is very high and consideration should be given to a more radical approach where extractions are indicated or full-mouth restorations under a general anaesthetic.

It is strongly advised not to start with restorations in the mandibular arch, no matter how badly broken down the lower teeth are, but allowing for the need to deal with severe pain as a priority. It is far better to dress teeth with temporary zinc-oxide restorations and concentrate on a sequenced introduction of local analgesia so that the child readily accepts the care provided.

Any treatment plan in paediatric dentistry has to have as its aim the most efficient way of completing all the necessary restorations in the fewest number of visits, but at the same time managing the child's behaviour in such a way that all dental care is readily accepted. Success in doing this is the hallmark of a paediatric dentist, or any dentist who cares for children.

Example of treatment plan

Below is an example of a treatment plan drawn up to complete a number of restorations in the mixed dentition of a 6-year-old child with extensive decay of many teeth. This is based upon an actual case and serves not only to illustrate the type of work to be described later in this book but also to show how we recommend drawing up a treatment plan.

- *Visit 1* Examination, charting, plaque disclosure, discussion and approval with parents
- *Visit 2* 65 PRR composite resin, distal pit, topical fluoride varnish, issue diet sheet
- *Visit 3* 64 Pulpotomy, SSC LA/RD needed
  63 Distal resin, disclose plaque, discuss diet sheet
- *Visit 4* 55 MO alloy LA/RD needed
  54 Pulpotomy, SSC
  53 Buccal composite
- *Visit 5* 36 Buccal-pit alloy + FS
  75 Pulpectomy, SSC LA/RD needed
  74 Pulpotomy, SSC
  73 Buccal-pit composite
- *Visit 6* 46 FS
  85 MO alloy LA/RD needed
  84 Pulpotomy, SSC
  Check OHI, review treatment
- *Visit 7* Review care, polish restorations
  Reinforce prevention, check on F use

References

Curzon M. E. J. and Duggal M. S. (1994) Treatment planning. In: *Restorative Techniques in Paediatric Dentistry*, ed. Duggal M. S. et al. London, Dunitz.

Duggal M. S. and Curzon M. E. J. (1989) Restoration of the broken down primary molar: I. pulpectomy technique. *Dental Update* **16**, 26.

Fayle S. A. and Pollard M. A. (1994) Local analgesia. In: *Restorative Techniques in Paediatric Dentistry*, ed. Duggal M. S. et al. London, Dunitz.

Roberts J. F. (1983) The open faced stainless steel crown for primary molars. *J. Dent. Child.* **15**, 262.

Stoner J. E. (1967). Dental caries in deciduous molars. *Br. Dent. J.* **123**, 130.

Pitts N. B. (1993) Current methods and criteria for caries diagnosis in Europe *J. Dent. Educ.* **57**, 409.

Wright G. Z., Starkey P. E. and Gardiner D. E. (1987) *Child Management in Dentistry*. Oxford, Butterworth-Heinemann.

Chapter 5

Radiographic techniques

Radiographs are essential for the accurate diagnosis of both caries and possible pulp pathology. The value of radiographs in paediatric operative dentistry is described in other parts of the book (Chapters 1, 7, 16 and 17 in particular). This chapter will emphasize the techniques for taking radiographs on young children. Specifically, intraoral and simple extraoral procedures will be described since these are commonly used by practitioners.

General considerations

Radiographic procedures may well be one of the first 'treatment services' a child will receive. The experience should be as pleasant as possible so that it can be used as a stepping-stone in properly guiding the child's behaviour through the dental experience. A brief explanation of the anticipated procedure is necessary. The 'tooth camera' and 'tooth film' are shown to the child, who is reassured that the camera will not touch his or her face. The child is encouraged to remain very still so that the 'tooth picture doesn't come out fuzzy'. The lead apron, if used, is described as a 'blanket to cover your tummy as we only want pictures of teeth, not of your tummy'. The easiest film should be taken first, leaving the most difficult until last. This usually means that the maxillary anterior occlusal film is the first and mandibular molar periapical films last. Alternatively, where the equipment is available, an orthopantomogram is a good radiograph to take for the preschool child. This provides a considerable amount of information, yet is easy to take.

The radiographic techniques used for children vary. Current thinking recommends rectangular collimation with a 30–40 cm focus–skin distance and D- and E-speed film. However, dental radiography in small, preschool children is difficult. One of the main problems in taking radiographs of children is that of film stabilization; whenever possible the film is stabilized by occlusal pressure using a film holder. The rectangular collimator with a parallel cone requires the use of a dental film holder, but experience shows that this is not well accepted by small children. Accordingly the technique illustrated here is the tried and tested one of bisecting angle. Both methods should be in the armamentarium of the dentist caring for children and are described in other textbooks (Bricker and Kasle, 1994). For older children the rectangular collimator is recommended once they are old enough to tolerate the cumbersome film holders. For the collimator techniques the reader is referred to the appropriate textbooks (Whaites, 1992; Goaz and White, 1994).

Until recently, there has been no uniform agreement on the number and type of radiographs that should be taken on children. Valachovic and Lurie (1980) stressed the need for high-yield criteria to be established for the radiological examination of paediatric dental patients. In 1993 the American Academy of Pediatric Dentistry published, in a reference manual, guidelines for prescribing dental radiographs for children. These recommend that for a new patient, with a primary dentition with teeth in contact, posterior bitewings should be taken. In the transitional dentition, periapical/occlusal views and posterior bitewings *or* panoramic examination and posterior bitewings are indicated, while in the permanent dentition selected periapical views and posterior bitewings should be used. Recall appointments will require posterior bitewing radiographs at various time intervals depending on the caries status of the child. However, the degree of co-operation of the individual child will vary. Accordingly no hard-and-fast rules can be laid down as to which radiographs are needed for any one child. Recognition has to be taken of the present and/or past history of oral disease, based on clinical examination and the co-operation of the child.

The recommendations for radiographs in paediatric dental patients are summarized in *Table* 5.1, modified from those given by the American Academy of Pediatric Dentistry. From the exhaustive material available on the subject the following recommendations can be made for clinical practice.

General recommendations

1. Exposure should be made only after taking a history and completing a clinical examination and should be to supplement and not substitute for this clinical examination. If the child is a new patient but has been earlier seen by another dentist then access to, or copies of, previous radiographs should be sought.
2. X-ray equipment and darkroom procedures should be well controlled to minimize unnecessary radiation and poor-quality processing.
3. Fast film and rectangular collimation should be used.
4. A long-cone technique with a 70–90 kVP is encouraged wherever possible. Where a child will not tolerate film holders in the mouth, then the bisecting-angle technique may be used.
5. Operators should be well trained to minimize the likelihood of unnecessary retakes.
6. Where required by statutory regulations, child patients should have a lead apron placed during exposure, which will protect the gonads. This also applies to the use of the thyroid collar (Bricker and Kasle, 1994).

Frequency of bitewing X-rays for dental caries diagnosis

Once posterior contacts have closed, bitewing radiographs should be taken to determine the presence or absence of decay. Based upon this, the child is then designated to a high-risk or a low-risk group as follows.

High-risk

A high risk for dental decay may be associated with:

(1) poor oral hygiene,
(2) fluoride deficiency,
(3) prolonged nursing (bottle or breast),
(4) high-frequency carbohydrate diet,
(5) poor family dental health,
(6) developmental enamel defects,
(7) developmental disability and acute or chronic medical problem,
(8) genetic abnormality.

If interproximal (approximal) caries is noted, the bitewing radiographs should be repeated half-yearly until the patient returns decay-free, and then can be classified as having a low risk for dental decay. Lesions identified as present only in enamel should be watched and monitored radiographically, another reason for 6-monthly radiographs, until the lesions have been stabilized in enamel for more than 2 years.

Low-risk

These patients do not exhibit interproximal decay. In the primary and mixed dentition, bitewing radiographs should be taken every 12–18 months when posterior contacts are closed. Due to the close proximity of the pulp to the external surface of primary teeth, a 12-month period is recommended. In the permanent dentition the frequency of repeated bitewing X-rays is every 18–24 months provided no new decay is found. Once interproximal decay is found, the patient reverts to a high-risk group.

Table 5.1 Guidelines for prescribing dental radiographs

Patient category	Child		Adolescent
	Primary dentition (prior to eruption of first permanent tooth)	Transitional dentition (following eruption of first permanent tooth)	Permanent dentition (prior to eruption of third molars)
*New patient** All new patients to assess dental diseases and growth and development	Posterior bitewing examination if proximal surfaces of primary teeth cannot be visualized or probed	Individualized radiographic examination consisting of periapical/occlusal views and posterior bitewings *or* panoramic examination and posterior bitewings	Individualized radiographic examination consisting of posterior bitewings and selected periapicals A full-mouth intraoral radiographic examination is appropriate when the patient presents with clinical evidence of generalized dental disease or a history of extensive dental treatment
*Recall patient** Clinical caries or high-risk factors for caries**	Posterior bite-wing examination at 6-month intervals *or* until no carious lesions are evident		Posterior bitewing examination at 6–12-month intervals *or* until no carious lesions are evident
No clinical caries and no high-risk factors for caries**	Posterior bitewing examination at 12–24-month intervals if proximal surfaces of primary teeth cannot be visualized or probed	Posterior bitewing examination at 12–24-month intervals	Posterior bitewing examination at 18–36-month intervals
Periodontal disease or a history of periodontal treatment	Individualized radiographic examination consisting of selected periapical and/or bitewing radiographs for areas where periodontal disease (other than non-specific gingivitis) can be demonstrated clinically		Individualized radiographic examination consisting of selected periapical and/or bitewing radiographs for areas where periodontal disease (other than non-specific gingivitis) can be demonstrated clinically
Growth and development assessment	Usually not indicated	Individualized radiographic examination consisting of a periapical/occlusal *or* panoramic examination	Periapical *or* panoramic examination to assess developing third molars

The recommendations contained in this table were developed by an expert dental panel comprised of representatives from the Academy of General Dentistry, American Academy of Dental Radiology, American Academy of Oral Medicine, American Academy of Pediatric Dentistry, American Academy of Periodontology, and the American Dental Association under the sponsorship of the Food and Drug Administration (FDA). The chart is being reproduced and distributed to the dental community by Eastman Kodak Company in co-operation with the FDA. It appears here modified from *Guidelines for Prescribing Dental Radiographs* (1993), p. 27, by courtesy of the American Academy of Pediatric Dentistry.

*Clinical situations for which radiographs may be indicated include: (A) positive historical findings – (1) previous periodontal or endodontic therapy, (2) history of pain or trauma, (3) familial history of dental anomalies, (4) postoperative evaluation of healing, (5) presence of implants; (B) positive clinical signs/symptoms – (1) clinical evidence of periodontal disease, (2) large or deep restorations, (3) deep carious lesions, (4) malposed or clinically impacted teeth, (5) swelling, (6) evidence of facial trauma, (7) mobility of teeth, (8) fistula or sinus tract infection, (9) clinically suspected sinus pathology, (10) growth abnormalities, (11) oral involvement in known or suspected systemic disease, (12) positive neurological findings in the head and neck, (13) evidence of foreign objects, (14) pain and/or dysfunction of the temporomandibular joint, (15) facial asymmetry, (16) abutment teeth for fixed or removable partial prosthesis, (17) unexplained bleeding, (18) unexplained sensitivity of teeth, (19) unusual eruption, spacing or migration of teeth, (20) unusual tooth morphology, calcification or colour, (21) missing teeth with unknown reason.

**Patients at high risk for caries may demonstrate any of the following: (1) high level of caries experience, (2) history of recurrent caries, (3) existing restoration of poor quality, (4) poor oral hygiene, (5) inadequate fluoride exposure, (6) prolonged nursing (bottle or breast), (7) diet with high sucrose frequency, (8) poor family dental health, (9) developmental enamel defects, (10) developmental disability, (11) xerostomia, (12) genetic abnormality of teeth, (13) many multisurface restorations, (14) chemo/radiation therapy.

Other indications for X-rays

1. Primary dentition (3–6 years)

A radiographic examination should be carried out, dependent on the co-operation of the child. Obviously, for the very young (under the age of 3 years) this will not usually be possible, or desirable, unless there is some specific indication such as in the case of trauma. At age 3 all primary teeth should be present in the mouth and in most cases there will be closure of the posterior contact points. Accordingly, small posterior bitewing radiographs are indicated once the contacts have closed. If co-operation is not very good and dental caries is suspected, then a panoramic view can be taken. Caries diagnosis is poor on such films, however.

Alternatively, posterior bitewings may be taken, together with an anterior occlusal view of the incisors (sometimes called the four-film series). This series is useful where pathology of the anterior segments is suspected and particularly where pulp therapy of the primary incisors has been carried out. Where there is evidence of dental caries in the incisors, then a film should be taken to determine the extent and depth of the lesions. At the same time an anterior occlusal view shows the structure of the alveolus around the incisors, presence of permanent incisors, and presence or absence of supernumerary teeth.

2. Early mixed dentition (6–9 years)

A complete radiographic examination, using a combination of bitewings, periapical films of appropriate teeth, panoramic radiograph or lateral oblique films, should be made to identify the developing permanent dentition and allow the diagnosis of developmental anomalies once permanent teeth are erupted. No specific recommendations (such as 8- or 16-film surveys) are indicated in the authors' opinion. Rather the necessary films should be obtained on the basis of history and clinical examination. Appropriate films should be taken to determine the eruption sequence of the permanent canines, premolars and second molars, and to aid in the management of the developing dentition.

3. Permanent dentition (12+ years)

Radiographs (panoramic or periapical) should be taken to assess the status of third molars within 2 years of the eruption of the second permanent molars.

4. Other reasons (that pertain to this text)

Periapical films, taken at appropriate intervals, are essential to detect pulp pathology whenever a carious lesion is close to the pulp; in the case of Class 2 lesions this occurs when the marginal ridge has spontaneously broken down. Anterior occlusal radiographs may assist in the diagnosis of Class 3 and 4 lesions, their proximity to the pulp, and the presence of physiological and pathological root resorption in primary incisors. Teeth treated with pulp therapy or those that have been traumatically injured require periodic radiographic evaluation, as do molar teeth treated with fissure sealants.

The practitioner must decide which radiographs are indicated for the individual child after making a clinical examination and considering previous radiographs. While it is convenient to describe preschool and mixed dentition surveys as total entities, the clinician must determine the number and type of radiographs that are appropriate for each child only after the clinical examination. Therefore, the reader is encouraged to select appropriate films from each survey that match the child's radiographic requirements. Myers et al. (1984) found that the size-2 bitewing can give valuable diagnostic information on the pulp and periapical tissues in mixed-dentition children who have extensive decay. Therefore, when co-operation permits, bitewings should be used routinely in the mixed dentition, so that the need for supplemental periapical films is reduced. The techniques described are appropriate for the primary and mixed dentitions; modifications are described for radiographic procedures on infants.

Specific aspects of technique

Head position

The ala–tragus line (ala of the nose to the tragus of the ear) is parallel to the floor for all maxillary films and the bitewings (*Fig.* 5.1). The tragus–angle-of-the-mouth line is parallel to the floor for all mandibular periapical films (*Fig.* 5.2). Head position for the mandibular anterior occlusal film and lateral jaw is considered later.

Individual films

All intraoral films are placed with one edge 2 mm beyond the incisal or occlusal surfaces of the teeth. All occlusal films are stabilized during exposure by having the child gently close the mouth to hold the film. Bitewings for children are identical to those for adults and use bite-tabs or adhesive bite-sponges. Maxillary posterior periapical films can be held by thumb pressure; alternatively a holder or suitably

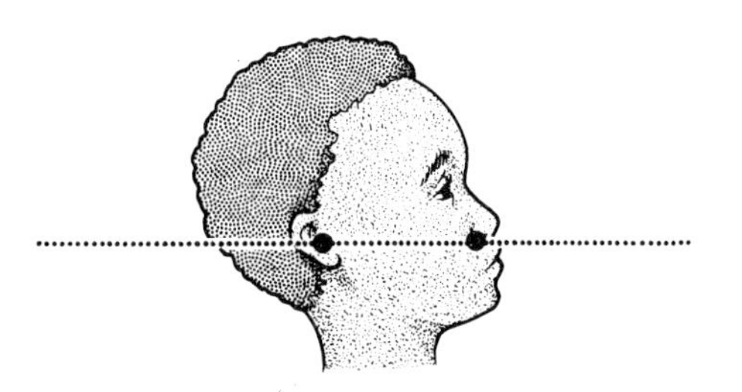

Fig. 5.1. Correct head position for all maxillary films and bitewings: ala–tragus line parallel to the floor.

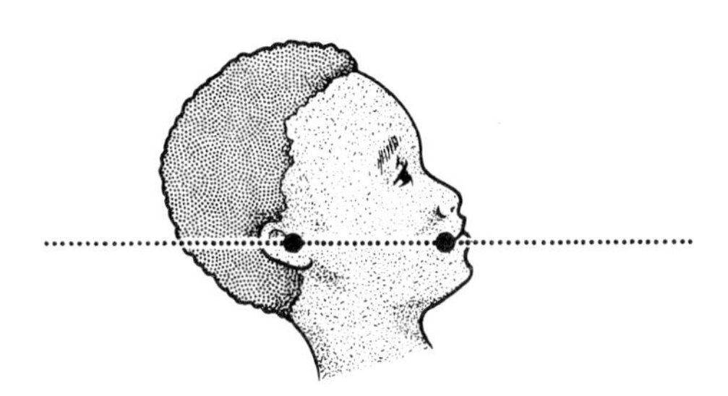

Fig. 5.2. Correct head position for mandibular molar films: tragus–angle-of-the-mouth parallel to floor.

positioned bite sponge can be used as with mandibular periapical films. Identification dots are placed towards the incisal edge or occlusal plane. The dots are placed in the anterior–superior corner for bitewings. This standardization prevents misinterpretation of radiographs.

Preschool survey: primary dentition

Where a panoramic radiograph is possible the ideal survey for the primary dentition is illustrated in *Fig.* 5.3, comprising a pair of bitewings with a panoramic view. The panoramic clearly shows the primary dentition and the developing secondary teeth, and the stage of development of the secondary teeth as well as their probable sequence of eruption. Dental caries can be seen but not as clearly as on the bitewings, which also show the depth of caries and where pulp therapy is likely to be indicated (as in teeth 84 and 64; *Fig.* 5.3).

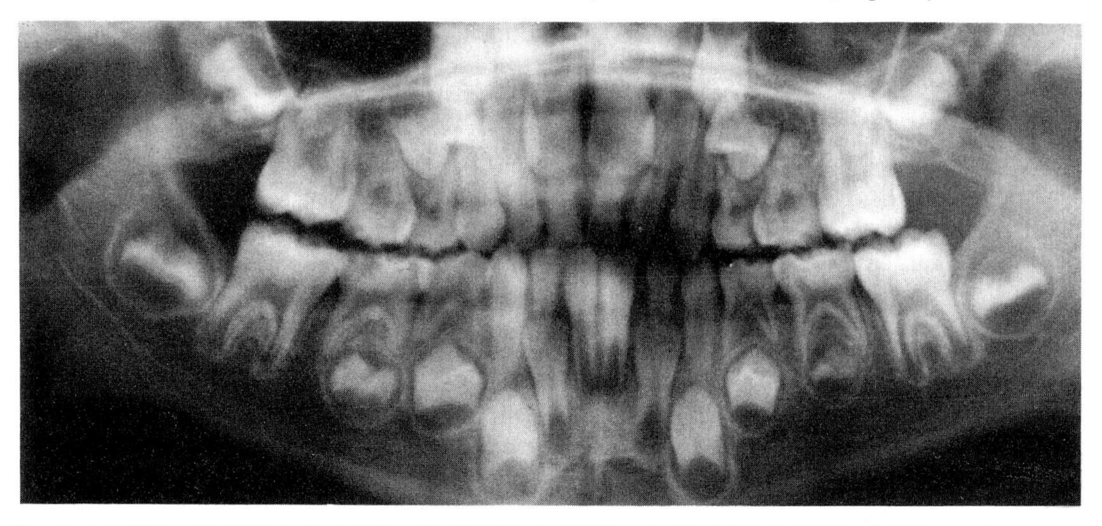

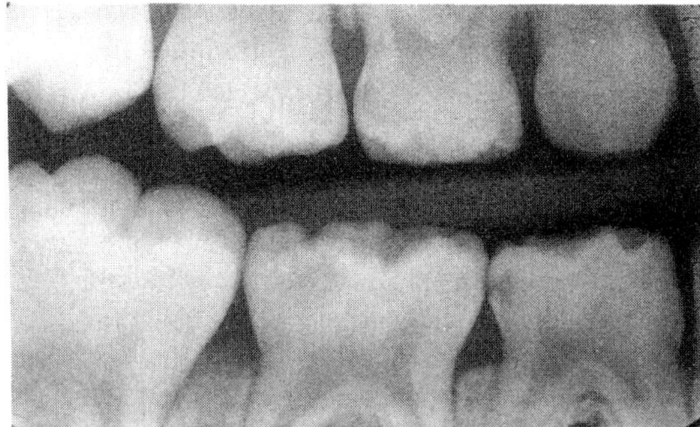

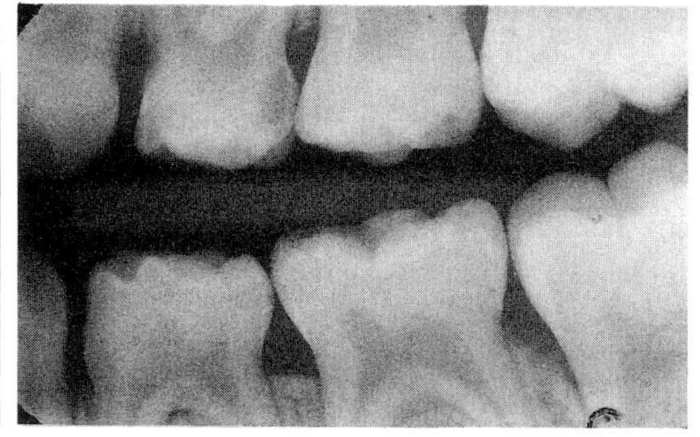

Fig. 5.3. Sequence of films for preschool children of panoramic view plus bitewings.

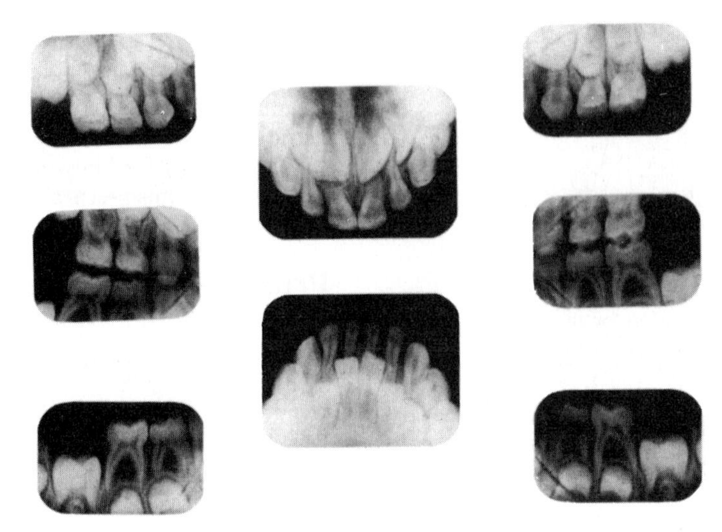

Fig. 5.4. Eight-film, preschool survey.

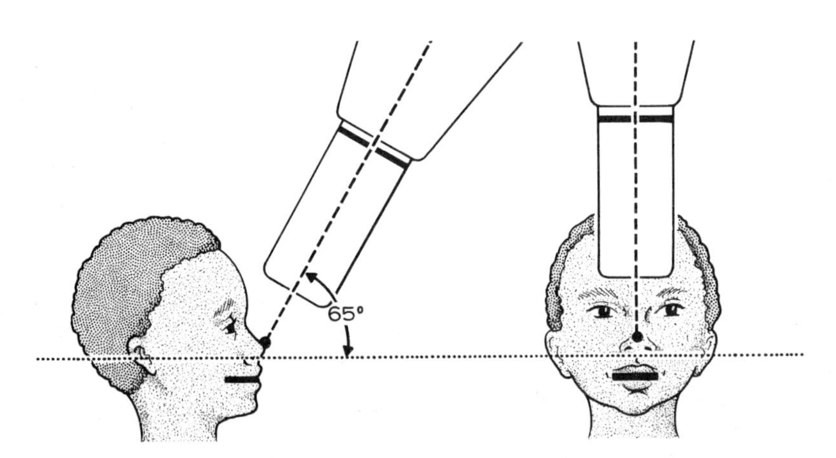

Fig. 5.5. Anterior maxillary occlusal film. Cone angled at +65°. Central ray enters at tip of nose in the midline.

A survey of up to eight intraoral films may be taken in the maxillary and mandibular anterior occlusals (using size-2 film, adult size), four molar periapical films and two posterior bite-wings (using size-0 film, child size) (*Fig.* 5.4) when a panoramic view is not possible. This is a lot of films to tolerate, particularly for the small child, and bilateral oblique films are a useful substitute.

Film placement, central-ray entry point and angulations are as described in the following subsections.

Anterior maxillary occlusal

Size-2 film is placed with its long axis running right to left and not anteroposteriorly. The anterior edge of the film is 2 mm in front of the incisal edge of the primary central incisors. It is placed symmetrically to the midline, the edges of the film extending to the primary canines. With the ala–tragus line parallel to the floor, the cone is placed at a +65° angulation so that the central ray enters at the midline half an inch (13 mm) above the tip of the nose (*Fig.* 5.5). The exposed developed film should demonstrate the crowns and roots of all maxillary primary incisors as well as the developing permanent incisors.

Anterior mandibular occlusal

The head is tilted backwards and upwards so that the occlusal plane is at 45° to the

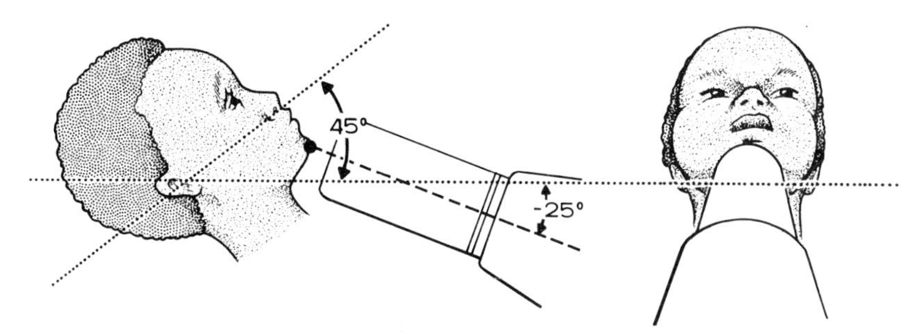

Fig. 5.6. Anterior mandibular occlusal film. Occlusal plane at 45°. Cone angled at −25°. Central ray enters 13 mm (or ½ in) above the lower border in the midline.

horizontal. This correct head position is obtained by placing the X-ray cone at 45° on the child's chest and moving the head until the occlusal plane is parallel to the end of the cone. Film placement is identical to the maxillary occlusal radiograph except that the film is upside down. Cone position is at 25° below the horizontal (*Fig.* 5.6), the central ray being directed at the apices of the mandibular incisors. The completed radiograph should demonstrate the crowns and roots of the mandibular primary incisors as well as the developing permanent mandibular incisors.

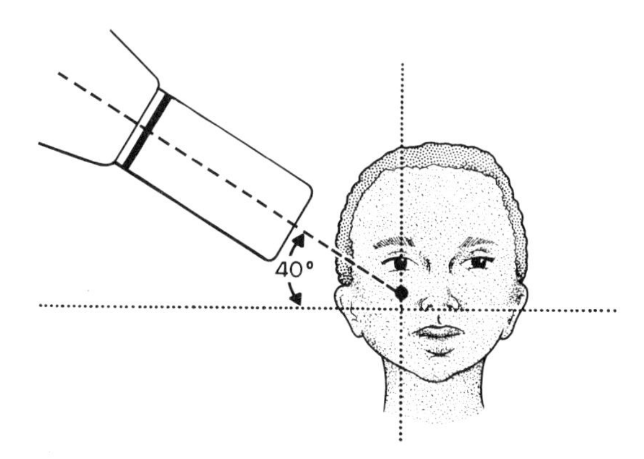

Fig. 5.7. Maxillary molar periapical film, stabilized by the thumb. Cone angled at +40°. Central ray enters on line with pupil of eye.

Maxillary molar periapicals

Ideally, radiographic films should be placed in a suitable holder; however, not all young children will tolerate this. Alternatively, the technique to be used takes a size-0 film bent sharply at the anterior corner, which will adapt to the hard palate. The long axis of the film runs anteroposteriorly with the edge located at the mesial surface of the primary canine. The film should extend an even 2 mm beyond the cusps of the primary molars. The film is stabilized during exposure by light thumb pressure from the hand opposite to the side being radiographed (i.e. right thumb for left-side film). The thumb is placed in the middle of the film, the fingers of the hand extending out of the X-ray source. A holder can also be used; the child then bites on the plastic. With the ala–tragus line parallel to the floor, the cone is angled at +40° so that the central ray enters below the pupil of the eye on the ala–tragus line (*Fig.* 5.7). The crowns and apices of primary canine and primary molars as well as their permanent successors should be seen on the exposed film.

Mandibular molar periapicals

Size-0 film is sharply bent at the anterior inferior corner to minimize impingement on the sublingual tissues. The film is symmetrically placed in a wooden, metal or plastic (Snap-a-Ray, Silverman's, Plymouth Meeting, PA; see *Fig.* 5.8) holder, or bite-sponges are used. The tongue is retracted and the film and bite-block are placed with the anterior edge extending to the mesial surface of the primary canine. The bite-block is usually stabilized by the first and second primary molars. The superior edge of the film should extend occlusally 2 mm from the cusps of the primary molars. As the child closes to stabilize the film, there is the danger of it tilting. With the tragus–angle of the mouth line parallel to the floor, the cone is angled at −5° so that the central ray passes about 13 mm (or half an inch) above the inferior border of the mandible in line with the pupil of the eye (*Fig.* 5.9). The crowns and apices of the primary

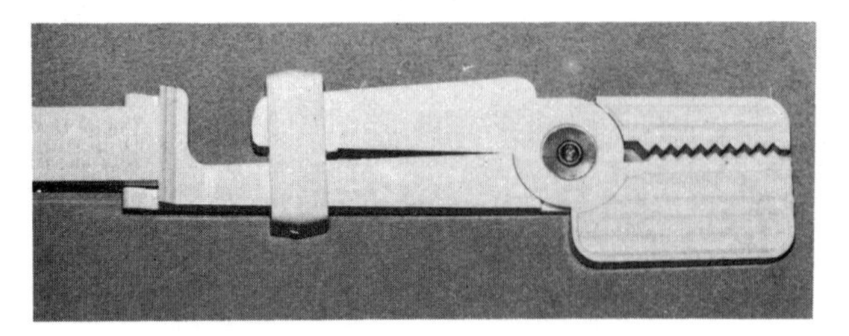

Fig. 5.8. Snap-a-Ray plastic filmholder.

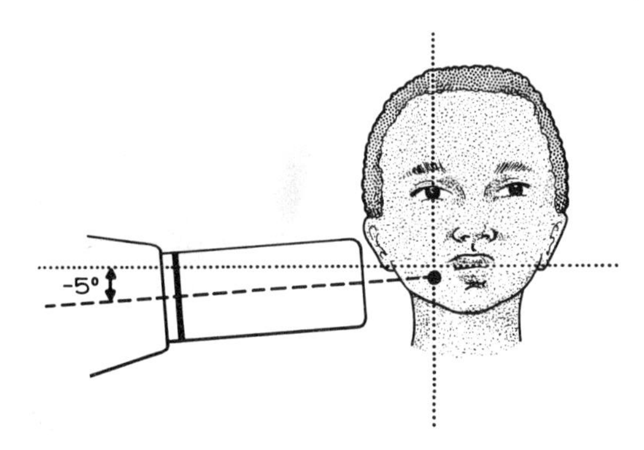

Fig. 5.9. Mandibular molar periapical film. Cone angled at $-5°$. Central ray enters 13 mm (or $\frac{1}{2}$ in) above lower border in line with pupil of eye.

canine, primary molars and developing permanent crowns should be seen on the radiograph.

Posterior bitewings

The posterosuperior and anteroinferior corners of a size-0 film are bent sharply to minimize impingement on the anterior hard palate and anterior lingual tissues, respectively. A bite-tab is added to the film prior to insertion into the mouth. When the film is placed slightly across the mouth so that the anterior part is close to the midline it will be more comfortable than if it is placed closely adjacent to the lingual tissues. The child is required to close on the bite-tab in centric occlusion. The anterior part of the film should extend to the primary canine. With the ala–tragus line parallel to the floor, the cone is angled at $+8°$ with the central ray passing between primary-molar contact areas (*Fig.* 5.10). The processed radiograph should demonstrate the maxillary and mandibular cheek teeth from primary canine to second primary molar in occlusion. The occlusal plane should be in the middle of the film so that equal amounts of mandibular and maxillary teeth are shown. All posterior contacts must be opened by the exposure to make the radiograph of diagnostic value. The most common error in exposed bitewing X-rays is overlap of the contact areas. Usually this occurs when the central X-ray point of entry is too far distally. Occasionally it is useful to use a size-0 film placed vertically to show clearly the furcation areas.

Modifications for infants

The child under 3 years of age will usually experience difficulty with any of the preschool survey radiographs. For these infants it may be necessary to obtain parental help in taking a film of diagnostic value. The parent should hold both the child and the film. Both child and parent face the same way with the child's head being cradled against the parent's shoulder. The parent's left hand restrains the child's body and arms while the right hand positions and holds the film. Alternatively, the parent's right hand stabilizes the head from upward movement (to look at the X-ray head). The left hand closes the lower jaw on the film (*Fig.* 5.11). If the

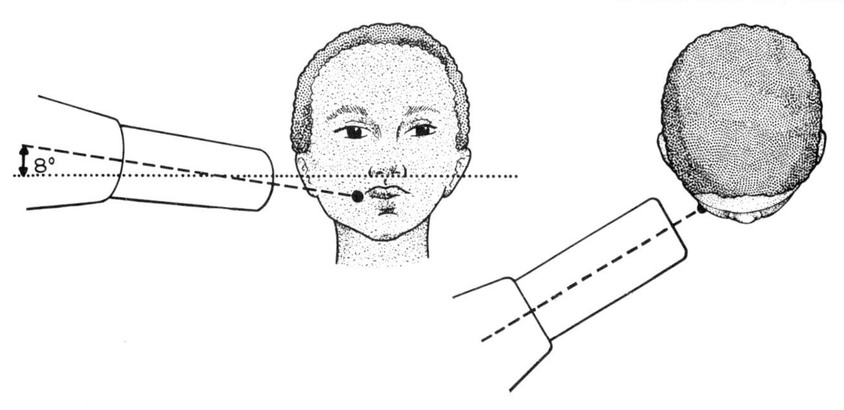

Fig. 5.10. Bitewings. *Left*, Cone angled at +8°. *Right*, Central ray enters between contact areas of primary molars.

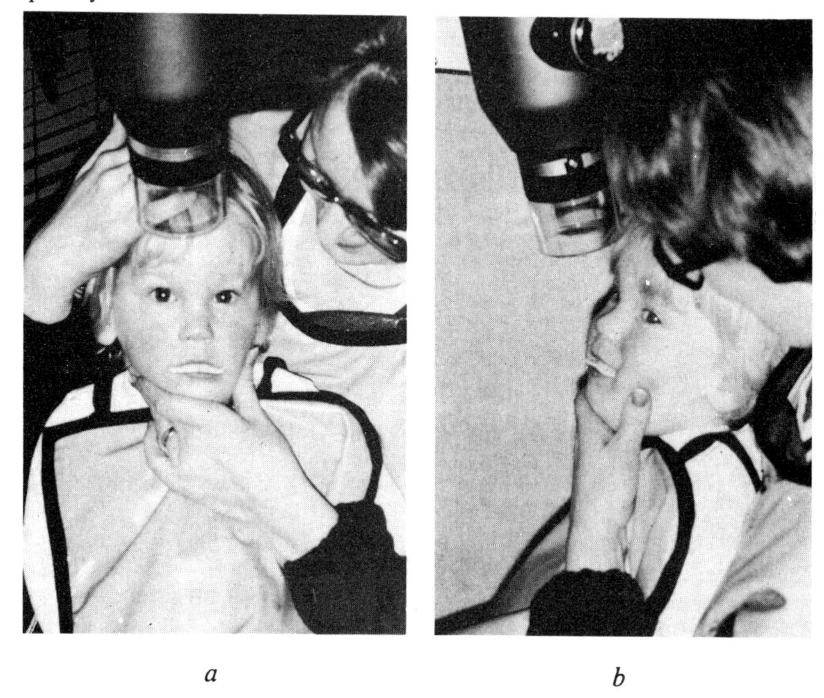

Fig. 5.11. Parent and infant positioned for maxillary anterior film. *a*, Anterior view. *b*, Lateral view.

attending adult is pregnant, someone else should hold the child.

Size-0 film should be used for all intraoral exposures in preference to the larger size 2. It will often be impossible for the young child to manage the molar periapical films and the posterior bitewings. He or she will be unable adequately to stabilize the maxillary molar film during exposure by digital pressure. Also, the mandibular molar film and bitewing impinge intolerably on the sublingual tissues in these young children. In these cases the panoramic film can be used, if available, as there is then no necessity to place films inside the child's mouth. Alternatively, oblique laterals can be used. While dental caries cannot be readily diagnosed on these films the lesions can be detected sufficiently well to be able to identify lesions and plan the treatment accordingly.

Posterior maxillary occlusal

Size-0 or size-2 film can be used, depending on the age of the child and what size they can tolerate. The long axis of the film runs anteroposteriorly with the anterior part of the film located between the maxillary primary lateral incisor and the primary canine. The film should extend 2 mm beyond the primary molar crowns. It is stabilized by having the child bite or by the parent's digital pressure. With the ala–tragus line parallel to the floor, the cone is angled at $+60^\circ$ so that the central ray passes through the apices of the primary molars (*Fig.* 5.12).

Lateral jaw

When a panoramic radiographic machine is not available then the oblique lateral jaw film may be taken instead for the very young child. The occlusal plane is parallel to the floor. The 5×7 lateral jaw film is held by the child's hand on the side that is being X-rayed. The film is placed perpendicular to the floor along the face adjacent to the primary molars. The head is rotated so that the nose and the chin touch the film. The vertical angulation of the cone is -17° with the central ray perpendicular to the film passing about 13 mm (half an inch) below and behind the angle of the mandible on the side opposite to the film. As the film is large enough to accommodate both right and left sides, metal markers should be used to identify the appropriate sides.

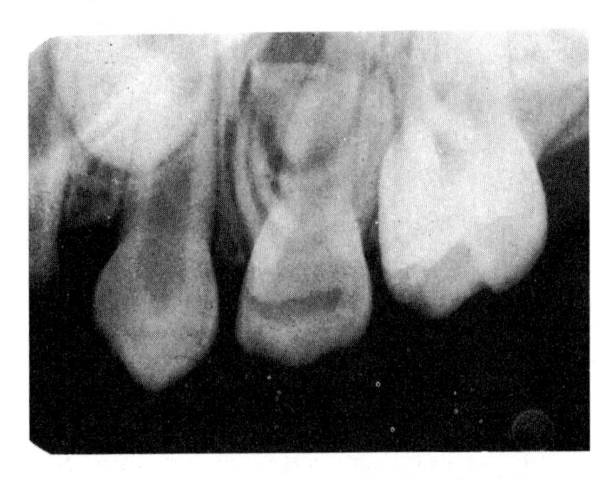

Fig. 5.12. Posterior maxillary occlusal film of an infant. Note deep lesion in the first primary molar.

Posterior bitewing modifications

A 'vertical bitewing' can also be taken, which is useful as it will show both furcation areas of the mandibular and maxillary molars, almost to the apices of the first permanent molar. Yet another variation is to place a bitewing (size 0) film in the buccal rather than the lingual sulcus with the bite-tab facing the occlusal surfaces of the teeth. The film is bent along its long axis so that it is easily tolerated. Head position, cone angulation and central ray entry point are identical to the lateral jaw. Essentially this is a reverse bitewing taken like a lateral jaw film.

The mixed dentition survey

For most children the panoramic radiograph, or lateral obliques, with bitewings are indicated in the mixed dentition. Other views may be taken as discussed below when needed.

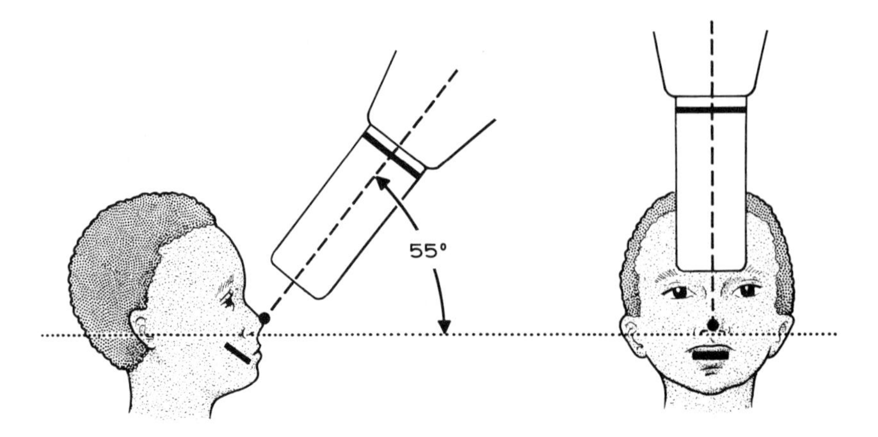

Fig. 5.13. Maxillary permanent incisor periapical. Cone at $+55^\circ$. Central ray enters at tip of the nose in the midline.

Maxillary permanent incisor periapical (*Fig*. 5.13)

Size-2 film is used with its long axis running anteroposteriorly; 2 mm of film shows anterior to the incisal edges of the permanent central incisors. The film is symmetrically placed with respect to the midline. The film is stabilized by thumb pressure as in the maxillary primary molar periapical. If the arch is narrow, the film can be bent along its length at its lateral border. With the ala–tragus line parallel to the floor, the cone angled at +55°, the central ray passes through the tip of the nose. The radiograph should demonstrate the undistorted crowns and apices of the maxillary permanent central incisors.

Maxillary primary canine periapical (*Fig*. 5.14)

Size-2 film is sharply bent at the corner, which will fit it into the midline of the palate. The film is placed in line with the lateral incisor and canine roots with 2mm showing anterior to their crowns. The mesial part of the film should extend to the midline. Thumb pressure holds the film, as with maxillary molar periapicals. Alternatively a film holder is used. The ala–tragus line is parallel to the floor, the cone angled at +50°, the central ray passing through the ala of the nose. The undistorted crowns and roots of lateral incisor and canine should be shown on the radiograph; there will, however, be some overlap of the first primary molar.

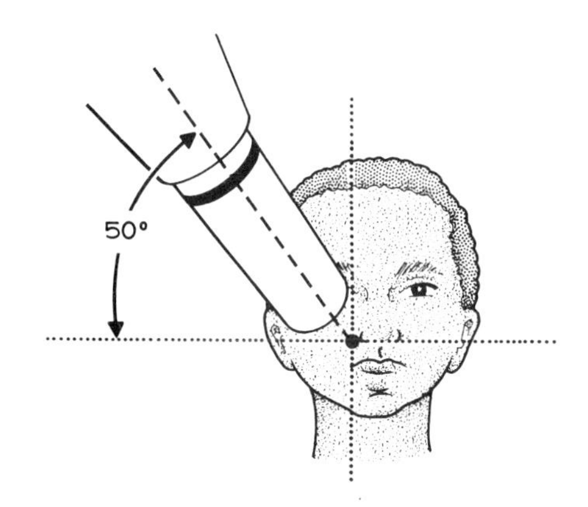

Fig. 5.14. Maxillary canine periapical. Cone at +50°. The central ray enters at ala of the nose.

Mandibular permanent incisor periapical (*Fig*. 5.15)

Size-2 film is bent sharply at the inferior corners to facilitate positioning of the film and to minimize impingement on the soft tissues. These bends are unnecessary if the smaller size-0 film is used. With the film symmetrically placed in the bite-holder, the inferior part is placed under the tongue as far back as possible. As the superior part of the film is placed, the sublingual tissues are depressed; the further back the inferior part is placed the more comfortable it is for the child. The film is stabilized by biting pressure from the permanent central incisors on the bite-block. The tragus–angle of the mouth line is parallel to the floor, the cone angled at −10° with the central ray entering 13 mm (or half an inch) above the lower border of the mandible at the midline. The processed radiograph should show the undistorted crown and roots of the permanent central incisors. This film, together with the mandibular primary canine film, is one of the most difficult for the child to tolerate. For this reason, many clinicians prefer to use a mandibular anterior occlusal film until the child reaches the age of the permanent dentition.

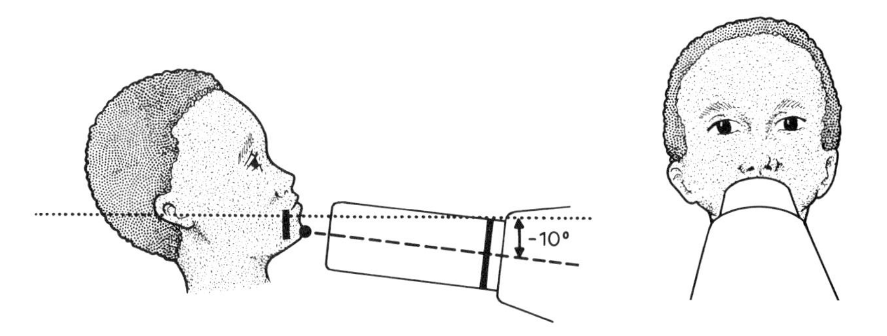

Fig. 5.15. Mandibular permanent canine periapical. Cone at −10°. Central ray enters 13 mm ($\frac{1}{2}$ in) above lower border in the midline.

Mandibular primary canine periapical (*Fig.* 5.16)

Size-2 film is sharply bent at the inferior corner that will be placed closest to the midline. Alternatively, unbent size-0 film is used. The inferior part of the film is positioned first as far under the tongue as possible; the film is placed in line with the crowns and roots of the lateral incisor and canine. The film is stabilized by biting pressure on the crowns of these teeth. The tragus–angle-of-the-mouth line is parallel to the floor. The cone is angled at -5° with the central ray passing 13 mm (half an inch) above the lower border of the mandible, through the roots of the primary canine; this will usually be in line with the ala of the nose.

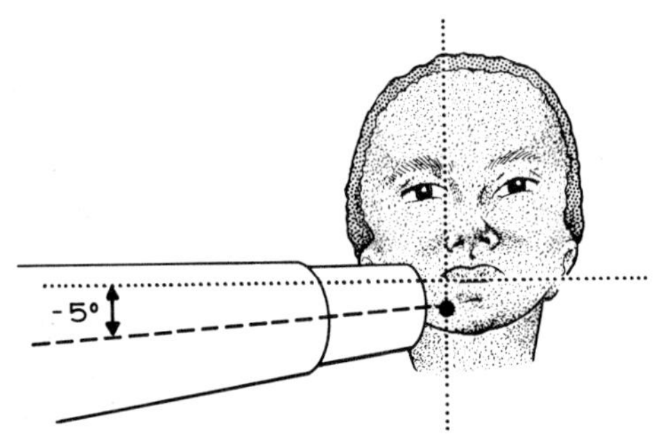

Fig. 5.16. Mandibular canine periapical. Cone at -5°. Central ray enters 13 mm ($\frac{1}{2}$ in) above lower border in line with the ala of the nose.

Other radiographs

In addition to the above there are other times when radiographs are indicated in children. When pulpotomies or pulpectomies have been carried out they need to be monitored clinically and radiographically at intervals. Pulp therapy requires a preoperative radiograph of diagnostic quality. If only bitewings have been taken, then a periapical radiograph of the tooth (teeth) for pulp therapy should be obtained if at all possible. These should show the periapical and furcation areas of the tooth to determine the presence or absence of pathology, and vertical bitewings can be used. Postoperatively a periapical radiograph should be taken to ensure that any root canal material has been properly placed and, ideally, not extruded through the apices. This should be taken at least within 1 month. Subsequent periapical radiographs are required after 6 months postoperatively and then at 1-year intervals until the primary tooth has exfoliated.

Exposure times and developing techniques

Successful radiographs are dependent on correct exposure times and developing techniques as well as film placement, cone positioning and central-ray entering points. Because of the variety of radiographic machines and the use of both short and long cones, no set rules will be given for exposure times and developing techniques. Rather, dental practitioners are encouraged to review the manufacturer's instructions for their individual machines. They are also referred to texts on radiology to help improve the quality of their X-rays. There is an ever-increasing trend to use automatic developers. These machines can be recommended from personal use since they standardize the quality of the processed radiograph. Bent films should be straightened prior to processing to minimize being caught in developer rollers.

References

American Academy of Pediatric Dentistry (1993) *Guidelines for Prescribing Dental Radiographs.* Chicago, American Academy of Pediatric Dentistry.

Bricker S. L. and Kasle M. J. (1994) Radiographic techniques. In: *Dentistry for the Child and Adolescent.* 6th edn, ed. McDonald R. E. and Avery D. R. St Louis, Mosby.

Goaz B. W. and White S. C. (1994) Dental radiography for children. In: *Oral Radiology.* 3rd edn, pp. 213–215. Philadelphia, Mosby.

Myers D. R., Barenie J. T. and Bell R. A. (1984) Requirements for supplemental periapical radiographs following No. 0 and No. 2 bite-wings. *Pediatr. Dent.* **6**, 235.

Valochovic R. W. and Lurie A. G. (1980) Risk–benefit ratio considerations in pedodontic radiology. *Pediatr. Dent.* **2**, 128.

Whaites E. (1992) *Essentials of Dental Radiography and Radiology.* London, Churchill-Livingstone.

Chapter 6

Behaviour management and pain control

Behaviour guidance

Correct guidance of the child's behaviour through the dental experience favourably influences both child and parent in their attitudes towards dentistry. The dentist's objective should be to lead a child through a pleasant dental experience so that he or she becomes a good dental patient, accepts treatment gracefully and therefore seeks and enjoys good dental health throughout life (Wright et al., 1983). Operators who are constantly evaluating their techniques of behaviour management will be able to provide the highest standard of care because the success of the treatment procedures depends in part upon an ability to manage the child. When conventional measures fail, the use of premedication, nitrous oxide analgesia, intravenous sedation and, in rare instances, general anaesthesia must be considered so that the necessary dentistry can be performed. No longer is it excusable to provide substandard or compromised care on the pretext that the child was 'impossible'. If a child proves resistant to dental care, then the dentist should either set about identifying the cause of the difficulty and devise a strategy for behaviour modification, or refer the child to another dentist, preferably a specialist paediatric dentist. In any case the end result must be the proper dental care for that child; the type of care dentists would want for their own children. Also, a compromise on standards of care for primary teeth on the basis that they will exfoliate ignores the duration required of the restorations and the value of the teeth in maintaining arch integrity. In addition, ignoring and neglecting dental caries in the primary dentition, which oftentimes the parent can easily see, sends the message that teeth are not important.

The objectives of this book do not include an elaborate account of child behaviour guidance. Indeed, no rigid rules can be given since both the child and the practitioner are individuals and their personal communication and interaction will be unique. The following generalizations, however, may be of practical value. The dentist's efforts should be directed to preventing behaviour problems (Wright et al., 1983). We should talk to children in terms that they can understand, and once communication is established the dentist should use a 'tell–show–do' approach. Anticipating the child's emotions will allow the dentist to explain the procedure to be performed and the sensations that the child should expect. The timing of explanations is very important and should serve as a foundation for building trust and confidence. The child's behaviour should be shaped by positively reinforcing appropriate, behaviour, which makes it more likely to be repeated. Inappropriate behaviour should be calmly discouraged or ignored, which reduces the likelihood of such behaviour recurring. A set of working rules should be established early and rigidly enforced so that the child knows the limits of acceptable behaviour. The calm, confident manner of the dentist conveys a sense of security to the child, who can quickly sense any nervousness, indecision or annoyance on the part of the operator. A sense of purpose, that an important health service is to be provided, should be transmitted to child and parent, who may respond by improved oral home care and punctual appointment keeping.

Some children may require a 'go-ahead' approach even if their behaviour is not amenable to reason. The astute operator reserves this approach for those children who must be made to realize that their fears are unfounded and that a certain procedure is within their ability to cope. The fearful child may require premedication to reduce anxiety to a level where treatment is no longer a major trauma. In contrast, the truly resistant or defiant child needs to realize early who is 'captain of the ship'; they may use temper tantrums to great advantage at home and not surprisingly will test out the dentist in an effort to get their own way. Once controlled, such children are often co-operative patients and faithful admirers of the dentist, who may have been the first person ever to limit their behaviour. The reader is referred to comprehensive textbooks on child management (for example, Wright et al., 1983) which also discuss the value of parental and sibling support.

Once managed, a child's behaviour must be consistently cared for and all procedures designed and carried out in such a way as to ensure there are no further unpleasant experiences. To this end, control of pain and discomfort becomes paramount. Today, there should be no excuse whatsoever for not providing dental care free of pain and discomfort as far as is professionally possible. The use of local analgesia (anaesthesia) should be as routine for the dentist treating children, in fact all patients, as is the dental examination.

Many textbooks on dentistry for children describe the technique for atraumatic injection (McDonald and Avery, 1994; Fayle and Pollard, 1994). Infiltrations provide adequate anaesthesia for maxillary but not for mandibular teeth, where an inferior alveolar block is indicated. However, except in the very young, small child under the age of 3 years the mandibular block may be used, although it is not always indicated (see below). Coupled with good topical analgesia the routine use of local analgesia is part and parcel of good behaviour management.

A child's co-operation is founded on trust and honesty. A hurt child may no longer trust a dentist, especially if that dentist fails to prepare the child for possible pain or, even worse, fails to recognize and acknowledge the discomfort the child has suffered. It is inconceivable to think that anyone would consider restoring a deep lesion without local analgesia, when caries removal could result in a possible pulp exposure. There is no evidence that primary teeth are any less sensitive than their permanent successors, although this has been claimed on the basis of clinical impressions.

Pain control with local analgesia is important to enable complete restoration of primary teeth within a reasonable period of time. In Chapter 4, treatment planning was described in relation to quadrant dentistry. Most children can tolerate quite long appointments (Lenchner, 1966) but this presupposes that local analgesia, sufficient even for pulp therapy, is achieved.

Pain control

The need for effective local analgesia was well documented in a study of the longevity of occlusal amalgam restorations in first permanent molars in children (Walls et al., 1985). Two factors – the lack of local analgesia and the age of the patient – significantly reduced the survival rate of these restorations. In 12-year-olds, 63% of occlusal amalgams survived 5 years, with the mean survival rate being 8 years 11 months, provided that the restoration was placed under local analgesia. This success is comparable to that in adult dentistry. By contrast, in 6-year-old children when the restoration was placed without local analgesia, only 30% lasted 5 years or more, and the mean survival rate was only 2 years 2 months.

Further, the dentist who works on primary teeth without local analgesia is placed in an impossible situation if the child becomes restless, for it can be difficult to decide whether the child is in pain or becoming fatigued – the treatment differing markedly for each case.

Topical analgesia

Because it is important to have profound analgesia of a tooth before restoring it, so it is necessary to be successful in giving local analgesia. The authors highly recommend first applying topical analgesic gel routinely to the mucous membrane before giving an injection.

There is now a variety of flavoured gels available and it is a good policy always to have two or three different flavours readily at hand.

There are two topical analgesic drugs available. Lignocaine-based gels have been on the market for many years but suffer from being very bitter. No matter what flavour is used the bitterness is a serious disadvantage, particularly in young children. The alternative drug is benzocaine, which has the disadvantage of a much shorter duration and depth of analgesia but the considerable advantage of its bitter taste being masked by flavourings. Thus there are presently several brands (for example, Sultan 'Topex', Englewood, NJ; Ultracane topical gel, Optident, Bingley, West Yorkshire) of topical analgesic gels with such flavours as 'mint', 'cherry', 'bubblegum', 'cinnamon' and 'pineapple/coconut'. More flavours will no doubt be developed and we do not recommend any one brand or flavour. Prior to giving an injection a child is given the choice: 'which flavour "magic cream" would you like today?'. By offering a choice the child is included in the procedure and is given a sense of control and participation. In fact, there is no choice in the sense of having local analgesia or not, but the dentist is structuring the procedure to include the choice of topical gel to facilitate this.

Local analgesia

It is not the remit of this book to describe in detail the techniques for local analgesia as these are well described (Roberts and Sowray, 1987; McDonald and Avery, 1994) and illustrated (Fayle and Pollard, 1994) elsewhere. The reader is referred to these texts to study the techniques. What is more important to us here is the philosophy of the need for routine local analgesia before performing most of the operative techniques described herein.

The overall approach should be a careful measured technique with full explanation to the child throughout the process. It cannot be emphasized too greatly the need to explain to the child, in simple language, why and how the tooth is being 'put to sleep with "magic sleepy water" ' so that the 'tooth can be mended quickly'. The use of what is known as 'Childrenese' is most appropriate for local analgesia.

Briefly, topical analgesia is allowed to work for about 40–60 s before an injection is given. The anaesthetic solution should be warmed to body temperature. We recommend the use of a cartridge warmer for this purpose. A fine-gauge needle, preferably 30G, is recommended for infiltration injections in most children up to the pre-teen age group. Once a child is well into the permanent dentition, then longer, wider-gauge needles may be required, especially where aspiration during a block injection technique is desired. The local analgesia technique should focus on:

- flavoured topical gel,
- fine-gauge needle,
- warmed analgesia solution,
- slow administration of the solution,
- constant reinforcement.

With care and attention to the needs of the child, all teeth can be adequately anaesthetized prior to any operative procedure.

The rule of '10'

There is a continuing argument as to whether local analgesia can be used on young, preschool children. There is no physiological, anatomical or behavioural reason not to give local analgesia. The one area of discussion is whether there is a need for an inferior dental nerve block for primary molars in the mandible. After all, the inferior dental nerve block is for many dentists the most difficult injection to give entirely painlessly. An argument is that a buccal (mental) infiltration is sufficient. This is so in most cases for preschool children.

A better approach is to use the 'rule of 10' to determine which injection is appropriate. The age of the child is added to the number of the tooth to be restored, the first incisor being numbered 1 and the second primary incisor 2 and so on. If the total is less than 10, a mental (buccal) nerve infiltration is sufficient. For example, if a filling is required in the second mandibular primary molar (tooth number 5) in a 4-year old child then 4 + 5 = 9 and therefore the infiltration is indicated. If the tooth is the first primary molar in a 7-year-old child, then 7 + 4 = 11 and a mandibular block is indicated. This simple approach works well in most cases. The only instance where the rule would indicate an infiltration but where it would be contraindicated would be where quadrant dentistry involving pulp treatment of two molars was planned. In this case the infiltration injection may not provide a sufficient depth of pulpal analgesia and a mandibular block would be preferred.

References

Fayle S. A. and Pollard M. A. (1994) Local analgesia. In: *Restorative Techniques in Paediatric Dentistry*, ed. Duggal M. S. et al. London, Dunitz.

Lenchner V. (1966) The effect of appointment length on behaviour of the pedodontic patient and his attitude towards dentistry. *J. Dent. Child.* **33**, 61.

McDonald R. E. and Avery D. R. (1994) Local anesthesia for the child and adolescent. In: *Dentistry for the Child and Adolescent*, 6th edn. St Louis, Mosby.

Roberts D. H. and Sowray J. H. (1987) *Local Anaesthesia in Dentistry*, 3rd edn. Bristol, Wright.

Walls A. W. G. et al (1985) The longevity of occlusal amalgam restorations in first permanent molars of child patients. *Br. Dent. J.* **158**, 133.

Wright G. Z., Starkey P. E. and Gardiner D. E. (1983) *Child Management in Dentistry*. 2nd edn. Oxford, Butterworth-Heinemann.

Chapter 7

Isolation – rubber dam

To restore primary teeth to a high standard the operating area has to be well isolated for two procedures: cavity preparation and placement of the restoration. Isolation improves access and visibility, and an uncontaminated field is essential for any form of pulp treatment. At its simplest, isolation may take the form of soft-tissue retraction by cotton rolls in the sulci and a mirror to retract the tongue. For the insertion of the restoration, isolation not only improves access but, more importantly, keeps the operating area dry. Many restorations fail due to faulty manipulation of the restorative material and insertion under less than optimal conditions. The practitioner must pay attention to the details of material handling, particularly for the newer materials such as composite resins, glass-ionomer cements and compomers, which are very sensitive to moisture. For the best results, effective isolation must be obtained.

There are several means of achieving isolation: rubber dam, cotton rolls or buccal absorbent pads, e.g. Dry Tips. As rubber dam provides the best isolation by far, the question arises as to why so few dentists use it (Marshall and Page, 1990). Many practitioners probably do not feel sufficiently practised in the use of the dam to place it confidently on a child. They may also feel that it takes too long to apply. The first reason for not using the rubber dam can be eliminated by practice, starting with simple cases. The objection that placing the dam takes too long is, in fact, inaccurate. Approximately 25% of an operative visit is spent unproductively in conversation, watching patients rinse, and waiting for them to reposition themselves. The child patient may use these as delaying tactics, and, in a 30-min appointment as many as 10 min can be wasted. Once practised, rubber dam takes less than 2 min to isolate a quadrant of two primary molars and a primary canine (Heise, 1971). If operative visits are approximately 30 min long, it is easy to see that the rubber dam is not time-consuming; in fact, it allows the operator to work faster because of lack of unproductive interruptions and therefore saves time. It permits safe, high-quality, quadrant dentistry to be performed efficiently at one visit.

There will never be uniform agreement about the use of the rubber dam in paediatric dentistry; the decision to use it or not must therefore lie with the individual practitioner. The results of clinical studies to examine whether restorations placed under the dam endure the insults of the mouth better than those placed under cotton roll isolation have been equivocal, with some showing improved longevity (Strickland, 1985) and others no effect (Smales, 1993). No long-term studies have been conducted on primary teeth to date. But it is well known that there is greater expansion and corrosion of alloys contaminated with saliva, which makes them more susceptible to failure.

Readers should not condemn the rubber dam without giving it a good trial of constant use over several months so that their technique is refined to the point when placing the dam is no longer a major hurdle. Only when this has been achieved can the operator properly evaluate the use of the rubber dam in paediatric dentistry. It is worth looking seriously at those many operators in exclusive paediatric dental practice who have worked both with and without it and asking why they are no longer using cotton-roll isolation in preference to the rubber dam. The acceptance of the rubber dam by children is directly related to the acceptance of the technique by the dentist (Curzon and Barenie, 1973). That was said over 20 years ago and still holds true.

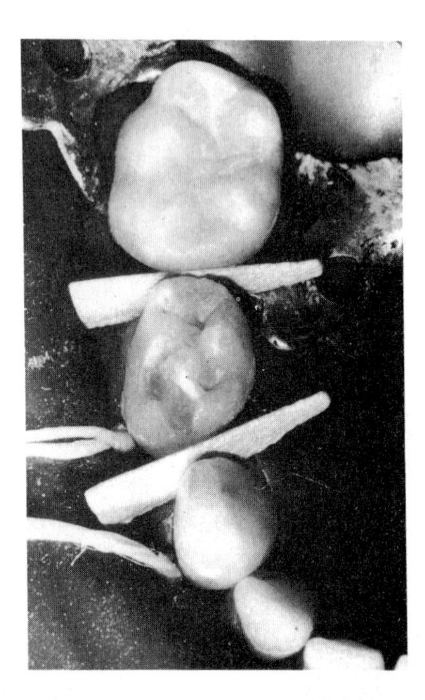

Fig. 7.1. Isolated mandibular right quadrant showing complete isolation and clear access for restorations in teeth 84 and 85.

Rubber dam

Advantages and indications

The advantages of the rubber dam can be listed as follows:

(1) improvement of access;
(2) retraction and protection of soft tissues;
(3) provision of a dry operating field;
(4) improved visibility;
(5) provision of an aseptic environment;
(6) prevention of the ingestion and inhalation of foreign bodies;
(7) aid to patient management;
(8) aid to cross-infection control by reducing aerosol spread of micro-organisms;
(9) minimization of mouth breathing during inhalation sedation procedures.

Improvement of access

Almost every dentist who has worked with children is familiar with the very inquisitive tongue that interferes when least wanted. The rubber dam improves access and visibility by eliminating the tongue, lips, cheeks and saliva from the operating field (*Fig.* 7.1). It allows the operator an unhindered access to the isolated area. Because of the improved access, details of cavity preparation can be refined; decalcification and minute pulpal exposures can be more readily reached and better manipulation of the instruments is possible.

Retraction and protection of soft tissues

Besides retracting the tongue and cheeks, the rubber dam both protects and retracts the gingiva. A criticism of the rubber dam is that the 'bur always catches in it'. This begs the question, 'where would the bur go if there were no rubber dam?' Answer: 'into the soft tissues'.

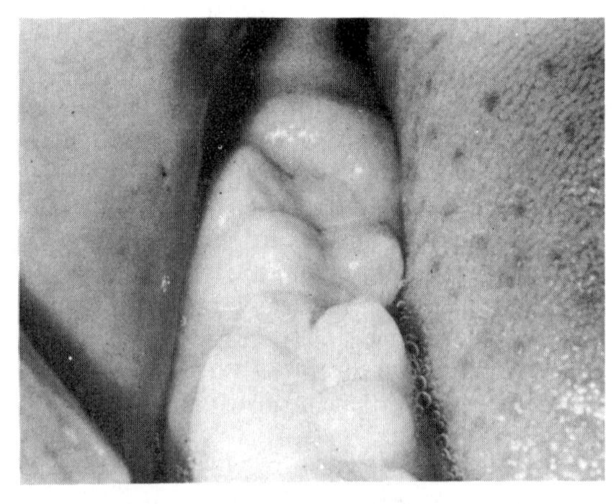

Fig. 7.2. Mandibular second permanent molar with soft-tissue operculum covering distal part of the occlusal surface.

Selective use of rubber-dam clamps and ligation facilitates access to deep subgingival caries, particularly in partially erupted teeth. The mandibular second permanent molar often exhibits a Class 1 lesion with an operculum of soft tissue partially covering the distal aspect of the tooth (*Fig.* 7.2). When the dam is not used in such an instance, the operator cannot extend the cavity for prevention, which means that the restoration may fail and need to be replaced. However, when rubber dam is used on a partially erupted molar it can be tucked between the operculum and the tooth to retract the operculum and allow an unhindered, uncontaminated field. The restoration can, therefore, be completed at one visit (*Fig.* 7.3). Any gingival trauma from the use of the dam is transient.

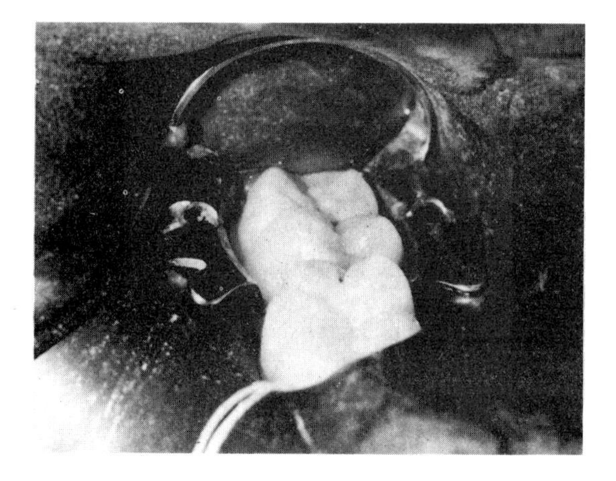

Fig. 7.3. Retraction of operculum allows correct cavity extension for prevention.

Provision of a dry operating field

The dam can be placed immediately after a local analgesic has been given and while it is taking effect. A dry field is impossible with the use of water-cooled, high-speed cutting instruments; however, high-velocity vacuum aspirators can either be used by the dental assistant or attached to a saliva ejector placed in a trough created by lifting the bottom of the dam up and attaching it to the rubber dam frame, as shown in *Fig.* 7.4. The improved access is a good reason for preparing the cavities under the dam. If the rubber dam is placed following cavity preparation, the sharp cavity walls may tear it and frustrate the clinician.

The correctly placed rubber dam ensures a dry field in which the restorative material can be placed. Only then can one hope to obtain the best properties of that material. Local anaesthesia and rubber-dam placement eliminate contamination from both saliva and gingival haemorrhage.

Improved visibility

The use of coloured rubber dam provides a contrast to the white/yellow teeth (*Fig.* 7.3). Because of this improved visibility, preparing and restoring teeth is that much easier. When restorative work has been completed the dam

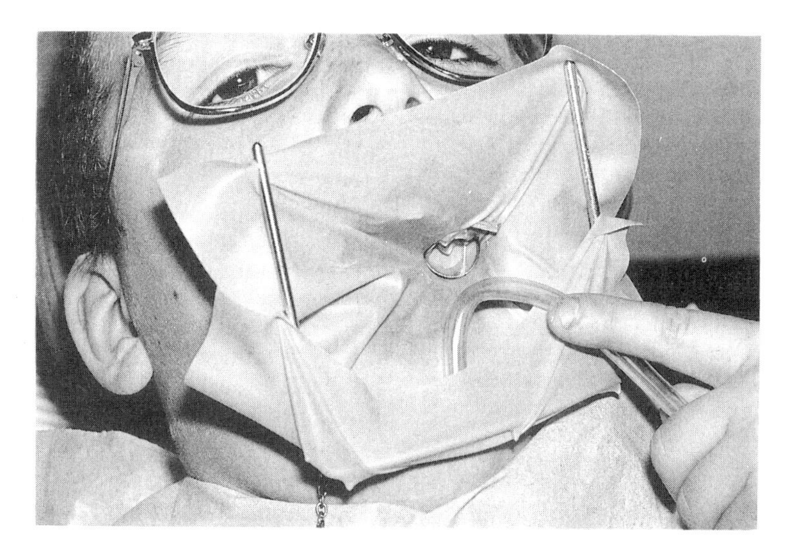

Fig. 7.4. Trough of rubber dam created by lifting the bottom of the dam and attaching it to the side of the frame with a saliva ejector placed to evacuate the water.

can be left in place and the parent(s) can be shown the restorations. Because of the contrast, as well as a clean, dry field, it is very easy to show the parent what has been achieved. It could therefore be said that the rubber dam is also useful for parent education.

Provision of an aseptic environment

Endodontists have recommended routine use of the rubber dam for all phases of root-canal work in permanent teeth. The pulp of primary teeth is made up of the same tissues as that of the permanent tooth, and the primary tooth should have the same aseptic environment as the permanent tooth for its pulp treatment. Stoner's conclusion (1967) that a primary molar with a broken-down marginal ridge will exhibit a carious pulp exposure, with irreversible damage, strongly emphasizes the need to use a rubber dam for restoring all extensively decayed primary molars, since endodontic treatment is a distinct possibility.

Reduction of aerosol spread

The use of rubber dam also improves the control of cross-infection. The dam will reduce contamination of the water spray by oral organisms when using a high-speed turbine, which will create an aerosol, so lessening the risk of contamination of the dental team (Samaranayke et al., 1989).

Prevention of the ingestion and inhalation of foreign bodies

Malpractice insurance companies unfortunately have many records of inhaled and ingested broaches, files, reamers, inlays and other foreign bodies. These serious and traumatic occurrences for both patient and dentist could have been avoided by use of the rubber dam (Grossman, 1977). Indeed, several anaesthetists in North America, and also now in the UK, refuse to assist dentists performing work under general anaesthesia unless they use the rubber dam, which serves as additional airway protection to the conventional throat-pack.

Conscious children do not take kindly to particles of alloy, cement and tooth fragments resting on their tongues, palate and cheeks. In addition to the increased salivation, the added aggravation does little to relax the patient, particularly where there is a danger of ingesting or inhaling these foreign bodies.

Patient management

Dentists who are inexperienced with the rubber dam find it difficult to believe that it aids the management of the patient, particularly the young preschool child. However, there must be a good reason why so many paediatric dentists use it routinely. Personal experience indicates that the upset child often settles down once the rubber dam is in place. It may be that the child mentally dissociates the tooth from the rest of the body, which could explain an improvement in behaviour (Jinks, 1966). More likely, the child realizes that he or she is in no danger of choking from the water of the high-speed air turbine; also, they are not embarrassed by the taste of particles and the like and thus respond favourably to the increased comfort afforded by the rubber dam.

Rubber-dam technique

Teeth to be clamped

This will depend on which teeth are to be restored. When a single-surface restoration is planned, only the affected tooth needs to be clamped. When a posterior quadrant is to be isolated, the most distal tooth should be clamped. Individual anterior teeth can be ligated or isolated by inversion of the rubber dam into the gingival sulcus, assisted where necessary by wedges (see *Fig*. 7.1). The isolation should include all teeth to be restored and the adjacent teeth when Class 2 lesions exist. Some clinicians prefer to extend isolation to the midline; this requires very little additional time but is seldom necessary in the child, especially since it is difficult to isolate mandibular primary incisors.

The experienced paediatric dentist knows that quadrant dentistry is the most efficient practice of dental care for children. Accordingly the placing of quadrant rubber dam should become routine. When this is so, the dental nurse can prepare ahead of time pre-punched sheets of dam suitable for quadrant dentistry, so saving even more chairside time.

Clamp selection

Individual operators develop their own preference for clamps, and a scientific approach to clamp selection has been described (Wiland,

Table 7.1 Rubber-dam clamps for paediatric applications

	QED[a]	Ash[b]	Hygenic[b]
Second primary molars	HAR 26	BW or DW	26
Upper first and second permanent molars	HAR W8A	AW	W8A
Lower first and second permanent molars	HAR 7A	K	7A
Partially erupted first and second permanent molars	—	FW	—
Premolars, first primary molars (occasional use)	HAR 27	DW	27

[a] QED Ltd, Bakewell Road, Orton, Southgate, Peterborough, England.
[b] Procare Dental Co, Bradford, England.

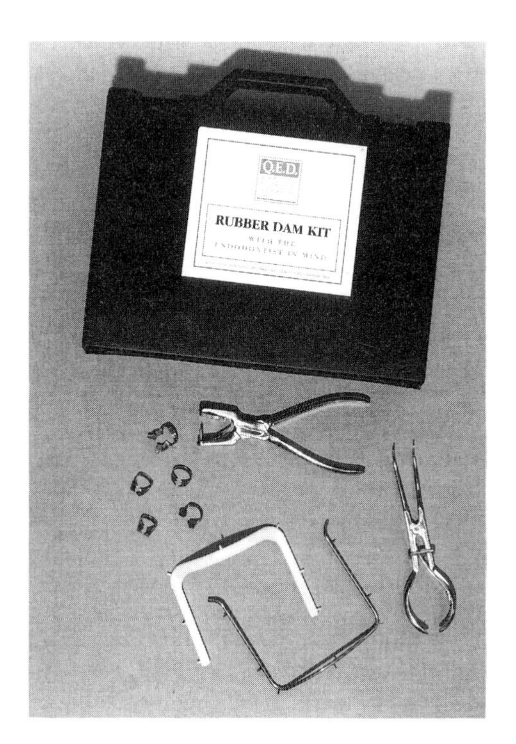

Fig. 7.5. Complete set of rubber-dam equipment suitable for use in paediatric dentistry. (Photograph courtesy of QED Co. Ltd., Peterborough.)

1973). Complete rubber-dam kits are now available (QED, Peterborough; Prestige, Bradford) that include a set of suitable clamps (*Fig.* 7.5). The clamps shown in *Table* 7.1 will suffice in a paedodontic practice.

In the majority of child patients (about 90%), for quadrant dentistry, the BW/26 clamp is used on second primary molars (see *Fig.* 7.4). The K/7A (lower) and AW/W8A (upper) are used in the mixed dentition when the first permanent molar is present. The other clamps are rarely used. Routine use of these clamps improves efficiency and reduces indecision and operating time. Analgesia is required buccally and occasionally lingually to place rubber dam. Wingless clamps are preferred for the application of rubber dam in children (see method I below). However, winged clamps are recommended by some authors when the application methods II and III (below) are used. Trial fitting of the clamp is recommended until the operator gains experience. Dental floss should be attached to the clamp so that it can be easily retrieved if dislodged.

Primary incisors, either in the maxilla or mandible, can be isolated with rubber dam by ligation of the teeth. However, the availablity of the 'Dry Dam' (Procare, Bradford) makes this much easier (*Fig.* 7.6).

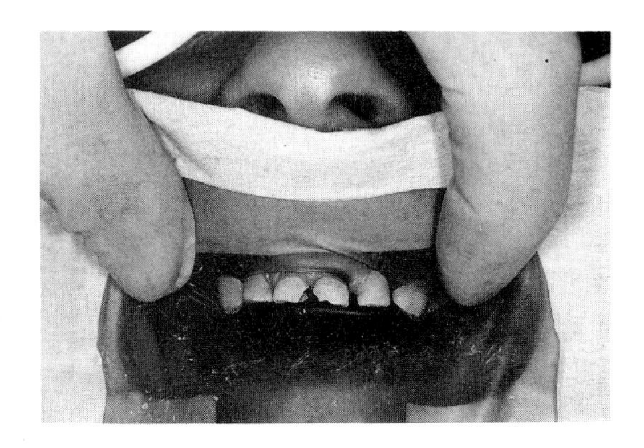

Fig. 7.6. Primary maxillary incisors isolated using Dry Dam.

Punching the holes

Placement of the holes for the teeth has been well described by Jinks (1966). Alternatively, a stamp for both primary and permanent dentitions can be stencilled on the dam to give the correct position of punch holes for every tooth. Individual variations in tooth position will determine the exact location of the holes.

It has usually been recommended that permanent molars warrant the largest hole, second primary molars the second largest and so on to the primary incisors, which have the smallest. However, in the authors' experience the largest hole suffices for most cases and saves unnecessary steps in changing the punch-hole size. The distance between holes should be about 2 mm. Intervals that are too small allow interproximal leakage while too much dam between the holes makes it difficult to pass the rubber through the broad and flat primary-molar contact areas. *Figure* 7.7 shows the correct position of the punch holes. Note that the posterior holes are on an angle of 45°. The dam can be mentally divided into four quadrants, right and left, upper and lower, and the holes punched appropriately. Posterior teeth are closest to the horizontal midline and the incisors are closest to the vertical midline. Any edentulous area should be accommodated by leaving greater space between punch holes. The trained dental nurse can punch the dam for the appropriate quadrant as indicated on the treatment plan. The nurse can determine which tooth will be clamped and therefore which clamp to select by looking at the treatment records and noting the patient's age. All this can and should be done before the patient arrives for the appointment, the rubber dam being incorporated into every operative tray set up. This is the key to efficient use of the rubber dam.

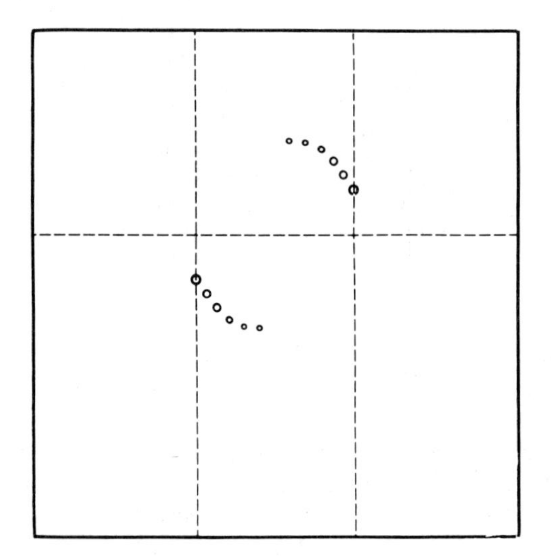

Fig, 7.7. Correct location of punch holes for maxillary left and mandibular right quadrant.

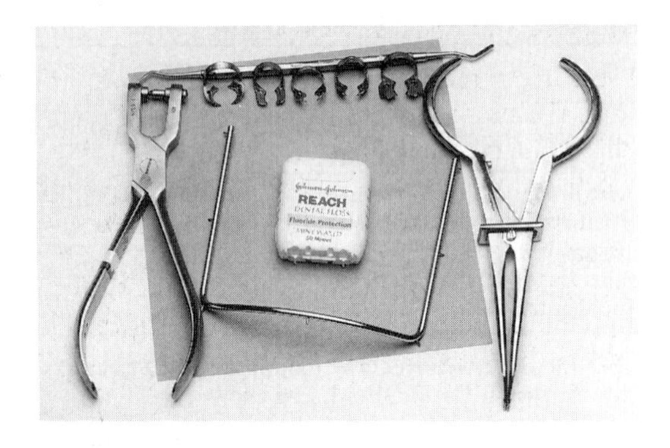

a

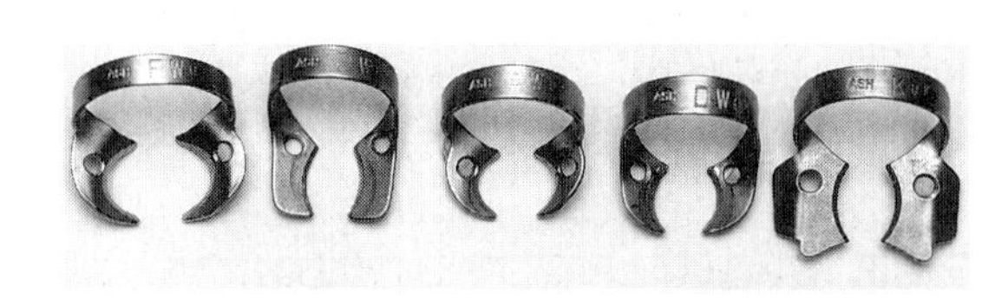

b

Fig. 7.8. *a*, Materials for rubber-dam placement: 6 × 6 in (150 × 150 mm) coloured rubber dam. Rubber-dam forceps, Young's frame (old style), waxed dental floss, plastic instrument, suitable rubber-dam clamps. *b*, Set of clamps for children: FW, BW, AW, DW, K.

Selection of materials (Fig. 7.8)

Young's rubber-dam frame is recommended, particularly the older, smaller style made of thin metal (Procare, Bradford) rather than the newer version made of thick plastic, as it holds the dam away from the child's face. Its size is commensurate with the dimensions of the child's face. Waxed dental floss is preferred for individual ligatures since it frays less than unwaxed floss on sharp edges. Dark, heavy- or extra heavy-bodied 6×6 in (approx. 150×150 mm) or 5×5 in (approx. 130×130 mm) (QED, Peterborough) rubber-dam squares are recommended. These days rubber dam comes in a variety of colours (pink, green, blue and burgundy) as well as flavours and thus provides yet another opportunity for the child to choose the colour they would like. As mentioned above, the coloured dam also provides a good contrast to the teeth. The heavy dam best retracts and protects the soft tissues but lighter-grade dam is more appropriate for the 'trough technique' (see below) where sufficient stretching of the dam is desired.

Methods of application

There are three methods of applying the rubber dam. Opinions vary as to which method is best suited, particularly to children. No one method is better than others, although in our experience method I, described below, is the easiest to use on children. All methods can be used single-handedly but application is easiest when working with a dental nurse. In all instances the rubber dam is punched beforehand.

Method I

Method I involves placing the clamp on the appropriate tooth first. The rubber dam, already punched, is stretched over the clamp and the frame is then placed. Wingless clamps mean less stretching and therefore less likelihood of tearing the dam or displacing the clamp. However, this method is possible with winged clamps also. It has the advantage of being able to place the clamp securely on the tooth before fitting the dam. Should the clamp not be secure or should the child suddenly move while the rubber dam is being stretched, the clamp could come loose and be either inhaled or swallowed (Alexander and Delholm, 1971). A dental-floss ligature will permit easy retrieval.

Individual teeth are then ligated if needed. Waxed dental floss passed through the contacts helps retract the dam through the broad, flat, primary molar contact areas. Primary canines provide good retraction of the dam and these teeth should be ligated first. Open carious lesions sometimes have jagged edges that repeatedly fray the floss, leaving interproximal wedging as an alternative to individual ligation.

'Trough Technique'. This is a variation on method I where a series of four to five holes is punched overlapping each other (Fayle and Pollard, 1994). Thus a 'trough' is made in the dam, which is fitted over the bow of the rubber-dam clamp, as described above, and the front of the 'trough' is fitted over the primary canine. Isolation of the teeth from saliva seepage is less effective but the technique is easier and slightly quicker to apply.

Method II

The clamp is placed in the appropriate punch hole in the dam which is already stretched on the frame. The dam can be stretched between thumb and forefinger as described by Jinks (1966) so that its wings are engaged by the rubber. The clamp is then placed on the appropriate tooth. The tension on the stretched dam should be eased by releasing it from the lower corner of the frame to the side to be clamped. Once the clamp is firmly secured, the rubber is eased off the wings with a plastic instrument.

This method is easier than method I to apply single-handedly, making it attractive in areas where dental laws allow the trained dental assistant to place and remove the dam.

Method III

This differs only slightly from the above-described method. The clamp can be placed in the dam as before; alternatively, the bow of the clamp only is engaged in the dam, which is held superior to the clamp. The clamp and dam are placed on the tooth and the frame is applied later. The advantage of this is that the dam is not under any tension when placed. However, Starkey (1957) recommends having a dental nurse hold the upper corners of the dam to improve visibility while placing the clamp.

Modifications

Some anterior teeth present problems with individual ligation. Partial eruption and active soft tissues may lead to poor stability of the dam. In these instances the dam can be stretched over a posterior tooth, which is then clamped. This secures the dam and permits easier isolation of anterior teeth. Occasionally, clamps may be required bilaterally.

A further alternative for anterior teeth in the child is the use of 'Dry Dam' when the teeth to be restored are isolated with the rubber dam. It is held in place by light-weight cords that are hooked around the child's ears (see *Fig.* 7.6).

Misadventures and disadvantages

Improperly directed clamp forceps can traumatize the lip of the arch opposite to the one being restored, and clamps and ligatures can impinge upon and/or traumatize the gingiva, but this injury is transient. It is also possible to catch either tongue or cheek tissues within the jaws of the clamp, but this can be avoided by sliding an index finger along the buccal sulcus while the clamp is placed. Insecurely placed or poorly selected clamps are prone to be dislodged easily; the dangers of inhalation and ingestion have already been mentioned. Poor retention of the clamp may also be caused by fatigue of its bow, resulting in loss of springiness. Worn-out clamps should be discarded. Weakened cusps could conceivably fracture should a clamp suddenly come off a tooth, although this has not been reported in the literature.

The rubber-dam frame can cause pressure marks on the face but this can easily be avoided by placing a cotton roll under the frame or a large cotton gauze under the dam. Incorrectly punched holes can move the frame and dam unnecessarily high on the face, with the frame coming close to the eyes and the dam covering the nose. The claustrophobic sensation which is sometimes experienced can be eliminated by cutting the dam away from the nostrils and, if necessary, cutting a hole in the centre of the rubber to allow an oral airway.

Once the rubber dam is in place, stimuli to salivary flow are decreased. If any build-up of saliva occurs, which may create a drowning feeling, it can be removed by high-speed suction. Personal experience with saliva ejectors has not been favourable since they tend to irritate the child (see next section). Build-up of saliva can also result in leakage should the clamp be incorrectly placed. This often occurs on the lingual surface of partially erupted mandibular molars. The problem is corrected by holding the dam down with finger pressure on the lingual and rolling the clamp buccally and occlusally, allowing the rubber dam to re-adapt to the lingual surface of the tooth at the same time. The clamp is then allowed to assume its original position. When this does not eliminate leakage, Cavit can be packed around the clamp to seal the area (Helpin and Michal, 1980).

Patient acceptance of the rubber dam should not be a problem to the experienced paediatric dentist when the child has never received dental care before. Rubber dam placement can be presented as a normal part of operative dentistry, just as local analgesia should be. It is explained as a tooth 'raincoat', the clamp being the raincoat's 'button'. When children are correctly managed they come to expect rubber dam application as normal since they know no other way. Routine use of the rubber dam is one of the greatest assets in paediatric operative dentistry, both to the clinician and to the child. It eliminates the problems of saliva contamination and interference by soft tissues that contribute to poor-quality restorations. Clinicians who object to the dam should ask themselves whether the quality of the restorations they are providing for children meets the standard required. They will be surprised how easy it is to apply the dam to a single molar and of the significant improvement in the behaviour of the child and quality of their restorative work. From easy cases they may progress to isolating quadrants and finally the most difficult teeth, the incisors (Curzon and Barenie, 1973).

Other isolation techniques

Cotton rolls placed in the buccal and lingual sulci can be used but are a poor substitute for rubber dam. Alternatively, cotton gauze (2×2 in; approx. 50×50 mm) can be rolled tightly and used. Maxillary teeth are easier to isolate than mandibular teeth since 70% of the saliva is produced by the submandibular gland. Thus a cotton roll placed opposite the parotid duct by the second primary molar, along with a saliva ejector, can be sufficient isolation for maxillary teeth. However, the cotton-wool roll does not keep the tongue under control nor does it provide safety and the other features of rubber dam. The authors only use cotton-wool rolls for the placement of temporary dressings for casual patients attending for the first time and requiring the quick sealing of open cavities.

The use of a saliva ejector in small children is not easy as it is not well tolerated. With practice in the use of rubber dam the caring dentist will soon find that he or she becomes so adept at its placement that it becomes uncomfortable when working without it. The alternative methods such as cotton-wool rolls become relegated to emergencies only. Cotton-wool rolls are useful for placing fissure sealants when no other restorative work is required, although even here some paediatric dentists advocate the quick placement of a rubber dam isolating only the tooth in question.

'Dry Dam' (Procare, Bradford) is marketed for the quick isolation of incisors and is very useful for this. Although mainly used in endodontics it has been found to be ideal for restoring primary incisor teeth. In Chapter 11 the use of strip crowns for decayed primary incisors is described. These restorations can be very effectively placed using 'Dry Dam'.

Yet a further approach is the use of 'Dry Tips' (Procare, Bradford). These small, heart-shaped discs absorb water into a wadding protected by a permeable membrane that allows saliva/water to go only one way. They are particularly useful for carrying out short restorative procedures such as fissure sealants or small occlusal restorations. 'Dry Guards' (Procare, Bradford), also heart shaped absorbent cards, may be similarly used.

References

Alexander R. E. and Delholm J. J. (1971) Rubber dam clamp ingestion, an operative risk: report of case. *J. Am. Dent. Assoc.* **82**, 1387.

Curzon M. E. J. and Barenie J. T. (1973) A simplified rubber dam technique for children's dentistry. *Br. Dent. J.* **135**, 532.

Fayle S. A. and Pollard M. A. (1994) Rubber dam. In *Restorative Techniques for Broken Down Primary Teeth*, ed. Duggal M. S. et al. London, Dunitz.

Grossman L. I. (1977) Prevention in endodontic practice. *J. Am. Dent. Assoc.* **82**, 395.

Heise A. L. (1971) Time required in rubber dam placement. *J. Dent. Child.* **38**, 116.

Helpin M. L. and Michal B. C. (1980) Improved moisture control with the rubber dam. A clinical technique. *Pediatr. Dent.* **2**, 59.

Jinks J. M. (1966) Rubber dam technique in pedodontics. *Dent. Clin. North Am.* **327**.

Marshall K. and Page J. (1990). The use of rubber dam in the UK: a survey. *Br. Dent. J.* **169**, 286.

Starkey P. E. (1957) The application of the rubber dam in the pre-school child. *J. Dent. Child.* **24**, 230.

Stoner J. E. (1967). Dental caries in deciduous molars. *Br. Dent. J.* **123**, 130.

Samaranayake L. P., Reid J. and Evans D. (1989) The efficacy of rubber dam isolation in reducing atmospheric bacterial contamination. *J. Dent. Child.* **56**, 442.

Smales R. J. (1993) Rubber dam usage related to restoration quality and survival. *Br. Dent. J.* **174**, 330.

Strickland C. (1985) *Art and Science of Operative Dentistry*, 2nd edn. St Louis, Mosby.

Wiland L. (1973) An evaluation of rubber dam clamps and a method for their selection. *J. Am. Dent. Assoc.* **87**, 160.

PART III

Restoration of teeth

Chapter 8

The Class 1 lesion, fissure sealants and preventive restorations

General considerations

Pit-and-fissure caries has not reduced at the same rate as caries on other surfaces (Bohanan and Bader, 1984). The depth and inclination of the occlusal fissures predispose these surfaces to plaque retention and subsequently to caries. The fissure may be impossible to cleanse properly since the diameter of a toothbrush bristle may exceed the diameter of the fissure orifice. This means that toothbrushing at best will remove superficial dental plaque and at worst will force debris into the depths of the fissure. Since these fissures often extend to the amelodentinal junction, it is not surprising that carious involvement of the dentine can occur soon after eruption. This rapid dentinal involvement poses a severe problem to the prevention-oriented clinician. If one believes that the carious lesion cannot arrest once the dentine is involved (indirect pulp treatment excepted, see Chapter 17), then it is imperative to apply preventive measures as soon as possible after eruption. At this time such measures are usually hindered by a young and sometimes apprehensive child, as well as by an incompletely erupted tooth which cannot be effectively isolated.

Another complicating factor is the lack of agreement on what an occlusal cavity is and what constitutes a stained fissure that could perhaps be observed rather than restored. Criteria such as decalcification, grey discoloration resulting from the undermining of enamel, or bitewing radiolucency assist in the diagnosis.

The presence of caries (either occlusal or interproximal) in the tooth is a contraindication to the use of preventive measures for protecting the occlusal surface. In the case of an interproximal radiolucency, the occlusal fissure would have to be removed to form the occlusal part of the cavity. Also, there is questionable value in sealing a permanent tooth that has an interproximal lesion confined to enamel if previous decay experience indicates that such a lesion will progress to dentine involvement.

The methods of protecting the occlusal surfaces from decay are in historical order:

(1) prophylactic odontotomy,
(2) reshaping the fissures,
(3) fluoride,
(4) sealants,
(5) restorations.

Prophylactic odontotomy

Hyatt (1923) recommended eliminating all susceptible fissures by cutting a shallow, minimal-width Class I cavity in enamel. Since the cavity floor is left in enamel, local anaesthesia is not required, but the outline form must include all deep fissures. The cavity is then filled with amalgam. This procedure has the following disadvantages: cutting instruments must be used; the tooth is always committed to a restoration; and there is a risk of sealing in caries if the preoperative diagnosis is inaccurate or if the fissure extends to the amelodentinal junction. For these reasons, and because of the encouraging results with fissure sealants, prophylactic odontotomy cannot be recommended.

Reshaping the fissures

It has been recommended that the fissures be reshaped by reducing the steep cuspal inclines so that the occlusal surface is more readily cleansed by the child (Bodecker, 1929). No studies indicate its success and the destructive nature of the procedure is irreversible. On these grounds the technique cannot be recommended.

Fluoride

Fluoride, either systemic or topical, is most effective in preventing caries on smooth surfaces; the least benefit is to the occlusal surface. Systemic fluoride may be responsible for producing teeth with less steep occlusal fissures (Lovius and Goose, 1969). However, epidemiological studies indicate that any modification of occlusal anatomy caused by systemic fluoride does not result in a significant reduction in occlusal caries. Some benefit will occur if the enamel in the depths of the fissure is exposed to fluoride topically. Marthaler (1969) found a 36% reduction in DMFT in children who chewed fluoride tablets; it is speculated that crushing the tablets can force fluoride into the embrasures and into the depths of the occlusal fissures to obtain a topical effect from this systemically directed agent.

Saturating the fissures with topical fluoride is an avenue that has been further investigated, but the minimal reduction in occlusal caries is disappointing. It is speculated that neither stannous nor acidulated fluoride is able to impregnate the enamel at the depths of the fissures. This disappointing finding has prompted the evaluation of fluorides in concentrated polyurethane coatings or fissure-protecting lacquers. These have limited effectiveness, especially when compared with pit-and-fissure sealants.

Sealants

Selection of teeth

Teeth with the greatest susceptibility to dental caries should be candidates for sealant use. First and second permanent molars are most susceptible to occlusal caries and these teeth should always be considered (NIH, 1984). Ripa (1990) claimed that first and second permanent molars continue to be the most caries-susceptible teeth, and that the change in the pattern of disease means that decay principally involves pits and fissures. He concluded that there is a greater need than ever before for sealing these teeth. The occlusal surfaces of premolars and primary molars should also be considered for pit-and-fissure sealants in children with a high decay rate.

For many years it has been suggested that sealant should be applied as close as possible to eruption time and that there was little value in sealing a tooth which had been erupted for 3 years or more. Ripa et al. (1988) argued otherwise; they followed for 3 years children who were 10–13 years old at the start of the study. The proportion of first permanent molars developing occlusal caries or having fillings placed increased throughout the study at an average rate of 10%. They concluded that it is not just in the first few years of the life of a tooth that we should consider sealants. The depth and inclination of the fissures, and the presence of fissure staining, must also be considered since they will determine the likelihood of developing caries. The child's previous decay experience will also help the clinician predict whether a tooth is at risk and if so would benefit from a sealant.

Selection of teeth on the basis of freedom from caries has already been described. These rigid criteria for application of sealants are in contradiction to the results with deliberately sealed deep carious lesions using Nuva-Seal (Handelman et al., 1973). A comparison of sealed and untreated non-sealed lesions revealed a marked reduction in cultivatable bacteria in the sealed lesions 6 months postoperatively. This speaks highly of the sealant's marginal integrity over the first 6 months, as it can be assumed that the bacteria within the lesion could no longer remain viable in the absence of nutrients and saliva, which were denied by the effectiveness of the seal. However, such findings should not encourage the clinician to seal active lesions. The temptation to do this is greater when the child presents as a behaviour problem, but application of the sealant may be more difficult in such a child and the clinical result imperfect. Should that sealant fail and decay progress in the tooth, the clinician is faced with the problem of treating a large lesion in a difficult child.

An ideal sealant should adhere to all sound tooth surfaces around a fissure, theoretically providing the key to prevention of bacterial invasion and subsequent caries formation. The problem of retention and adaptation is magnified by the irregular anatomy of the occlusal surface, both at a macroscopic and microscopic level. Acid conditioning of the enamel surface before the sealant is applied improves the resin's retention. This conditioning is universally used in all present-day sealants to enhance retention and improve the marginal seal. Recently, Ripa (1993) has reviewed the effectiveness of pit-and-fissure sealants and noted that retention was clinically greater for second-generation (autopolymerized) compared with first-generation (ultraviolet light-initiated) sealants. After 5–7 years following application, approximately one-third of the teeth were fully protected with first-generation sealants compared with two-thirds with second-generation sealants. Third-generation sealants (visible light-cured) appear to have similar retention rates to the second-generation ones.

Enamel conditioning

Buonocore (1955) demonstrated the improved retention of simple acrylic resin to enamel that had been conditioned by acid. Since that time, acid conditioning or etching of enamel has been used in the retention of pit-and-fissure sealants, the attachment of orthodontic brackets directly to teeth, the restoration of fractured incisors, splinting of mobile teeth and to increase enamel fluoride uptake. Various types and concentrations of acid and durations of application have been studied. Silverstone (1974) found that a 60-s application of an unbuffered solution of 37% phosphoric acid produced the most favourable conditions for bonding. Fuks et al. (1984) and Eidelman et al. (1984) showed, respectively, that a 20-s etch provided similar leakage resistance and retention rates when compared to a 60-s etch. This has very obvious implications for the management of young children when sealing their teeth, and therefore upon the success of the sealant itself. Acid-etching has two distinct actions on human enamel. Firstly, it removes superficial plaque, debris and a very shallow layer of enamel, including chemically inert enamel crystallites. Secondly, it renders the enamel surface more porous. A honey-combed lattice-work is produced within the remaining superficial enamel, where enamel tags are left projecting in different planes and at different angles (*Figs* 8.1–8.3). There is differential demineralization of the prisms because the primary attack occurs on the cores of enamel rods to produce the microspaces. However, this depends on the incident angulation of the enamel rods to the tooth surface. On an average, the etching is about 25 μm deep in permanent teeth.

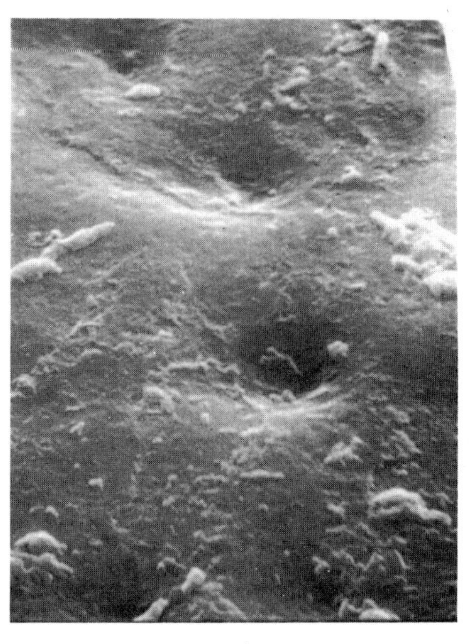

Fig. 8.1. Photomicrograph of normal enamel: permanent tooth (× 2400). (Courtesy of Dr H. Lee, South El Monte, California.)

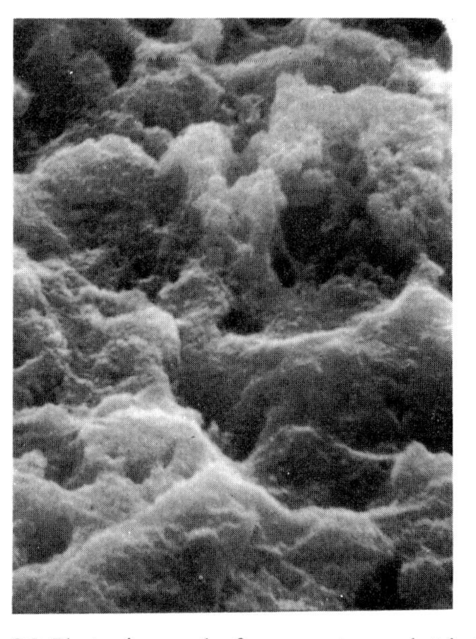

Fig. 8.2. Photomicrograph of permanent enamel etched by 50% phosphoric acid (× 2400). Note the honeycomb effect. (Courtesy of Dr H. Lee, South El Monte, California.)

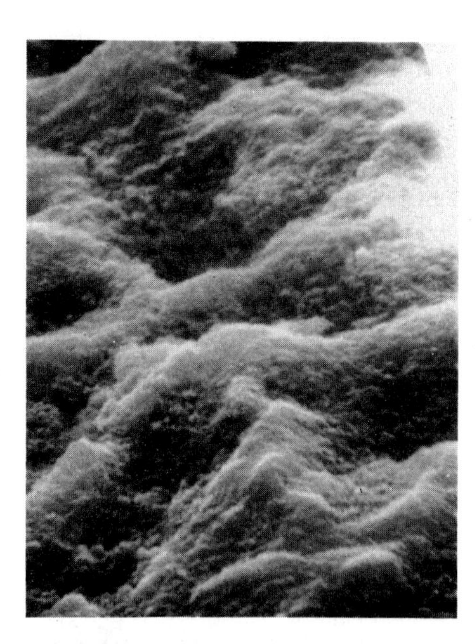

Fig. 8.3. Photomicrograph of primary enamel etched by 50% phosphoric acid (× 2400). Note that the etching is considerably different from that in *Fig.* 8.2. (Courtesy of Dr H. Lee, South El Monte, California.)

It was thought that the outer prismless layer of primary enamel (Ripa, 1966) prevented the penetration of resins in the surface of etched primary enamel (Sheykholeslam and Buonocore, 1972; Hinding and Sveen, 1974). There is no universal agreement that prismless enamel occurs in all surfaces of all primary teeth (Mortimer, 1970; Silverstone, 1970). To obtain a pattern of etching comparable to that found in permanent teeth, Silverstone and Dogon (1976) found it necessary to etch for 120 s. However, Redford et al. (1986) looked at the effect of different etch times on the sealant bond strength, etch depth and pattern, on primary teeth. They found that the bond strength was no greater at 60 or 120 s than at 15 or 30 s, but the standard deviation was greater at the two shorter times; the etch depth was not very different at the three shorter times but was five times greater at 120 s. They felt unable to recommend an etch time for primary enamel of less than 60 s because of the greater variability of bond strength at 15 and 20 s. Our clinical experience is of good results with a 30-s etch.

Retention of the sealant is by mechanical locking into the microspaces produced in the outer enamel surface by etching. This occurs on the inclined planes and not at the depth of the fissures (*Fig.* 8.4). Differential dissolution of the enamel of teeth treated with fissure sealants reveals tags of resin penetrating into the enamel; this confirms the mechanical locking that produces retention. The depth of the resin tags is related to the strength of the bond. The factors which influence the sealant's retention to the etched enamel of the pits and fissures are those which influence etching, and the viscosity and handling of the sealant itself.

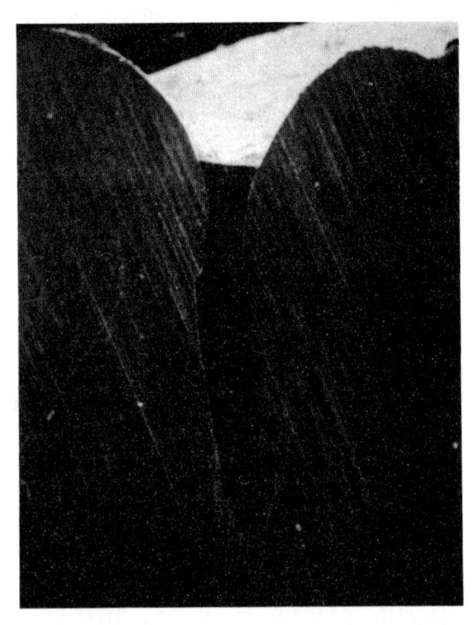

Fig. 8.4. Cross-sectional view of a sealed fissure. Note incomplete extension into the fissure: the retention is mainly from the inclined planes of the fissure. (Courtesy of Dr H. Lee, South El Monte, California.)

Factors that influence etching

Prior to etching, the recommendation has historically been to clean thoroughly the surface of the tooth with an oil-free prophylactic paste, to remove plaque and other organic material that may prevent the normal etching process. Donnan and Ball (1988) found, in a double-blind study, no significant differences in the retention rates of sealants with or without a pre-etch pumice prophylaxis. However, there is insufficient corroborating evidence to advise the omission of this stage. Brown et al. (1988) determined that the inability of the acid, liquid or gel to penetrate the fissure completely was dependent upon the presence of debris within the fissure. It should not be imagined that the prophylaxis cleans into the fissures to allow deeper penetration of the resin; Taylor and Gwinnett (1973) showed that the pumice particles became lodged and impacted into the fissures and therefore did not improve the length of resin tags. Brocklehurst et al. (1992) showed that air-polishing the surface before sealing produced a significantly greater depth of penetration of sealant resin into the fissure itself. They recommended air-polishing as a standard cleaning method before sealing pits and fissures, but the cost of the equipment may prove to be prohibitive at present.

When the etched surface is contaminated with saliva before the sealant is applied, the result is reduced bond strength for the sealant. The contamination prevents adaptation of the sealant, and causes remineralization of etched enamel. Buonocore (1971) reports good retention of the sealant with cotton-roll rather than rubber-dam isolation. Moisture-absorbing buccal pads such as 'Dry-Tips' (see Chapter 7) can be easier to use than cotton rolls. There is a strong indication for the routine use of the rubber dam during application, even though it requires additional time; when the procedure is not being done in conjunction with operative work, cost-effectiveness is reduced. However, we feel that once the technique has been mastered, and using winged clamps inserted into the dam (Chapter 7, method II) a rubber dam can easily and quickly be used for sealant placement.

Oil contamination of the etched surface can occur from a faulty air delivery system, and reduces the bond strength of the sealant. It is therefore advisable to clear the air hose into a cotton roll to observe whether any oil droplets stain the white cotton before drying the etched surface. Once contamination occurs, the tooth must be re-etched for 10 s. There is conflicting advice regarding the wash time after etching. To wash for the same time as to etch could mean 60 s of washing, simultaneously trying to prevent salivary contamination if rubber dam is not being used. This could prove difficult in a young child. Mixson et al. (1988) found there were no significant differences in the bond strengths of composite resin to enamel with wash times of 10 s or more. Turner et al. (1987) analysed the rinse times of liquid and gel etchants using ^{32}P labelling, evaluating the time necessary to remove the residual soluble and insoluble radiolabel from the enamel surface. No significant soluble residues were present after 2.5 s, and all insoluble residues were gone after 7.5 s. There seems little advantage to be gained from rinsing for more than 7–10 s.

Viscosity and handling of the sealant

The strength of the bond depends on the sealant's ability to flow both into the microspaces produced by acid etching and into the depths of pits and fissures. The more viscous materials will not flow and their retention is consequently reduced. Improper mixing or application will make the material porous, and if this occurs adjacent to the etched surface, the seal will be imperfect.

Sealant application and polymerization

After etching, rinsing and drying, the treated enamel should appear chalky, dull and opaque with loss of natural lustre (*Fig.* 8.5). If this appearance is not observed, the etching process should be repeated before the resin is applied and then polymerized. Chemically cured systems have largely been superseded by third-generation, visible light-cured systems, owing to their ease of handling and command-set properties, which increase the working time of the resin. The light source is held 1–2 mm from the surface for 20 s to obtain polymerization. Cured resin should appear smooth and shiny, with an uncured air-inhibition layer on the surface; this layer is thicker with chemically cured systems than with light-cured ones, and in either case can be wiped away with a cotton roll. Air bubbles in the surface should be covered with more resin in case they penetrate to the enamel. The margins of the resin should blend imperceptibly with the tooth surface.

Postoperative evaluation

The retention of the sealant should be tested immediately after curing by trying to prise it off (Houpt and Shey, 1983). This approach may identify those sealants that would have been lost early due to inadequate bonding. This retention testing should become routine. There is frequently occlusal interference from a newly applied resin. Tillis et al. (1992) looked at the effects of occlusal discrepancies arising from filled and unfilled sealants. They found that when unfilled sealant led to premature contact, natural abrasion quickly returned the occlusion to normal in 2–7 days; when filled sealants containing 50% particles were applied, the

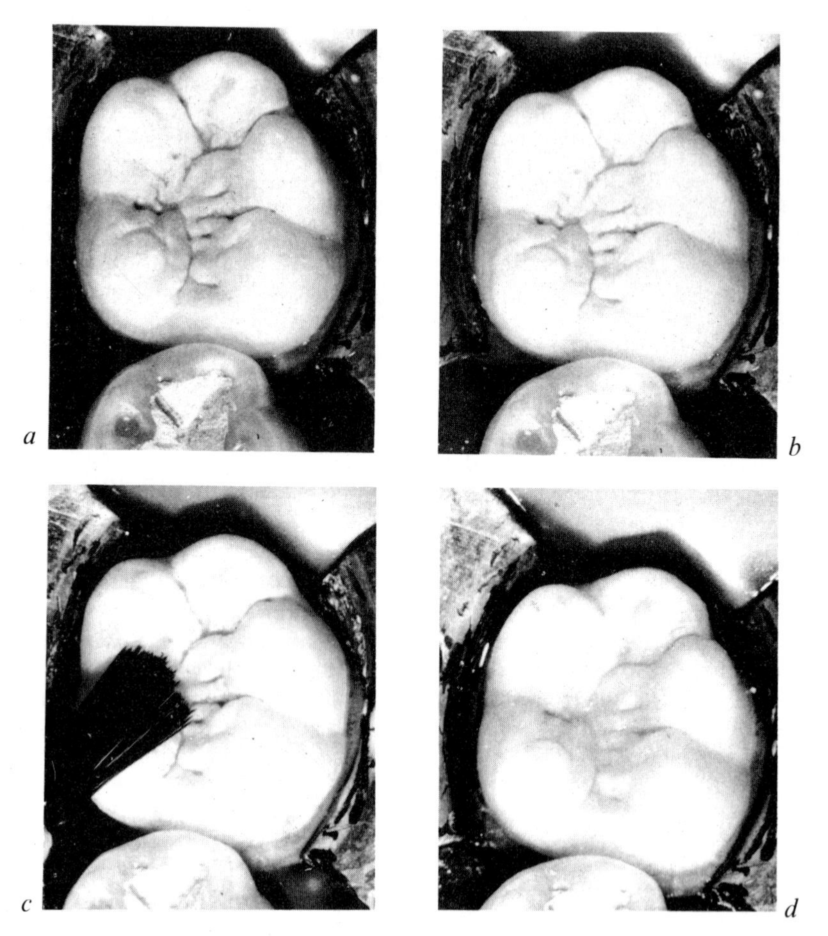

Fig. 8.5. *a*, Preoperative view of isolated tooth suitable for fissure sealant. Note absence of caries. *b*, After etching with phosphoric acid the occlusal surface appears chalky. *c*, The sealant is applied with a camel-hair brush. *d*, Completed fissure sealant.

occlusion had still not returned to normal after 7 days, and participants asked for adjustment because of discomfort. It would seem prudent to adjust gross interferences when using filled sealants, but to allow minor ones to adjust spontaneously.

Clear sealants are more difficult to evaluate than opaque or coloured ones, but any enamel surface changes beneath the sealant caused, for instance, by leakage are more readily identified through clear sealants. Bitewing radiographs taken at appropriate intervals should be compared to the pre-sealant ones to check for changes beneath the sealant. Any alteration in radiographic appearance should prompt removal of the sealant and restorative treatment of the occlusal surface. In the absence of any such radiolucency, re-application of the sealant is indicated if the margins are deficient and no lesion is apparent clinically.

Sealant failure

Most sealant failures occur at the enamel–resin interface. They are usually caused by insufficient etching or contamination of the etched enamel prior to sealant application, and would not occur if a meticulous technique was followed. When contamination does occur, the tooth should be re-etched for 10 s.

The highest number of sealant failures occur on second molars with an operculum covering the distal marginal ridge (Dennison et al., 1990) and especially in the distal pit of maxillary molars (Ripa, 1980). With the patient in the supine position, the distal pit of the maxillary molar is the least accessible, especially in the presence of an operculum distal to a partially erupted tooth. Furthermore, gravity may cause the sealant to flow distal to the marginal ridge, and the resulting ledge easily becomes dislodged as it is not on etched enamel. When sealants are lost, the clinician is faced with the dilemma of whether to replace them or to observe. Extended protection against caries is provided to occlusal surfaces which have lost sealants (Hinding, 1974; Rock, 1974). Retention of resin tags within the superficial enamel may be responsible for this. However, we feel that it is appropriate to replace lost or defective sealants. Using the post-insertion retention test recommended by Houpt and Shey (1983), as described above, this early loss of sealants is significantly reduced.

It is disappointing to observe decay formation on the lingual and buccal pits and grooves of permanent molars when the occlusal surface has been effectively sealed. Therefore, as a routine, the lingual and buccal pits and grooves of maxillary and mandibular molars should be sealed. In newly erupted mandibular second permanent molars, the buccal pits may be very deep due to incompletely coalesced enamel. When partial eruption precludes proper sealant application, the patient may require a more frequent recall schedule so that these areas can be properly managed.

Sealant effectiveness

Study periods of at least 2–3 years are required to assess sealant effectiveness (Ripa, 1993). This allows detailed evaluation of retention, sealant leakage, the need for sealant re-application, and of subsequent carious formation both occlusally and interproximally.

Long-term studies of sealants over varying periods have been reported, such as 10 years in Canada (Romcke et al., 1990) and 15 years in the USA (Simonsen, 1991). These all report a reduction in the level of caries compared to unsealed teeth. Recently, however, it has been considered unethical to leave a tooth untreated to compare with a sealed tooth; instead, attention has focused on sealant retention and by implication its effectiveness against dental caries.

In general terms, the retention of the sealant equates proportionately to the reduction in occlusal caries, especially in the first 2 years after application. As the time from initial placement increases, there is a gradual increase in sealant loss; accordingly the sealant's effectiveness is reduced (Mertz-Fairhurst et al., 1982; Houpt and Shey, 1983). Buonocore (1971) reported 87% retention of Nuva-Seal to permanent teeth after 2 years. However, caries reduction was 99%, indicating that despite sealant loss, teeth have extended protection against caries from the retention of resin tags within the superficial enamel.

Fluoride release from sealants

A number of fluoride-releasing sealants have been tested and marketed (Cooley et al., 1990). Fluoride release is rapid and occurs mostly within 2 days. Retention of the sealant appears to be good, although only short-term studies have been reported. The clinical benefit from the use of such sealants remains to be adequately demonstrated.

Pit-and-fissure caries

Diagnosis

Pit-and-fissure involvement was the most frequent caries experience for children in the primary dentition in the study by Greenwell et al. (1990). The depth and inclination of the fissures determine that the second primary molar is affected more often than the first primary molar. For this same reason, mandibular teeth are carious more often than their maxillary counterparts. This trend is also seen in the first and second permanent molars (Walsh and Smart, 1948). Dental caries of the 1980s was felt to be a pit-and-fissure disease, and there is reason to believe that this still holds true in the 1990s (Ripa, 1990), particularly where water supplies are fluoridated. This should be borne in mind when examining the child patient.

The following should be available for the diagnostic examination:

- an explorer,
- a source of good light,
- a source of air to dry the tooth,
- current bitewing radiographs,
- an assessment of the patient's past and projected caries experience.

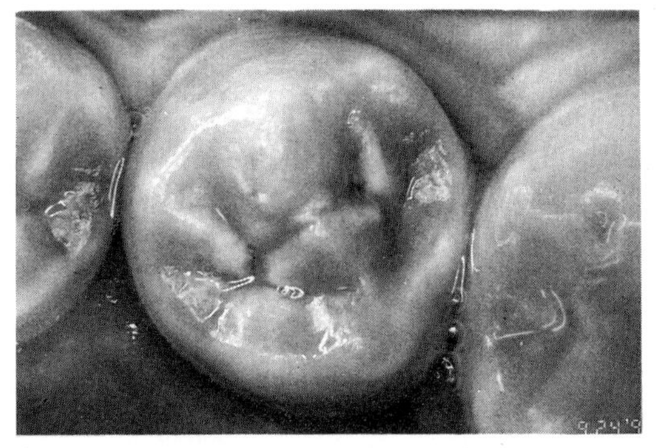

a

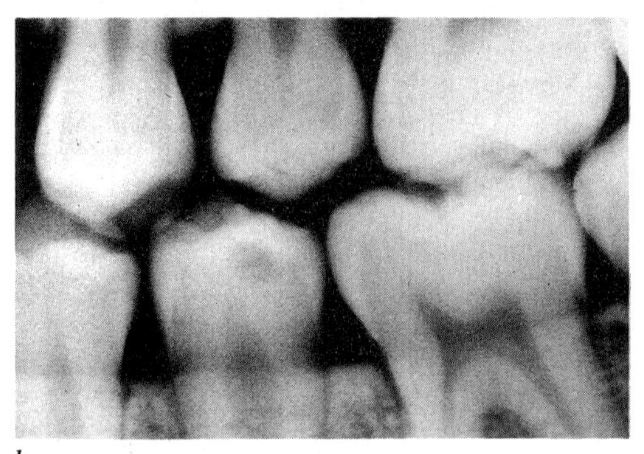

b

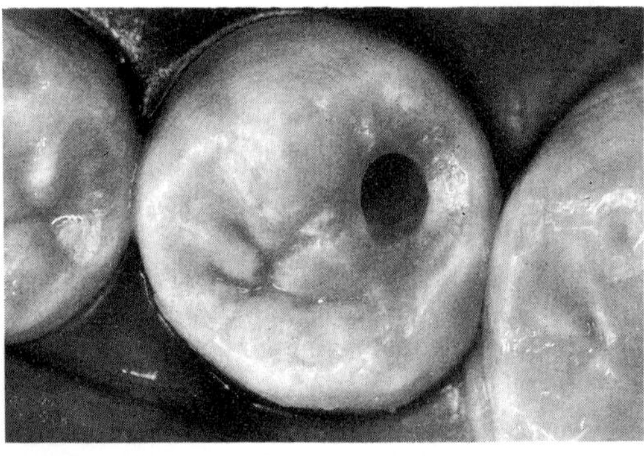

c

Fig. 8.6. Covert caries. *a*, Occlusal view of a premolar with little indication of caries except slight discoloration of the distal occlusal pit. *b*, Bitewing radiograph clearly shows the caries penetrating into dentine. *c*, Cavity prepared and showing extent of the caries.

Exploration of a gross lesion is contraindicated since it is unnecessary in establishing the diagnosis and it may distress the child. This is not the case with the incipient lesion. However, care should be exercised not to apply heavy pressure to a recently erupted permanent molar whose pit-and-fissure enamel may be incompletely coalesced or immature because of lack of saliva contact. Such action, especially with a sharp explorer, may actually create cavitation where deep fissures exist (Ekstrand et al., 1987). The term 'sticky fissure' was historically used to describe early occlusal fissure caries; unfortunately, besides the potential damage caused by the heavy probing of such a fissure, its interpretation can lead to confusion. To say that a fissure is 'sticky' indicates that an explorer will catch in the depths of the fissure; it may or may not be carious. Other diagnostic criteria (the grey discoloration, the radiographic appearance and the previous decay experience) are needed to confirm the diagnosis.

The grey discoloration that results from the undermining of enamel by caries is best seen on a well-illuminated, dry tooth. The occlusal lesion may sometimes be observed on a bitewing radiograph as two radiolucent triangles, one in the enamel and one in the dentine. The bases of the two triangles are coincident at the amelodentinal junction and the apices are towards the fissure and the pulp, respectively. The fissure may extend very close to the amelodentinal junction, which helps account for the rapid onset of occlusal caries after the tooth's eruption into the mouth. Also, the shape of the fissure may defy any attempt at cleansing because its orifice is finer than a toothbrush bristle (Cawson, 1972).

The use of topical fluoride has lulled the clinician into a sense of false security in the diagnosis of pit-and-fissure caries (Sawle and Andlaw, 1988). Topical fluorides, though least effective on the occlusal surface, seem to have the ability to make the pits and fissures hard and firm to exploration. This can occur after a lesion has reached dentine (*Fig.* 8.6). Careful examination of bitewing radiographs may reveal extensive caries involving the dentine that is not observable clinically. In fact, the lesion may progress to the pulp without showing any enamel surface breakdown. The term 'covert caries' has been used to describe this condition (Lavin, 1983). Therefore, special care should be taken in the diagnosis of occlusal lesions in patients who are regularly receiving topical fluoride. The same applies to patients with pit-and-fissure sealants; their use in the prevention of Class 1 lesions has been discussed earlier.

Another consideration in the diagnosis of Class 1 lesions is the past and projected caries experience of the patient. The astute clinician should always be alert to the possibility of a clinically unobservable but radiographically apparent Class 2 lesion in a tooth with occlusal caries. There is little value in spending an operative visit restoring a Class 1 lesion, only to spend more time 6 months later replacing it with a Class 2 alloy, when a Class 2 lesion existed from the outset but was undiagnosed.

The preventive resin restoration

Concept

Despite the various methods discussed above, the diagnosis of early occlusal caries remains less than perfect. There are times when no treatment is carried out or an inadequate sealant placed and undiagnosed caries progresses; on other occasions a conventional Class 1 cavity is cut where no caries existed.

When the clinician is confident that the occlusal surface is sound and the potential for early onset of caries is low, the correct treatment would be application of topical fluoride and a further period of observation; if confident that a stained fissure is not carious but simply poorly coalesced, then a fissure sealant is indicated; when most or all of the occlusal pits and fissures show definite signs of decay, then a conventional Class 1 cavity should be cut, as described later in this chapter. However, on many occasions the condition of the tooth will not be so clear-cut, and reasonable doubt will exist in the mind of even the best diagnostician concerning the presence or absence of caries.

If doubt exists, then it should be removed; either by removing just enough tooth substance to show that the fissure is not carious, or by removing just enough tooth substance to get access to the caries that does exist. Handelman et al. (1973) showed that caries will not progress beneath a well-applied sealant; fissure sealing is not a treatment for caries, however, and if the clinician suspects the presence of caries, then the diseased part(s) of the tooth should be removed.

Rather than extend the cavity preparation to include all pits and fissures, whether carious or not, the preventive resin restoration employs the concept of decay removal and resin placement, followed by prevention by sealing all other susceptible fissures. Due to the excellent results obtained with pit-and-fissure sealants, and the establishment of wear-resistant composite resins, the preventive resin restoration is a conservative approach to pit-and-fissure caries, which has shown to be very successful in 15-year studies (Simonsen, 1991). To date, the preventive resin restoration has only been studied in permanent teeth.

Technique (*Fig.* 8.7)

Preventive resin restorations are indicated for teeth with minimal pit-and-fissure decay or questionable decay. In these minimal situations, a small bur, in a fast or slow handpiece, is used to remove stained or carious material as conservatively as possible. If the decay does not extend into dentine the cavity is limited to enamel, and there will be no need for local analgesia. No base is required, and after etching, rinsing and drying the cavity is filled before the remaining etched areas are sealed in the conventional manner. Raadal (1978) pointed out that the consistency of the composite used for the filling part of the restoration is not of primary importance; sometimes it is convenient to use sealant throughout and at other times it is easier to condense a normal composite or glass-ionomer cement before sealing the remaining susceptible fissures.

When the decay is into the dentine, under local analgesia and with rubber dam, the decay is removed within a conservative outline form. Care should be taken to identify and remove caries spreading laterally along the amelodentinal junction; it is easily missed with such small cavities. A calcium hydroxide base is placed before filling the cavity and then applying sealant.

Clinical considerations

The significant reduction in dental caries (see Chapter 1), together with the long-term clinical success of pit-and-fissure sealants and advances in resin technology have prompted reassessment of the conventional Class 1 amalgam restoration. Since conventional cavity preparation dictates extension for prevention, there is considerable destruction of tooth structure, perhaps needlessly. The first restoration placed in a tooth dictates the minimum size of any subsequent restoration, be it a replacement or as a result of new decay on an approximal

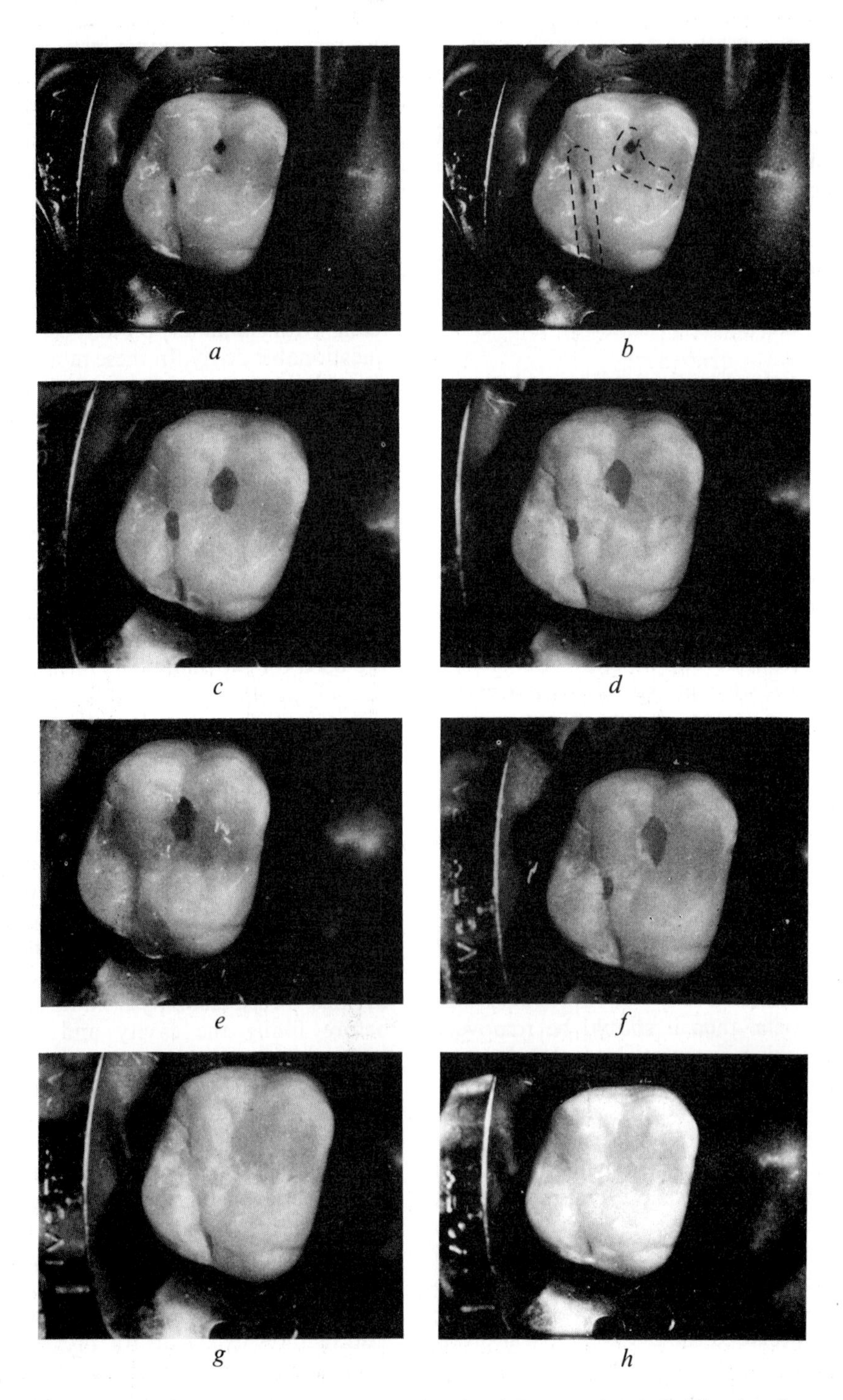

Fig. 8.7. Preventive resin restoration. *a*, Preoperative view. *b*, Preoperative: dashed line describes the extent of what would be a typical Class 1 amalgam cavity. *c*, Minimal cavity preparation. *d*, Calcium hydroxide lining. *e*, Etching with 37% phosphoric acid gel. *f*, Etched enamel. *g*, Filled resin placed in cavity preparation. *h*, Sealant applied.

surface. Elderton (1985a,b) suggested a thorough reassessment of the management of carious lesions due to the marked decline in decay rates. He encouraged the clinician to look at, rather than probe, lesions in order to protect the demineralized enamel surface from needless traumatic and iatrogenic cavitations. Wherever possible he recommended a non-invasive approach and suggested sealing questionable fissures. The conservative aspects of preventive resin restorations address concern about unnecessary tooth destruction and delay the possibility of cuspal fracture several years into the future. If the preventive resin restoration fails, then conventional, less conservative, measures can be used.

Limitations

We are not aware of any studies to date that have explored the limits of the preventive resin restoration, i.e. when the amount or location of the prepared cavity dictates that a conventional Class 1 amalgam or composite resin would be more suitable. The ability of resin to withstand occlusal pressures must be addressed. Fortunately, the central pits are most commonly decayed, and these areas do not occlude heavily. Our clinical experience suggests that when all or most of the occlusal pit-and-fissure system is decayed and the proportion of cavosurface in areas of potential occlusion is more than minimal, then amalgam should be placed. Clinicians need more guidance from research to help in their judgements. However, we believe that given the reported success of the preventive resin restoration, it should be strongly recommended to clinicians wherever possible, rather than the more destructive, conventional Class 1 preparation.

The class 1 conventional cavity

General considerations

The outline form should include all areas susceptible to further decay. That is, the cavity should be extended for prevention, which usually means including all deep pits and fissures in the preparation so that the margins can be easily finished and can be readily cleaned by the patient. The actual amount of fissure extension is determined by the anatomy of the fissure, the presence of caries and stain, and the patient's previous caries experience. It is better to err on the side of overextension of fissure elimination for safety. This does not mean that overdestruction of tooth structure intercuspally is acceptable. When incipient lesions are being treated the preoperative occlusal anatomy seldom requires gross reduction; the maximum intercuspal cavity width should be one-quarter to one-third of the intercuspal width. The buccal and lingual extension of the Class 1 cavity, both mesially and distally, determines the isthmus width of any Class 2 cavity which is subsequently prepared in that tooth; this justifies conservative preparations. A small, fissure, turbine bur (No. 330) should be used to prepare the cavity.

Class 1 cavities should be extended at least 0.5 mm pulpally to the amelodentinal junction to provide sufficient bulk of amalgam to withstand occlusal forces. Any remaining caries can be removed with round burs run at slow speed. The pulpal floor should be flat wherever possible. The deeper portions of the cavity are lined with a pulp-protecting base, although it is not necessary to replace all carious material with a base. Internal line angles should be rounded to reduce any stresses in the set amalgam. The cavosurface margin should approximate 90° to render both amalgam–surface and cavosurface angles strong enough to avoid marginal deterioration. The extension and depth of the cavity will be determined by the amount and location of caries and preoperative occlusal anatomy. Every effort should be made to retain as much well-supported enamel as possible.

The first primary molar

The central pit of lower first primary molars usually becomes carious before the mesial pit, which decays less frequently. Thus the outline form should be limited to the central pit and its adjacent buccal and lingual developmental grooves and distal triangular fossa (*Fig.* 8.8). Seldom is it necessary to cross the ridge of enamel joining the mesiobuccal and mesiolingual cusp to eliminate caries. In fact, it is inadvisable to do so because of the proximity of the mesiobuccal pulp horn, and because of the strength imparted to the tooth by that central ridge remaining intact.

The occlusal surface of the first primary

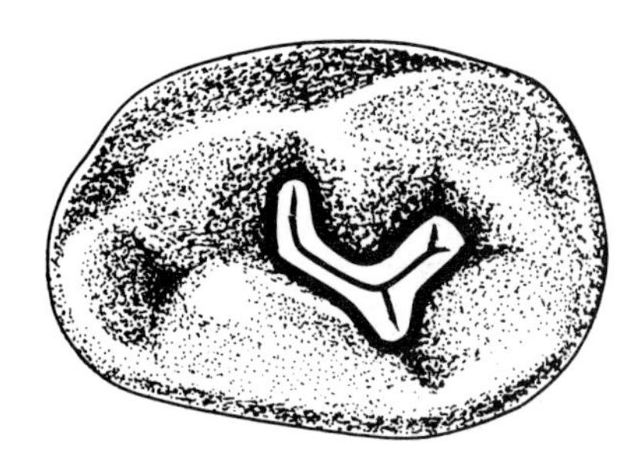

Fig. 8.8. Correct cavity outline form in mandibular right first primary molar. It is unnecessary to cross the central ridge.

molar may be extensively destroyed at a young age by nursing-bottle caries (described in Chapter 1). The young age of the child and the extensive lesions that are seen warrant special consideration that differs from the previously recommended principles. The extent and depth of decay may necessitate a wider outline form and even pulp therapy. When treating these lesions, the clinician must also consider the prognosis for improvement in home care, which is in part determined by the parent's ability to break the child's feeding habit and the child's taste for sugars. If the parent is unsuccessful, the tooth may be subject to further decay. For this reason a temporary 'treatment filling' may be used while the home care is being assessed.

Resin-bonded zinc oxides are suitable intermediate restorative materials as their durability has been clinically proven (Hutchins and Parker, 1972; Weaver et al., 1972). The bland qualities of these materials may eliminate the need for a pulp-protecting base and their ease of manipulation makes them attractive for use in the very young child when working time and co-operation may be at a premium. Also useful in the treatment of nursing caries are fluoride-releasing glass-ionomer cements. However, the need for moisture control means that these materials are less desirable as restorations. It is important to inform the parent that 'treatment fillings' have been placed and that they will need replacement later. The term 'treatment filling' is preferred to 'temporary filling' as it implies such fillings have a purpose and serves as a means of educating the parent. The treatment restorations can be replaced after a minimum of 6–8 weeks. However, a longer interval (6 months to 1 year) is advisable before replacement, to permit further assessment of the home care. Also the child may mature to the extent that he or she will accept more extensive treatment.

Sometimes the caries is so extensive that the whole occlusal surface is destroyed. In such instances, a stainless-steel crown will probably be the treatment of choice.

Second primary and first permanent molars

These teeth are considered together because of their almost identical anatomy. The outline form should include the fissures throughout the occlusal surface (*Figs* 8.9 and 8.10). However, the intercuspal dimensions of the cavity should be kept small, as previously described.

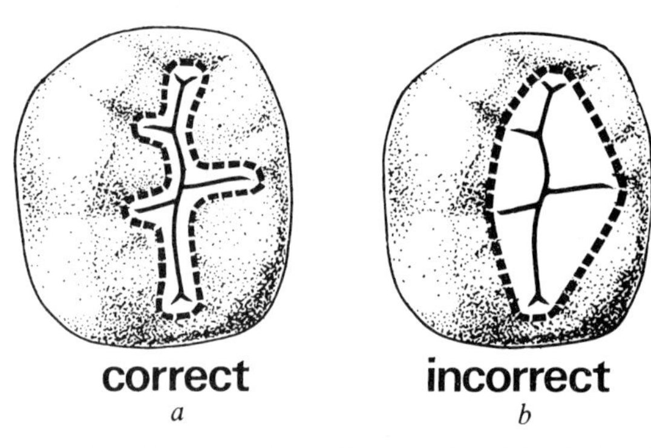

Fig. 8.9. *a*, Correct cavity outline form for minimal Class 1 lesion in mandibular first permanent molar. Note the extension into fissures and maintenance of intercuspal width. *b*, Incorrect cavity form for minimal Class 1 lesion in mandibular first permanent molar. Excessive destruction of tooth will result in weakening of cusps if ever a Class 2 restoration is placed in this tooth.

1. Mandibular

The danger areas for underextension and the development of recurrent caries seem to be at the extremities of the lingual and buccal fissures. It will be necessary in some instances to extend the cavity preparation to include a poorly supported, or carious, buccal or lingual fissure which would make an occlusobuccal or occlusolingual cavity (*Fig.* 8.10), although the tooth remains stronger if the fissure remains intact, with separate buccal or lingual restorations being placed. If the extension is made, the buccal or lingual cavity walls should be straight and either parallel or converging occlusally with square external line angles. The extension should be cut 0.5 mm into dentine and should

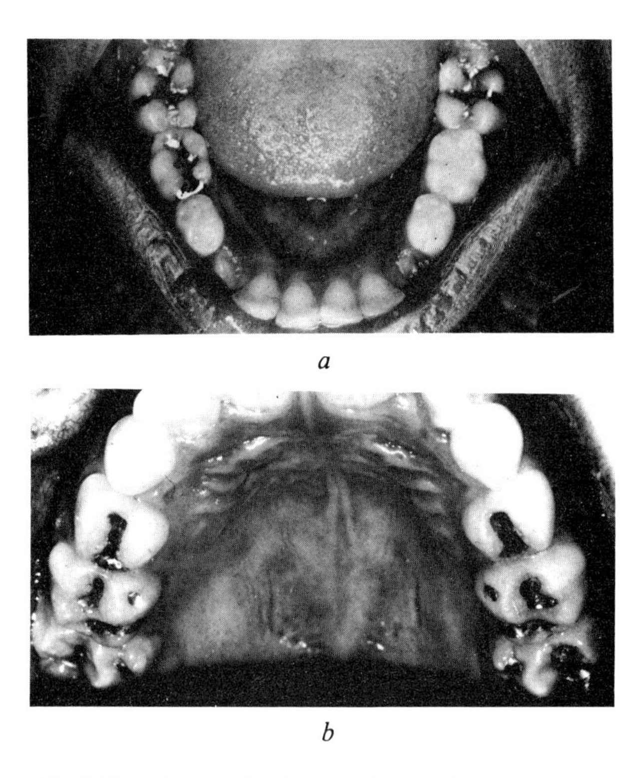

Fig. 8.10. *a*, Completed occlusobuccal restorations in mandibular first permanent molars. *b*, Completed occlusal and occlusolingual restorations in second primary molars.

extend gingivally to include the buccal developmental pit. Retention grooves can be placed in dentine if considered necessary. The 'isthmus' area where the extension meets the occlusal section can be rounded or bevelled to increase the bulk of amalgam, which is subjected to heavy stresses during lateral movements.

2. Maxillary

Carious attack is usually limited to the central pit, distal pit, lingual pit and the groove separating the cusp of Carabelli from the mesiolingual cusp. Therefore it is seldom necessary to cross the oblique ridge which joins the mesiolingual and distobuccal cusps when treating small lesions (*Fig.* 8.10); it should only be done when caries undermines the oblique ridge.

The depth of the lingual developmental groove and its continuity with the distal pit and distal developmental groove frequently necessitate the placement of an occlusolingual restoration in maxillary molars. Inclusion of the lingual developmental groove and lingual pit can be regarded as extension for prevention, just as with the mandibular buccal extension. The outline and depth of this lingual extension are similar to those of the buccal extension seen in the mandibular molar. Occasionally an accessory groove runs from the lingual developmental groove to the groove separating the cusp of Carabelli and mesiolingual cusp; when this fissure is carious or pre-carious it may have to be included in the cavity preparation as 'extension for prevention'. The width of the lingual extension should be minimal, with alloy bulk being compensated for by deepening the cavity. The reason for this is that excessive tooth removal would weaken the distolingual and mesiolingual cusps should a Class 2 lesion ever require restoration subsequently. Straight cavity margins at the buccal and lingual extensions with square external line angles are easy to prepare and they also facilitate finishing of the restoration.

It is seldom necessary to place a matrix band to help condense the alloy; direct condensation is advised. A common fault is to underpack and overcarve at the junction of the occlusal and lingual extensions (or buccal in mandibular teeth).

The second permanent molar

The principles outlined for first permanent molars apply also for the second permanent molars. The occlusal anatomy differs, particularly in the maxillary arch when the distolingual cusp may be absent or rudimentary. The central developmental groove may extend distally across a very flat oblique ridge, joining up with the distal pit and distal developmental groove. Also, the absence of a distolingual cusp may eliminate the lingual developmental groove. Since cavity design should be related to the occlusal anatomy, it may be unnecessary to include a lingual extension in the cavity design. Two separate occlusal pits (mesially and distally) may require separate occlusal cavities. However, the presence of an extended central developmental groove may require that the outline form encompass both central and distal pits, crossing a rudimentary or absent oblique ridge.

The mandibular second permanent molar sometimes presents a unique problem. This tooth may become carious very shortly after eruption and the caries seems to spread very rapidly. Questionable occlusal fissures in mandibular second permanent molars should be restored. To add to the problem, the tooth may be only partially erupted, the distal aspect being covered by an operculum of tissue that persists for as long as a year following initial eruption into the oral cavity. *Figures* 7.2 and 7.3 (Chapter 7) demonstrate the use of the rubber dam to solve the problem of partial eruption. The extensive caries that is sometimes seen may require indirect pulp treatment (Chapter 20) to avoid pulp exposure.

Developmental pits

These can occur in four areas:

(1) midway down the mesiobuccal developmental groove in mandibular second primary, first and second permanent molars;
(2) midway down the lingual developmental groove in maxillary second primary, first and second permanent molars;
(3) between the fifth cusp (cusp of Carabelli) and the mesiolingual cusp of second primary and first permanent molars;
(4) the lingual pit in maxillary permanent incisors and, rarely, in maxillary permanent canines; the permanent lateral incisor is most frequently affected.

The developmental pit and any accessory developmental groove should be included in the outline form if they are considered to be carious or caries-prone. Other requirements for cavity preparation have already been mentioned.

A lingual pit and an accessory lingual cusp on a maxillary permanent lateral incisor represent just one step towards a dens in dente. Caries in this area may lead to a non-vital pulp in a tooth with an open apex, the endodontic treatment of which is not straightforward. These pits should be sealed as a prophylactic measure. A maxillary anterior radiograph at age 6 years may alert the astute paediatric dentist to deep developmental pits on developing maxillary permanent lateral incisors.

References

Bodecker C. F. (1929) The eradication of enamel fissures. *Dent. Items Int.* **51**, 859.

Bohanan H. M. and Bader J. D. (1984) Future impacts of public health and preventive methods on the incidence of dental caries. *J. Can. Dent. Assoc.* **50**, 229.

Buonocore M. G. (1955) A simple method of increasing the adhesion of acrylic filling materials to enamel surfaces. *J. Dent. Res.* **34**, 849.

Buonocore M. G. (1971) Caries prevention in pits and fissures sealed with an adhesive resin polymerized by ultraviolet light: a ten-year study of a single adhesive application. *J. Am. Dent. Assoc.* **82**, 1090.

Brocklehurst P. R., Joshi R. I. and Northeast S. E. (1992) The effect of air-polishing occlusal surfaces on the penetration of fissures by a sealant. *Int. J. Paed. Dent.* **2**, 157.

Brown M. R., Foreman F. J., Burgess J. O. and Summitt J. B. (1988) Penetration of gel and soluble etchants in occlusal fissures. *J. Dent. Child.* **55**, 265.

Cawson R. A. (1972) *Essentials of Dental Surgery and Pathology*, 2nd edn, p. 14. London, Churchill.

Cooley R. L., McCourt J. W., Huddleston A. M. and Casmedes H.P. (1990) Evaluation of a fluoride-containing sealant by SEM, microleakage and fluoride release. *Pediatr. Dent.* **12**, 38.

Dennison J. B., Straffon L. H. and More F. G. (1990)

Evaluating tooth eruption on sealant efficacy. *J. Am. Dent. Assoc.* **121**, 610.

Donnan M. F. and Ball I. A. (1988) A double-blind clinical trial to determine the importance of pumice prophylaxis on fissure sealant retention. *Br. Dent. J.* **165**, 283.

Eidelman E., Shapira J. and Houpt M. (1984) The retention of fissure sealants using twenty-second etching time. *J. Dent. Child.* **51**, 422.

Ekstrand K., Qvist V. and Thylstrup A. (1987) Light microscope study of the effect of probing on occlusal surfaces. *Caries Res.* **21**, 368.

Elderton R. J. (1985a) Management of early dental caries in fissures with fissure sealant. *Br. Dent. J.* **15**, 254.

Elderton R. J. (1985b) Assessment and clinical management of early caries in young adults: invasive versus non-invasive methods. *Br. Dent. J.* **158**, 440.

Fuks A. B., Grajower R. and Shapira J. (1984) *In vitro* assessment of marginal leakage of sealants placed in permanent molars with different etching times. *J. Dent. Child.* **51**, 425.

Greenwell A. L. *et al.* (1990) Longitudinal evaluation of caries patterns from the primary to the mixed dentition. *Pediatr. Dent.* **12**, 278.

Handelman S. L., Buonocore M. G. and Schoute P. C. (1973) Progress report on the effect of a fissure sealant on bacteria in dental caries. *J. Am. Dent. Assoc.* **87**, 1189.

Hinding J. (1974) Extended cariostasis following loss of pit and fissure sealant from human teeth. *J. Dent. Child.* **41**, 201.

Hinding J. H. and Sveen O. B. (1974) A scanning electron microscope study of the effects of acid conditioning on occlusal enamel of human permanent and deciduous teeth. *Archs Oral Biol.* **19**, 573.

Houpt M. and Shey Z. (1983) The effectiveness of a fissure sealant after 6 years. *Pediatr. Dent.* **5**, 104.

Hutchins V. W. and Parker W. A. (1972) Indirect pulp capping: clinical evaluation using polymethyl methacrylate reinforced zinc oxide-eugenol cement. *J. Dent. Child.* **39**, 55.

Hyatt T. P. (1923) Prophylactic odontotomy. *Dent. Cosmos* **65**, 234.

Lavin A. J. (1983) Covert caries detection. (Letter.) *Br. Dent. J.* **155**, 111.

Lovius B. B. J. and Goose D. H. (1969) The effect of fluoridation of water on tooth morphology. *Br. Dent. J.* **127**, 322.

Marthaler T. M. (1969) Caries-inhibiting effect of fluoride tablets. *Helv. Odontol. Acta.* **13**, 1.

Mertz-Fairhurst E. J. *et al.* (1982) A comparative clinical study of two pit and fissure sealants; 6 year results in Augusta, Georgia. *J. Am. Dent. Assoc.* **105**, 237.

Mixson J. M., Eick J. D., Tira D. E. and Moore D. L. (1988) The effect of variable wash times and techniques on enamel-composite resin bond strengths. *Quintessence Int.* **19**, 279.

Mortimer K. V. (1970) The relationship of deciduous enamel structure to dental disease. *Caries Res.* **4**, 206.

National Institute of Health (1984) Dental sealants in the prevention of tooth decay. Consensus Development Conference.

Raadal M. (1978) Microleakage around preventive composite fillings in occlusal fissures. *Scand. J. Dent. Res.* **86**, 495.

Redford D. A., Clarkson B. H. and Jensen M. (1986) The effect of different etching times on the sealant bond strength, etch depth, and pattern in primary teeth. *Pediatr. Dent.* **8**, 11.

Ripa L. W. (1966) The histology of the early carious lesion in primary teeth with special reference to a 'prismless' outer layer of primary enamel. *J. Dent. Res.* **45**, 5.

Ripa L. W. (1980) Occlusal sealants: Rationale and review of clinical trials. *Int. Dent. J.* **30**, 127.

Ripa L. W. (1990) Has the decline in caries prevalence reduced the need for fissure sealants? A review. *J. Paediatr. Dent.* **6**, 79.

Ripa L. W. (1993) Sealants revisited: an update of the effectiveness of pit and fissure sealants? *Caries Res.* **27** (suppl. 1), 77.

Ripa L. W., Leske G. S. and Varna A. D. (1988) Longitudinal study of the caries susceptibility of occlusal and proximal surfaces of the first permanent molars. *J. Public Health Dent.* **48**, 8.

Rock W. P. (1974) Fissure sealants: further results of clinical trials. *Br. Dent. J.* **136**, 317.

Romcke R. G. *et al.* (1990) Retention and maintenance of fissure sealants over 10 years. *J. Can. Dent. Assoc.* **56**, 235.

Sawle R. F. and Andlaw R. J. (1988) Has occlusal caries become more difficult to diagnose? *Br. Dent. J.* **164**, 209.

Sheykholeslam Z. and Buonocore M. G. (1972) Bonding of resins to phosphoric acid-etched enamel surfaces of permanent and deciduous teeth. *J. Dent. Res.* **51**, 1572.

Silverstone L. M. (1970) The histopathology of early approximal caries in the enamel of primary teeth. *J. Dent. Child.* **37**, 17.

Silverstone L. M. (1974) Fissure sealants: laboratory studies. *Caries Res.* **8**, 26.

Silverstone L. M. and Dogon I. L. (1976) The effect of phosphoric acid on human deciduous enamel surfaces *in vitro*. *J. Int. Assoc. Dent. Child.* **7**, 11.

Simonsen R. J. (1991) Retention and effectiveness of fissure sealants after 15 years. *J. Am. Dent. Assoc.* **122**, 34.

Taylor C. L. and Gwinnett A. J. (1973) A comparative study of the penetration of sealants into pits and fissures. *J. Am. Dent. Assoc.* **87**, 1181.

Tillis T. S. I., Stach D. J. and Hatch R. A., Cross-Poline G. N. (1992) Occlusal discrepancies after sealant therapy. *J. Prosthet. Dent.* **68**, 223.

Turner C., Courts F. J. and Gombola G. G. (1987) The removal of phosphoric acid and calcium phosphate precipitates: an analysis of rinse time. *Pediatr. Dent.* **9**, 208.

Walsh J. P. and Smart R. S. (1948) Relative susceptibility of tooth surfaces to dental caries and other comparative studies. *NZ Dent. J.* **44**, 17.

Weaver R. G. *et al.* (1972) Clinical evaluation of intermediate restorative materials. *J. Dent. Child.* **39**, 1892.

Chapter 9

The Class 2 lesion

Diagnosis (primary teeth)

The Class 2 lesion occurs after primary molar contacts have been established. Therefore, occlusal lesions are more prevalent than interproximal lesions in the very young child (under 4 years) prior to the establishment of primary molar contacts; this pattern is reversed in older children prior to the eruption of permanent molars (Parfitt, 1956).

Incipient Class 2 lesions in primary molars can be diagnosed only with bitewing radiographs. The flat, broad, elliptical contact areas of these teeth defy clinical exploration. Once primary molar contacts have been established, the taking of bitewings should not be delayed in the hope of detecting the lesion clinically, either by exploration or by observation of grey discoloration of the marginal ridge. In children whose proximal surfaces could not be examined by probe, proximal lesions were detectable only by radiographs in 28%, 47% and 64% of 4-, 5- and 6-year-old children, respectively (Steckson-Blicks and Wahlin, 1983). Transillumination has been suggested as an adjunct to radiography for the detection of proximal lesions, but the results have been variable. Although it provides information beyond clinical examination, transillumination needs further development before replacing bitwings for identifying proximal caries (Sidi and Naylor, 1988). Grey discoloration of the marginal ridge suggests an already extensive lesion. It has been shown that the pulp will frequently become exposed during excavation of Class 2 lesions in primary molars where the marginal ridge is broken down (Stoner, 1967).

Early diagnosis of the Class 2 lesion enables the clinician to prepare a cavity of conservative extension and dimensions. In such cases the resulting well-supported margins will give the best chance for the restoration to endure for the life of the tooth. If the Class 2 cavity in primary molars becomes appreciably larger than the minimal classical dimensions to be described here, then the tooth would be better served by a stainless-steel crown. However, although the lesion needs to be diagnosed and treated early for a successful intracoronal restoration, work by Kidd et al. (1992) has shown the potential of the tooth for remineralization of the early lesion. Thus radiographic lesions confined to enamel can be observed, either by longitudinal radiography or by direct vision when an adjacent proximal lesion is being restored, until cavitation occurs. When this philosophy of approach is explained to the child's parents, it may provide the necessary motivation for the behavioural change needed to control the decay process, namely a reduction in the ingestion of refined carbohydrates, plaque control, and fluoride supplementation.

The rate of progress of the lesion needs to be considered. In a longitudinal analysis of bitewing radiographs, lesions progressed through enamel in 24 months for primary teeth and 48 months for permanent teeth (Shwartz et al., 1984). When monitoring the progress of lesions in this way, however, it is important to have standardized beam angulation and film development. The clinician must also recognize the location and nature of interproximal lesions on radiographs. The lesion will appear as a radiolucent triangle in enamel whose apex points toward the amelodentinal junction with the base at or just below the contact area. If the lesion has progressed to dentine, a second radiolucent triangle will be seen whose base is at the amelodentinal junction and whose apex is towards the pulp. Critical analysis of bitewing radiographs, including when necessary the use of magnification, is essential to the early diagnosis of proximal lesions.

Materials

Dental amalgam has been the material of choice to restore the proximal lesion in primary and permanent molars for many years. With the better aesthetics afforded by resin-based composites, and the advantages of dentine adhesion and local fluoride release of glass-ionomer cements, the choice is now between these three materials. For the permanent dentition, ideally a restoration lasts the lifetime of the patient; for the primary dentition it only has to last the lifetime of the tooth. At 3 years the survival of composite Class 2 restorations is equal to that of amalgam, but at 6 years the failure of composites is much greater (Varpio, 1985). Although the use of rubber dam is strongly advised for all restorations, it has to be accepted that most practitioners do not use it, especially in the UK (Marshall and Page, 1990). Dental amalgam is more forgiving of poor moisture control than the other materials. Amalgam is also much easier than composite and glass-ionomer materials to pack effectively into the proximal box without leaving defects that can lead to further decay. Croll et al. (1993) describe a fine-tipped syringe system for use with a light-cured glass-ionomer/composite material to overcome potential defects in the proximal box. Further development of this type of material, with a suitable delivery system, may show it to be a worthy successor to dental amalgam for Class 2 cavities. However, until clinical research demonstrates otherwise, dental amalgam is still the restorative material of choice for Class 2 primary and permanent molar restorations in children.

Cavity preparation

Cavity preparation will be described in relation to the use of dental amalgam as the restorative material.

1. Primary molars

As with the Class 1 lesion, the cavity design depends largely upon two principles – the presence of caries and the potential for further caries to develop. Beyond that, the overriding concern is the preservation of sound tooth substance to leave the tooth as strong as possible. Frequently the Class 2 cavity consists of a proximal box, joined by an isthmus to an occlusal extension. However, if the occlusal surface is caries-free with well-coalesced fissures, it need not be prepared and the proximal box can be made to stand alone. The outline form is prepared with a turbine handpiece using a small, pear-shaped (No. 330 pattern) bur.

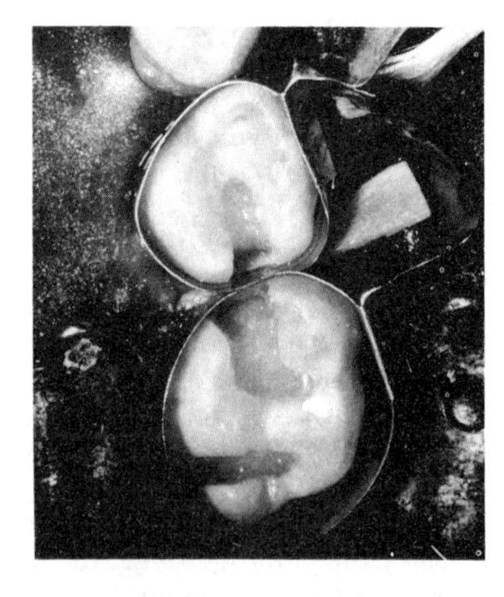

Fig. 9.1. Completed Class 2 cavity preparations in maxillary primary molars. Banded and wedged ready for amalgam.

The occlusal part has the same outline form as the Class 1 cavity (*Fig.* 9.1). That is, all carious, stained and poorly coalesced fissures are included in the preparation. The criteria used for determining whether to cross an oblique or central ridge have been described in Chapter 8. Minimum cavity depth is 1.5 mm, i.e. 0.5 mm pulpal to the amelodentinal junction to provide sufficient bulk of amalgam, to withstand occlusal loading without fracture. In width it can be as narrow as the No. 330 bur, widening with the dictates of caries. The pulpal

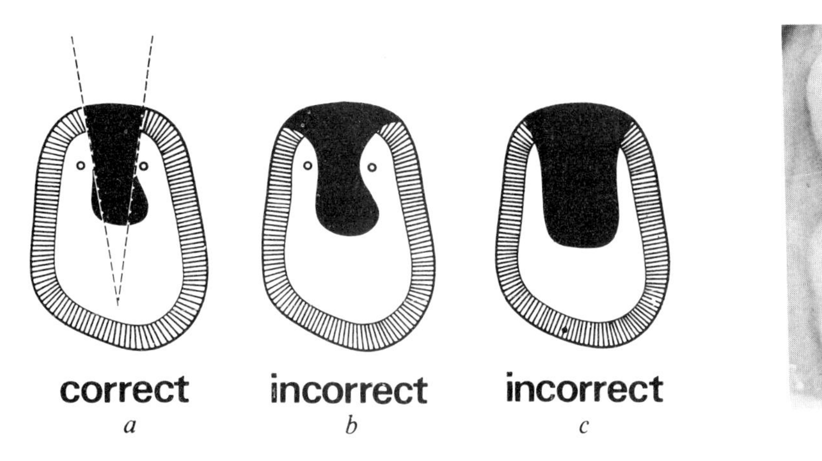

Fig. 9.2. Occlusal view of Class 2 preparations in the primary molar. *a*, Correct diagram demonstrates absence of flaring or proximal box walls. Imaginary extensions of the walls meet at the opposite marginal ridge. *b*, Widely flaring walls of proximal box cannot parallel enamel rods, predisposing the restoration to failure. *c*, Wide isthmus results in weakening of cusps and possible pulp exposure if the cavity floor is taken too deep. *d*, Marginal deterioration resulting from poorly supported proximal walls. (○ = pulp horns.)

floor is therefore flat mesiodistally, and in the buccolingual direction it will be rounded if very narrow, becoming flatter as the cavity widens, with rounded internal line angles. If any caries remains, it can be removed with slowly revolving round burs or excavators, and then the cavity walls further modified to remove any resulting unsupported enamel. The idea of a 'dovetail lock', cut at the opposite end of the occlusal part to the proximal box, is outdated. Its purpose was to increase the retention of the restoration by preventing flow of the set amalgam out of the cavity. However, when the occlusal fissures are prepared this does not result in a straight-line cavity that would require extra retention; instead it produces a curved shape that naturally resists any flow that might occur in the set amalgam. To destroy tooth substance further by producing a 'lock' would only serve to weaken the tooth unnecessarily.

The narrow occlusal aspect of the proximal box is prepared with the No. 330 bur, placing the buccal and lingual margins where they can be easily accessed for cleaning. The approach to the surface needs to be at approximately 90° when viewed from the occlusal aspect (*Fig.* 9.2a). With this correct design, if the buccal–lingual proximal walls were to be continued they would meet at approximately the opposite marginal ridge. If the occlusal part of the box is prepared too flared to the embrasure, acute amalgam–surface angles are the result, leading to possible amalgam fracture (*Fig.* 9.2b). This situation can sometimes be saved by a limited increase in the width of the isthmus alone. The resultant cavosurface angles of the proximobuccal and proximolingual walls may then approach the acceptable 70°, while still leaving the cusps strong enough to withstand occlusal stresses. However, if the flaring was initially very wide, then probably a preformed crown would be a better option.

Overextension of the buccolingual width of the box at the occlusal aspect results in poor support of the proximal walls and in turn to marginal deterioration. When the walls of the gingival aspect of the proximal box are being prepared, the clinician may be concentrating on the gingival position of the bur while the opposite proximal wall is being overextended by the bur's inclination. The operator is then tempted to correct the error by further extension. The pulp horns will be at risk of exposure, and the cusps will be weakened. Often the enamel rods are unsupported at the proximobuccal and proximolingual margins (*Fig.* 9.3b); this will eventually result in failure of the restoration (Castaldi, 1957; MacRae et al., 1962); and there will be unsupported enamel rods leading to possible tooth fracture (*Fig.* 9.2c). Commonly, the failure occurs at the distobuccal margin of mandibular first primary molars.

The gingival aspect of the proximal box is prepared next. When looking from above, the operator can judge the necessary angulation of the bur to the long axis of the tooth that will

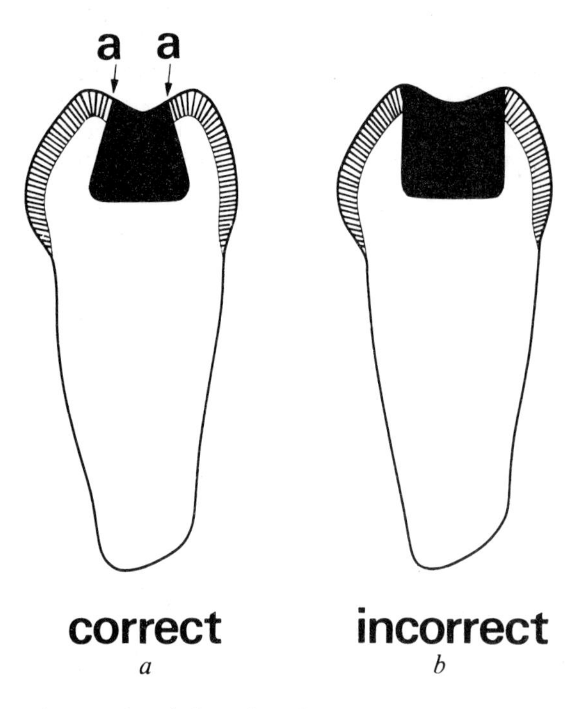

Fig. 9.3. *a*, Mesiodistal view of correct Class 2 preparation in a primary molar. The walls of the proximal box parallel the external surfaces. Areas (a) are easily overextended by improper use of burs. *b*, Incorrect Class 2 preparation in a primary molar: mesiodistal view. Overextension of the occlusal width of the proximal box weakens the cusps and leaves both enamel and amalgam poorly supported.

clear the contact with the adjacent tooth either buccally or lingually. At that angle of approach, the bur is advanced towards the gingiva, simultaneously maintaining a slight mesiodistal movement at 90° to the surface.

The whole length of the margins of the proximal box is placed in areas that are easily cleaned, and where marginal integrity can subsequently be checked by the operator. The anatomy of primary molars produces broad, elliptical, gingivally located contact areas. Decay is initiated at or just below that contact area, therefore the gingival seat of the box needs to be extended past this contact to remove the caries. Clearance from the opposing tooth will also allow the matrix band to be passed easily beyond the cavity margin. Buccal and lingual limits of the gingival seat are also placed clear of the contact with the adjacent tooth, so that the margins of the restoration can be cleaned. Thus, the gingival aspect of the box is very wide. The occlusal table of primary molars is narrow compared with that of permanent molars, and the contact with the adjacent tooth here is small. The occlusal aspect of the proximal box must therefore be kept narrow while still allowing access to the margins of the restoration for cleaning. The cusps are therefore not unduly weakened. The broad base and narrow occlusal aspects of the proximal box produce the characteristic flared shape. The buccal and lingual cavosurface angles of the box should be approximately 90° (range 70–110°) to have both cavosurface and amalgam–surface angles large enough to withstand fracture.

There needs to be sufficient bulk of amalgam in the box. Although 1.5 mm has been suggested for Class 1 cavities, this depth could be perilously close to a mesiobuccal pulp horn in a proximal box. Rodda (1972) suggested approximately 1.0 mm is sufficient for the proximal box. Primary enamel is generally uniformly thick at 1.0 mm, so the gingival seat and thus the axial wall need to be placed into dentine. Also, if proximal retention grooves are to be placed (see later), they must definitely be entirely within dentine to avoid unsupported enamel. If this principle of optimum thickness of amalgam is carried across the whole of the gingival seat, the resultant position of the axial wall will parallel the outer surface of the tooth. The enamel rods at the gingival aspect are either horizontal or inclined occlusally, rather

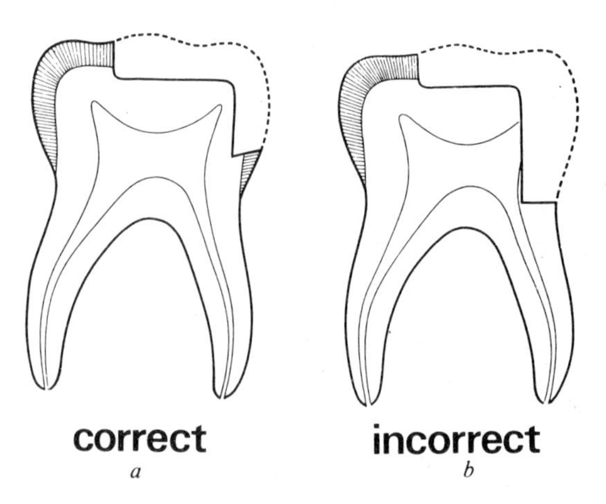

Fig. 9.4. *a*, Cross-sectional view of Class 2 cavity preparation in a primary molar in the buccolingual plane. Note correct rounded axiopulpal line angle, minimum cavity depth and occlusal inclination of the floor of proximal box. *b*, Incorrect Class 2 preparation in the buccolingual plane. The floor of the interproximal box is taken too far gingivally: when it is widened the axial wall exposes the pulp.

than gingivally as occurs in permanent molars. The gingival seat of the box should follow the line of the enamel rods, and so conventional margin trimmers are not used. (*Figs* 9.4 and 9.5).

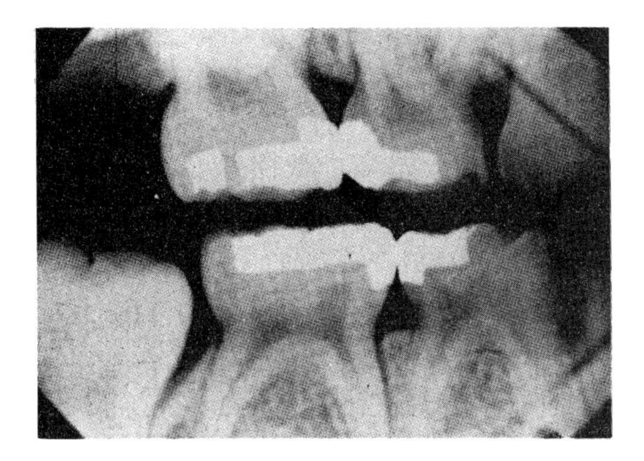

Fig. 9.5. Bitewing radiograph demonstrates Class 2 alloys in adjacent primary molars. Note minimal depth, extension of proximal box into a self-cleansing area gingivally, occlusal inclination of cervical seat and good contour.

The isthmus is at the junction of occlusal part and interproximal box. In the 1950s, Lampshire (1955) recommended a wide isthmus to provide bulk of alloy at a point of weakness. A very wide isthmus can lead to fracture (*Fig.* 9.6). Current trends (Law et al., 1966; McDonald and Avery, 1994) are to narrow this isthmus and obtain the bulk of alloy by making the cavity deeper (*Fig.* 9.7). Ideally, the isthmus width should not exceed one-third of the intercuspal width in primary molars. Fracture of the isthmus between the occlusal and proximal components has been reported as a common failure. Almquist et al. (1973) stated that the width of the isthmus is not critical in prevention of amalgam fracture as some had suggested. In their study an adequate depth of amalgam and non-coincidence of the axiopulpal line angle with the isthmus was more important. The width of the isthmus is important, though, in prevention of tooth fracture. A narrow isthmus gave greater fracture resistance to the tooth and better marginal integrity to the restoration. Davies and King (1961) claimed that the strength of the isthmus is proportional to the cube of its depth but only to the first power of its width. The pulpoaxial line angle can be rounded, tunnelled, or grooved to provide sufficient bulk at this weak isthmus area. While the student may be fearful of exposing the pulp horns when doing this, it should be re-emphasized that the pulp horns are located beneath the cusps. Thus, provided the isthmus width is conservative, there is no danger of exposure; the danger arises as the isthmus width increases.

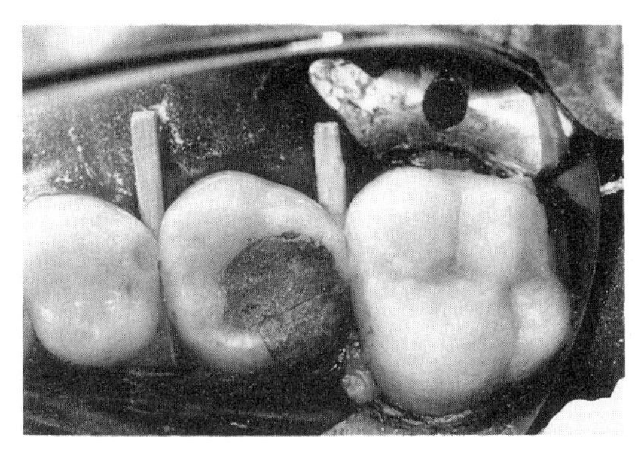

Fig. 9.6. Fractured isthmus. This resulted in a leaking amalgam and an abscess.

Retention

Retention of the restoration results from the mechanical undercut obtained by the extension into the fissures of the occlusal part and the diverging walls of the interproximal box. It is important that retention of the interproximal box and the occlusal part are independent of each other, as each may be subjected to different displacement forces. Additional retention can be obtained by placing a U-shaped retention groove within the dentine of the buccal and lingual walls of the proximal box. A No. 1 or 2, round fissure bur is used. These grooves do not contribute to marginal deterioration (Mathewson et al., 1974). Some suggest additional retention by placing a groove within the dentine of the gingival seat. Gilmore (1971) said that provided the entire gingival seat was not sloping apically (it would not do so for the reasons discussed earlier), then this 'gingival lock' is unnecessary.

Finishing the cavity

Final refinement of the cavity walls and ginigival seat is made with hatchets and chisels. This is especially important because many failures occur at the proximal margins.

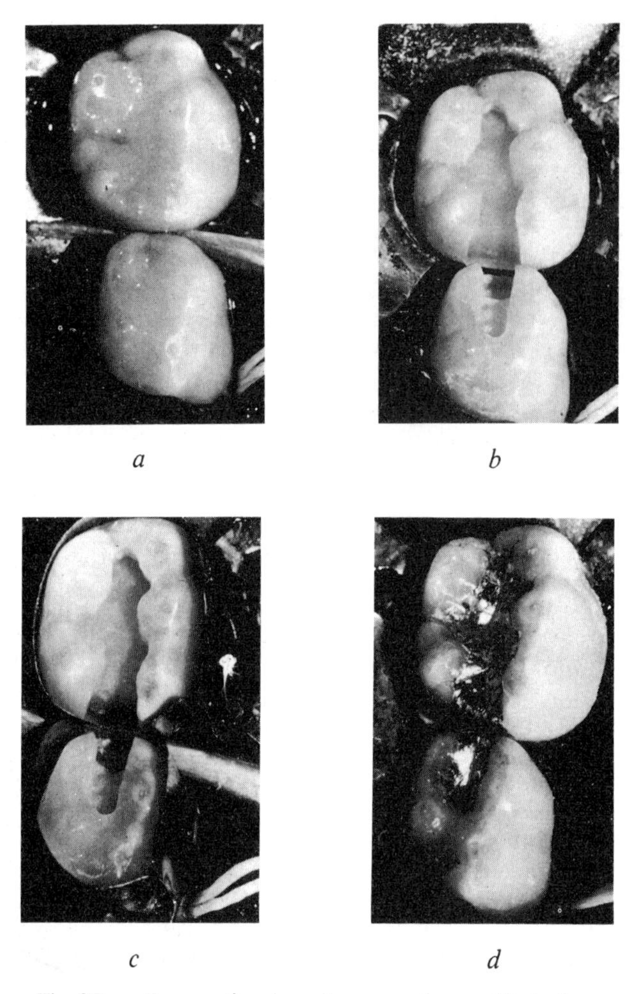

a *b* *c* *d*

Fig. 9.7. *a*, Preoperative. *b*, cavity preparations. *c*, Wedged matrices. *d*, Completed restorations. [From *Current Therapy in Dentistry* (1977) Vol. 6; St Louis, Mosby.]

Further considerations

When interproximal lesions occur both mesially and distally on the same tooth, it must be decided whether separate Class 2 cavities are indicated or whether a stainless-steel crown would be preferable. The occlusal anatomy and extent of occlusal decay are the determining factors, together with the age of the patient. It should be borne in mind that many investigations have reported that the failure of amalgams in primary molars is higher the younger the patient when the restoration was placed. In the maxillary second primary molar, an intact oblique ridge would allow the placement of two two-surface restorations. When caries undermines this ridge, or when retention is in doubt, a stainless-steel crown is placed. Therefore, in very young patients, and in all other primary molars, a stainless-steel crown is indicated when both proximal surfaces are carious.

2. The large lesion in primary molars

Unless the Class 2 lesion in a primary molar is diagnosed at the incipient stage from accurate bitewing radiographs, it will progress to undermine the marginal ridge. Eventually this will break down to present the clinician with a large Class 2 lesion closely approximating the pulp (Stoner, 1967). Because of the broad, gingivally located contact areas, undiagnosed and/or untreated Class 2 lesions will undermine the proximobuccal and proximolingual cusps before the marginal ridge finally breaks down.

Using conventional Class 2 cavity design in these large lesions invites subsequent failure since it will be impossible to maintain adequate support proximobuccally and proximolingually. Widely flaring walls (see *Fig.* 9.3b) from a narrow isthmus cannot be prevented.

Therefore the clinician must look beyond conventional cavity preparations. Castaldi (1957) and MacRae et al. (1962) recommended reduction of a weakened cusp and overlaying it with amalgam. However, with the simplicity and reportedly high success rates of stainless-steel crowns (Roberts and Sherriff, 1990), the cuspal overlay is very rarely used today.

Amalgam failures

The frequency of failure in multisurface amalgam restorations of primary molars is alarmingly high. In mandibular first primary molars, the distobuccal margin was defective in 29% of teeth evaluated after 1 year (MacRae et al., 1962). Braff (1975) found that only about 11% of multisurface amalgams lasted over 4 years without the need for further care. Of the remaining 89%, the majority required replacement; this reflects a need for a critical review of our attention to detail in restorative procedures.

The common failures are:

(1) deterioration at the proximal margins,
(2) isthmus fracture,
(3) recurrent caries,
(4) inadvertent pulp exposure.

1. Marginal deterioration

This is due to inadequate enamel support and faulty manipulation, and selection of the restorative material (see *Fig.* 9.2d). The means of ensuring adequate proximal wall support by conservative cavity preparation and cusp overlay have been described. Although marginal discrepancy usually becomes apparent several months or even years following restoration, the clinician may sometimes be faced with this immediately after the matrix has been removed. The amalgam has probably been insufficiently carved prior to matrix removal. Ditching (marginal discrepancy) at this early stage may also be due to faulty cavity design.

Severe discrepancies occur when the marginal ridge is fractured and removed together with the matrix band or when the child bites down hard before the restoration has been carved. Attempts to add amalgam should be discouraged as the strength of the bond with existing amalgam is less than desirable. Instead, the restoration should be removed in the partially set state and replaced using a new matrix.

Fracture of the marginal ridge during band removal can casily be prevented by placing the end of a large amalgam plugger on to the ridge as the matrix band is removed (*Fig.* 9.8). The use of rubber dam, as we strongly recommend throughout this book, will prevent the child biting on to the uncarved amalgam. Once the matrix has been removed, as shown, and the amalgam properly carved, then the rubber dam can be removed and the occlusion gently checked with articulating paper.

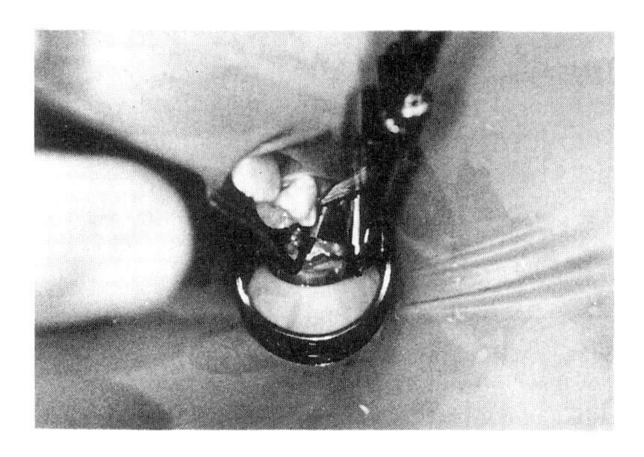

Fig. 9.8. Technique of holding marginal ridge in place with an amalgam plugger while removing the matrix.

Marginal deterioration that occurs years after the placement of the restoration may be due to clinical variation in the material's performance, or to wear from occlusal interference. The first problem will be discussed in Chapter 15. The problem of occlusal wear can be minimized by using articulating paper prior to cavity preparation. In this manner the margins can be placed away from occlusal interference. At recall appointments, the occlusion can be rearticulated and the restorations repolished where necessary to eliminate occlusal interference.

2. Isthmus fracture

This can be avoided by providing sufficient effective bulk of amalgam at the axiopulpal line angle. Grooving that angle increases amalgam bulk, while grinding the opposing cusp reduces the trauma from occlusion. The fractured isthmus will be apparent clinically (see *Fig.* 9.6b); when the interproximal part of the restoration is devoid of retention it may be displaced, giving the radiographic appearance of an overhang. Ingress of saliva, bacteria and food encourages the development of recurrent caries. It is not uncommon to see a very deep lesion closely approximating the pulp after isthmus fracture; direct pulp therapy is often required.

3. Recurrent caries

This can occur after isthmus fracture, as indicated earlier. Inadequate extension of the interproximal margins into a cleansable area also encourages development of recurrent caries. This also occurs at the gingivolabial and gingivolingual line angles of the proximal box when the amalgam has been poorly condensed.

4. Inadvertent pulp exposure

This occurs because of deepening of the occlusal or axial wall beyond the limits of the lesion. Frequently the pulp horn is exposed at the axial wall; the mesiobuccal pulp horn in primary molars is commonly closest to the surface and special care should be exercised when preparing this area. The distance between pulp horn and external enamel surface may be as little as 1.8 mm. The effects of inadvertent pulp exposure may not become apparent until the child's recall examination, when a fistula may be seen; alternatively, internal or external resorption are observed radiographically. This assumes, of course, that any base which was placed was not successful in direct pulp capping. Once this pathological process has occurred, the tooth can be saved only with pulpectomy procedures; otherwise it must be extracted (see Chapter 17). Either action does little to enhance the image of the profession or the individual dentist. When this repeatedly occurs, it is not surprising for parents to develop the attitude that primary teeth cannot be filled and, as a result, for children to be denied the benefits of regular care.

3. The permanent molar

Current trends in permanent molar preparations have been described by Kidd and Smith (1994). The tendency towards narrower and deeper cavity preparations is more conservative of sound tooth structure. Principles of cavity design already described for primary molars also apply to permanent molars. The following variations are recommended, however.

The occlusal part should be as narrow as possible, commensurate with the philosophy of extension for prevention. Minimal cavity depth is 0.5 mm into dentine; it may be advisable to deepen this to provide more bulk of amalgam in depth, due to the minimal cavity width. The isthmus should not exceed one-fourth of the intercuspal dimensions. The margins of the interproximal box should be accessible for easy cleaning.

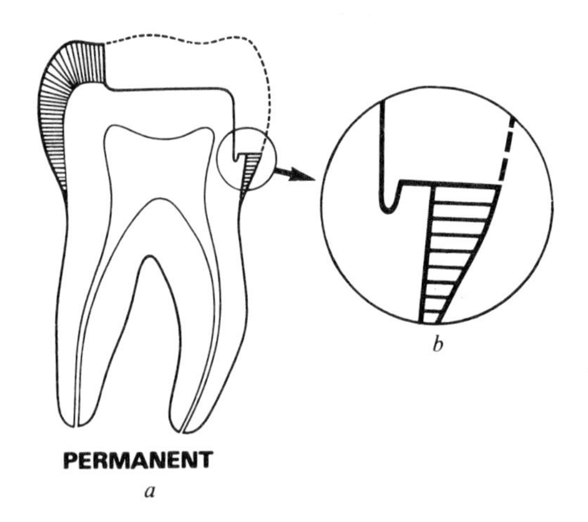

Fig. 9.9. *a*, Cross-sectional view of Class 2 preparation in a permanent molar in the buccolingual plane. Note rounded axiopulpal line angle, inclination of the proximal box floor and retention groove. *b*, Enlarged view of floor of proximal box. Note that when a margin trimmer is used to bevel the floor, the enamel rods are supported by dentine.

The gingival seat of the proximal box must be prepared with a gingival margin trimmer to ensure that all weakened enamel is removed (*Fig.* 9.9). Retention grooves are recommended for these 'modern' preparations to ensure independent retention of occlusal lock and proximal box. It should be re-emphasized that these retention grooves do not contribute to marginal deterioration. The clinician should be extremely careful to avoid unnecessary overextension of minimal lesions. Although any restoration placed in a young child's permanent molar has a potential lifetime of use ahead of it, clinical experience shows the need for replacing restorations due to marginal deterioration. Each time a restoration has to be replaced there is the danger of further tooth destruction. This should encourage a conservative approach in young children.

References

Almquist T. C., Cowan R. D. and Lambert R. L. (1973) Conservative amalgam restorations. *J. Prosthet. Dent.* **29**, 524

Braff M. H. (1975) A comparison between stainless steel crowns and multi-surface amalgams. *J. Dent. Child.* **42**, 474.

Castaldi C. R. (1957) Analysis of some operative procedures currently being used in paedodontics. *J. Can. Dent. Assoc.* **23**, 377.

Croll T. P., Killiam C. M. and Helpin M. L. (1993) A restorative dentistry renaissance for children: light-hardened glass ionomer/resin cements. *J. Dent. Child.* **35**, 89.

Davies G. N. and King R. M. (1961) *Dentistry for the Pre-school Child*, p. 237. London, Livingstone.

Gilmore H. W. (1971) Restorative materials and cavity preparation design. *Dent. Clin. North Am.* **15**, 99.

Kidd E. A. and Smith B. G. N. (1994) *Pickard's Manual of Operative Dentistry*, 6th edn, Oxford University Press.

Kidd E. A., Naylor M. N. N. and Wilson R. P. (1992) Prevalence of clinically undetected and untreated molar occlusal dental caries in adolescents of the Isle of Wight. *Caries Res.* **26**, 397.

Lampshire E. L. (1955) Evaluation of cavity preparations in primary molars. *J. Dent. Child.* **22**, 3.

Law D. B., Sim J. M. and Simon J. F. (1966) A new look at Class II restorations in primary molars. *Dent. Clin. North Am.* **341**.

McDonald R. E. and Avery D. R. (1994) *Dentistry for the Child and Adolescent*, 6th edn. St Louis, Mosby.

MacRae P. D., Zacherl W. and Castaldi C. R. (1962) Study of defects in Class II dental amalgam restorations in deciduous molars. *J. Can. Dent. Assoc.* **28**, 491.

Marshall K. and Page J. (1990). The use of rubber dam in the UK: a survey. *Br. Dent. J*, **169**, 286.

Mathewson R. J., Retzloff A. E. and Porter D. R. (1974) Marginal failure of amalgam in deciduous teeth: a two-year report. *J. Am. Dent. Assoc.* **88**, 134.

Parfitt G. J. (1956) Conditions influencing the incidence of occlusal and interstitial caries in children. *J. Dent. Child.* **23**, 31.

Roberts J. F. and Sherriff M. (1990) The fate and survival of amalgam and preformed crown molar restorations placed in a specialist paediatric dental practice. *Br. Dent. J.* **169**, 237.

Rodda J. C. (1972) Modern Class 2 amalgam preparations. *NZ Dent. J.* **66**, 132.

Sidi A. D. and Naylor M. N. N. (1988) A comparison of bitewing radiographs and interdental transillumination as adjuncts to the clinical identification of approximal caries in posterior teeth. *Br. Dent. J.* **164**, 15.

Steckson-Blicks C. and Wahlin Y. B. (1983) Diagnosis of approximal caries in preschool children. *Swed. Dent. J.* **7**, 179.

Stoner J. E. (1967) Dental caries in deciduous molars. *Br. Dent. J.* **123**, 130.

Swartz M. et al. (1984) A longitudinal analysis from bitewing radiographs of the rate of progression of approximal caries lesions through human dental enamel. *Archs Oral Biol.* **29**, 529.

Varpio M. (1985) Proximoocclusal composite resins in primary molars. A six-year follow up. *J. Dent. Child.* **52**, 435.

Chapter 10

The Class 3 lesion

Diagnosis

The most common site for a Class 3 lesion in the primary dentition is the mesial surface of the primary incisors; the maxillary arch is affected more than the mandibular. In the 18–39-month age group, the mesial surfaces of both primary central and lateral incisors are more frequently carious than the distal surfaces, coupled with buccal surfaces. This predilection for the mesial and buccal surfaces occurs in classic nursing caries (Ripa, 1988) and requires restoring if the teeth are to be saved.

The distal surface of the primary canine is commonly affected by caries in the mixed dentition. Not surprisingly, this lesion occurs when the contact area between the primary canine and first primary molar has closed. Thus the presence of this lesion is in part determined by the absence of a primate space; in the mandibular arch the eruption of the first permanent molars may obliterate the primate space. The changes that occur in the occlusion as the first permanent molar erupts and closes the spaces on either side of the primary canine result in the Class 3 lesion occurring to a lesser degree on the mesial surface of the primary canine rather than on the distal surface. In addition, the exfoliation of the primary incisors also means that the mesial surface of the primary canine becomes available for easy cleansing and hence is less likely to decay.

The Class 3 lesion in the primary incisors is often diagnosed by clinical means alone, particularly when the contact areas are open or when the lesion is larger than incipient. In primary canines the bitewing radiograph is invaluable in the diagnosis of the early Class 3 lesions when posterior contacts are closed, although bitewings (or, alternatively, periapical or anterior occlusal radiographs) of incisors are not taken as often as they should be. Bitewing radiographs for preschool children should normally include the posterior arch from primary canine to developing first permanent molar. This enables the practitioner to see all interproximal contact areas, as well as any developing abnormalities in first permanent molar eruption. Likewise the clinical diagnosis of Class 3 lesions in primary incisors may be supplemented by a maxillary anterior occlusal radiograph which can also determine the presence of some abnormalities in the developing permanent incisors. The Class 3 lesion may be accompanied by an adjacent Class 5 lesion on the same tooth. This is commonly seen on the maxillary primary incisors in the nursing-bottle mouth syndrome. Here the Class 3 and Class 5 lesions often blend into one to produce a circumferential pattern of decay. The untreated Class 3 lesion will progress to undermine the incisal edge. This occurs at a faster rate in the primary than in the permanent dentition because of the relatively small inciso-gingival height of the clinical crown of the primary incisor. In effect, the Class 3 lesion has now progressed to a Class 4 lesion and will be discussed in Chapter 11.

The Class 3 cavity

Primary incisor teeth

When the contact areas are open and the lesion is incipient the cavity can be prepared directly; therefore there is no need for a dovetail lock to improve access and retention. The outline form should be triangular, with the base of the triangle at the gingival aspect of the cavity. The buccal and lingual cavity walls should parallel the respective external surfaces of the tooth to meet at the apex of the triangle. The pear-shaped bur (No. 330) is suitable for preparing the cavity. The gingival cavity wall should incline slightly occlusally, thereby paralleling the enamel rod/prism structure. This also provides an undercut for mechanical retention. The incisal aspect of the cavity should not be undercut since this will undermine incisal enamel which is later subject to occlusal wear. Cavity depth should be 0.5 mm pulpal to the amelodentinal junction. Retention grooves can be placed along the amelodentinal junction with a small, No. 2 round bur.

With closed contacts an indirect approach to the caries has to be adopted. For aesthetic reasons, this is usually from the palatal surface of the tooth. Some clinicians advocate a lock or dovetail to facilitate access to the carious lesion and to aid in the retention of the restoration. However, with new materials and the acid-etch technique we can rely on chemical bonding for retention.

When used the lock needs to extend only to the middle of the tooth and should be dovetail-shaped to provide resistance to lateral displacement of the restoration (*Fig.* 10.1). Because of ease of access and the minimal aesthetic requirements of the restoration, the lock is placed on the labial surface in the mandibular primary anteriors. For aesthetic reasons, it is commonly placed on the lingual surface in the maxillary anteriors. Also, because of the location of caries less sound tooth structure is destroyed by the lingually placed maxillary dovetail.

The interproximal area of the cavity should be shaped like the letter 'C' when observed directly. The open end of the 'C' meets the retentive lock (*Fig.* 10.1). In some ways the cavity is similar to the Class 2 lying on its side. The width and location of the lock are partly determined by the extent and position of the caries. The inclination of the incisal and gingival enamel walls should be towards the incisal edge, paralleling the enamel rods. This recommendation applies to the walls of both the retentive lock and the interproximal area.

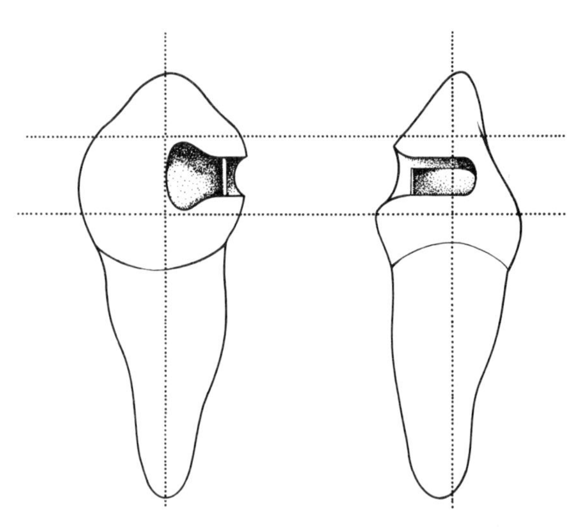

Fig. 10.1. Class 3 preparation in a primary maxillary canine with retentive lock: view from the palatal and the interproximal surfaces. The lock is in the middle one-third of the tooth and does not extend across the midline.

The Class 3 restoration requires the use of a celulloid matrix strip. This is inserted interproximally and wedged firmly underneath the gingival seat. Access to the cavity for the filling material is easy; it can be packed into the cavity with a suitable instrument. Once filled the matrix strip is held against the palatal surface of the tooth and pulled to condense the filling material into the cavity. At the same time this action provides a surface to the filling flush with the enamel. The resin is then cured either with a curing light or allowed to set chemically.

Deviation from this set pattern is indicated by the presence of both a Class 3 and a Class 5 lesion on the same tooth. In this instance, the Class 5 cavity becomes the retentive lock. However, in this type of situation the extent of the caries is such that a strip crown (Chapter 11) is the restoration of choice.

In the past the Class 3 cavity might have been restored with amalgam alloy but a high polish was required so as not to be unaesthetic at the front of the child's mouth. However, the quality of composite resin material is now so good that it is the material of choice. Almost ideal colour matching and biological compatibility can be achieved with simple, direct-filling composite resins. They are the material of choice since they provide good retention, minimum tooth destruction, and maximum tooth support.

Primary canine teeth

While the dovetail lock is no longer required for the restoration of the primary incisor, it is still occasionally useful in restoring the primary canine. Where the distal cavity in a canine is quite large, a palatal or facial lock is an advantage. It is prepared as described above and filled with an appropriate material. Because of the occlusion it is recommended that where a dovetail lock is used it should be a palatal lock for the maxillary canine and a facial lock for the mandibular canine. The reason for this is apparent when the occlusion and biting surfaces are taken into account. The biting forces will then tend to push the material into the cavity. When there is a Class III occlusal relationship of the canine (rare in the primary dentition), then the order of cutting palatal or facial locks is reversed.

Reference

Ripa L. W. (1988) Nursing caries: a comprehensive review. *Pediatr. Dent.* **10**, 268–79.

Chapter 11

Restoration of primary incisors – strip crowns

Diagnosis

The most common sites for caries in the maxillary central incisors are the mesial and buccal surfaces followed in frequency by the mesio-incisal corner of the maxillary primary lateral incisor. The small vertical height of the primary incisor crown, which is further reduced by attrition as the child grows older, may account for the rapid spread of a Class 3 to a Class 4 lesion. The disto-incisal corners of the maxillary primary central and lateral incisors seldom appear to be carious in the same frequency and degree as the mesio-incisal corners (Hennon et al., 1969). While buccal and distal caries occurs in mandibular primary incisors and primary canines (either maxillary or mandibular), Class 4 lesions are less common. No doubt the anatomical shape of the primary canine excludes this tooth from the possibility of a Class 4 lesion. Loss of incisal corners may also occur in young permanent incisors as a result of trauma.

Nursing caries is often associated with caries affecting the mesial, distal and buccal surfaces of the incisors as well as the occlusal surfaces of the first primary molars. In these cases the molars often need restoring with preformed stainless-steel crowns, leaving the clinician with the problem of dealing with carious maxillary incisors. Until recently the solution was either to extract them, leaving the child for a number of years without front teeth, or restoring them with various Class 3 and 5 restorations. Sometimes the caries was so extensive that Class 4 restorations (Doyle, 1967; Kennedy, 1986) were required. The longer-term survival of these restorations was poor and dentists were reluctant to undertake them. Furthermore, these tiny restorations in small teeth are difficult. The advent of the celluloid strip crown for primary incisors has now meant that these teeth can be easily restored with a good prognosis (O'Sullivan and Curzon, 1991).

The diagnosis of the Class 4 lesion should present no problem since the lesion is obvious. As there is always the possibility that the lesion may progress close to the pulp, the preoperative evaluation should include an assessment of the pulp status (Chapter 17). A preoperative radiograph will indicate the presence of any resorption (internal and external), which can either be pathological or physiological. The anticipated longevity of the tooth can be determined by the child's age and the radiographic extent of physiological root resorption. An investment of time in the comprehensive restorative treatment of Class 4 lesions may not be justified if the tooth will exfoliate within 18 months and a permanent successor is present.

Parental attitudes towards dental health should be evaluated. It may be that heroic efforts to save extensively broken down primary incisors are contraindicated because of parental apathy, poor appointment keeping, and lack of good oral hygiene and concern for dental health. In such instances the extraction of these teeth may be required; failure to perform any treatment will eventually result in acute or chronic abscess formation and increase the

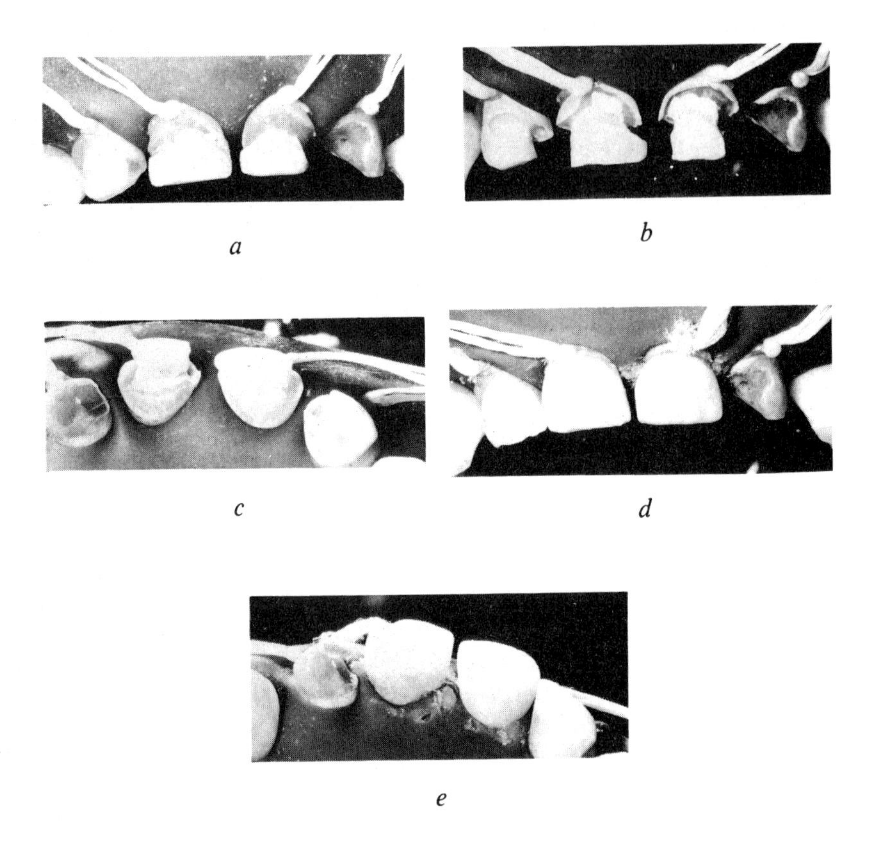

Fig. 11.1. Class 4 preparations. *a*, Preoperative. *b*, Mesial incisal 52 (B|); distal incisal mesial 51 (A|); mesial incisal distal incisal 61 (|A); buccal view. Preparations lined. *c*, Lingual view. *d*, *e*, Completed restorations. *d*, buccal view; *e*, lingual view – Adaptic was used.

likelihood of hypoplastic or hypocalcified defects occurring on the developing permanent incisors. Should the parents subsequently become more dentally aware and the child become concerned about aesthetics, a partial denture can be fabricated at a later date. This should be deferred until a good response to preventive care has been obtained.

Sometimes one or two maxillary primary incisors, often the central, may be non-vital while the remainder are vital but also extensively carious. Should the non-vital incisors be unsuitable candidates for pulp therapy and require removal, the remaining incisors should also be considered for extraction. However, pulp therapy may be desirable in many instances in order to retain the teeth and preserve the child's appearance. In these cases sufficient time should be allowed so that the pulp therapy can be performed within the appropriate appointment.

Treatment

For many years, paediatric dentists have sought the ideal treatment of mixed Class 3, 4 and 5 lesions in the primary incisors. This indicates that there are a few hard-and-fast rules to be followed and also explains the many different treatment techniques that have been recommended, none of which until recently has been ideal. However, the ideal restoration in these instances is the strip crown using composite resin.

The main problems in restorative treatment for primary incisors are:

(1) that insufficient tooth is left, following

caries removal, to retain a restoration;
(2) that the patients selected for treatment are very young since the teeth to be restored need to be maintained in the mouth for several years; the child's age may result in working conditions being less than ideal.

The following possibilities of treatment exist in order of desirability:

- anterior crowns (strip crowns and others),
- Class 4 restoration,
- discing.

The Class 4 lesion is often accompanied by a Class 5 lesion on the same tooth, with the two merging. In such instances the ideal treatment consists of the strip crown. However, the dental age of the patient and anticipated longevity of the tooth may encourage the operator to perform a compromise treatment consisting of a Class 5 restoration and a self-cleansing interproximal slice. This is a great mistake. Since the Class 5 lesion cannot be made self-cleansing, it must be conventionally restored as described in Chapter 12. However, the Class 5 cavity must exhibit resistance to displacement in the direction of the interproximal slice. But where the two lesions meet, the Class 5 cavity will in effect have no cavity wall or margin; the restorative material will not hold and the restoration is bound to fail. There is no substitute in these instances for the full-coverage, light-cured resin crown.

The Class 4 restoration

The cavity preparation for the Class 4 restoration includes an interproximal slice and labial and lingual retentive dovetails, as shown in Chapter 10 (*Fig*. 10.1) in the Class 3 primary anterior cavity. The retentive dovetails are located in the middle one-third of the tooth, extending up to but not across the midline (*Fig*. 11.1). These should be placed to a depth of 0.5 mm pulpal to the amelodentinal junction with a small, inverted-cone bur (No. 2, British; No. 35, American). Obviously they should include any Class 5 lesions that may be present, in which case the position of the lock will be determined by the location of the Class 5 lesion. If both interproximal areas are carious, the retentive locks should extend across the midline and serve both lesions, but here again the restoration will fail in the longer term and a strip crown should be placed as soon as possible.

The carious lesion is partially eliminated by an interproximal slice. This leaves a finite labial and lingual margin. At the gingival aspect of the slice there should be a definite interproximal shoulder or gingival seat rather than a chamfer; this will facilitate finishing of the restoration. Any remaining caries can be removed with a slow-running, No. 2 round bur. A calcium hydroxide, pulp-protecting base should be placed in the deepest parts of the cavity. Eugenol-containing bases are not used since the resin will be discoloured by the eugenol. Most calcium hydroxide bases are white and tend to show through the translucent resin to spoil the appearance of the finished restoration. Therefore the base should be avoided on the labial surface whenever possible.

The initial postoperative appearance (*Fig*. 11.1*d*) may be impressive but staining, marginal deterioration, fracture or discoloration are to be expected. This type of restoration is most suitable for the small Class 4 lesion in a co-operative 3- or 4-year-old whose parents have demonstrated their interest in dental health by improving the child's oral environment during treatment, and when strip crowns are not immediately available. The anteriors should be treated only after completing posterior restorations because of the importance of the primary molars in maintaining arch length. In the primary dentition, aesthetic restorations are secondary in importance to the maintenance of arch length.

Anterior strip crown

Severe tooth destruction, the anticipated longevity of the tooth, and a strong desire by the patients to save the teeth encourage the use of primary anterior crowns (Pollard and Fayle, 1994). Primary incisors with loss of mesial and distal incisal corners, as well as circumferential Class 5 lesions such as may occur in nursing-bottle mouth, are most suitable candidates for crowning (*Fig*. 11.2).

Other indications are children with disfiguring dental hypoplasias. Before the advent of the polycarbonate crown the stainless-steel crown was used exclusively, although a processed aesthetic facing was recommended (Kennedy, 1986). The polycarbonate crown has now been

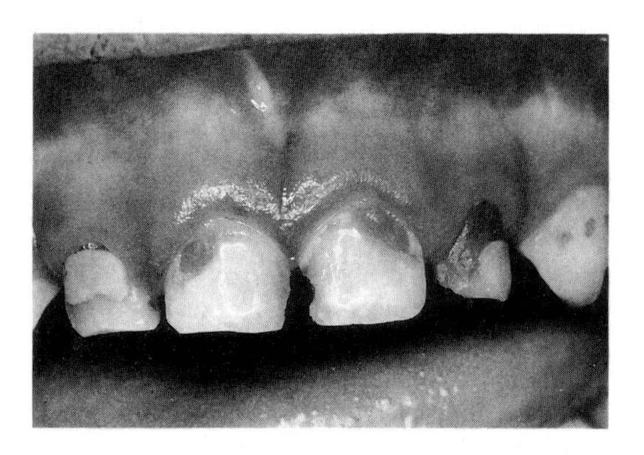

Fig. 11.2. Maxillary incisors affected by nursing caries and suitable for restoration with strip crowns. (Courtesy of Dr M. Pollard; reproduced with permission of Martin Dunitz Ltd., London.)

superseded by the strip crown and its use will not be described here.

Recent advances include appropriately sized celluloid crown forms for primary incisors, which can be used in conjunction with composite resin; retention can be obtained by mechanical undercuts and enhanced by acid-etching. The most recent addition in this area has been the availability of metal crowns with bonded plastic facings (discussed later).

Strip crown technique (Fig. 11.3)

Step 1. Isolation is desirable, although not essential, and can be achieved with rubber dam, 'Dry Dam' or cotton-wool rolls. Local analgesia may also be required. All caries is removed using a small round bur in a slow-speed handpiece. Care must be taken to remove all caries from both Class 3 and 5 lesions. It is advisable to restore all four incisors (if carious) at the same time. If this is not possible, but all four incisors need treatment, then the two central incisors should be treated on one visit and the lateral incisors at the next.

Step 2. The teeth need to be prepared as for a crown to allow for the bulk of resin in the final crown form. Using a high-speed, tapered diamond or tungsten-carbide bur, the length of the crown is reduced incisorly. Mesial and distal slices are cut tapering to a knife edge at the gingival margins (*Fig.* 11.3*a*). If there is a deep overbite it may be necessary to reduce the palatal bulk of the enamel also at this stage, but this is very rare. A calcium hydroxide lining material is applied to the pulpal wall of any exposed dentine (*Fig.* 11.3*b*).

Step 3. The shade of composite resin is now chosen, usually a very light shade to match the existing tooth if there is still sufficient enamel left, or the adjacent teeth. If all incisors are quite badly decayed, then one light shade should be chosen for all four teeth.

Step 4. Celluloid strip-crown forms are selected of the right size and trimmed using fine curved scissors (*Fig* 11.3*c*,*d*). The crowns are thin and easily split if care is not taken at this stage.

Step 5. Vent holes at the incisal-edge corners of the crown form allow air to escape when it is filled with composite resin. The crown(s) are trial-fitted for length and cervical fit (*Fig.* 11.3*e*).

Step 6. The teeth are etched for 1 min with an appropriate etchant, washed and dried (*Fig.* 11.3*f*). A bonding agent is then applied and cured for 15 s, if applicable, according to manufacturer's instructions.

Step 7. The crown form is then filled with composite resin, ensuring that resin is squeezed into all its corners. The resin should be hollowed out in the centre to reduce the amount of excess (*Fig.* 11.3*g*).

Step 8. The crown form(s) with composite resin are firmly seated on to the prepared teeth (*Fig.* 11.3*h*). If more than one incisor is being restored the crowns should be seated together. Care should be taken to remove excess resin with a probe or small Hollenback carver, as it will make final finishing easier and quicker. Excess pressure can result in the crown form splitting so the amount of pressure required is that to seat the crown only.

Step 9. The composite resin is cured for 1 min, taking care to cure thoroughly both labially and palatally.

Step 10. An excavator or probe is inserted beneath the edge of the celluloid and the crown form(s) stripped off (*Fig.* 11.3*i*). Reduction of the incisal length may be needed, in which case it should be done with the crown form *in situ*, facilitating its final removal.

Final Step. The cured crown is smoothed and polished, although usually minimal finishing is required with Soflex discs (3M). Fine diamonds or Baker–Curson high-speed burs can also be used. The finished crown(s) restore the aesthetics and avoid extractions with all the pain and discomfort entailed (*Fig.* 11.3*j*).

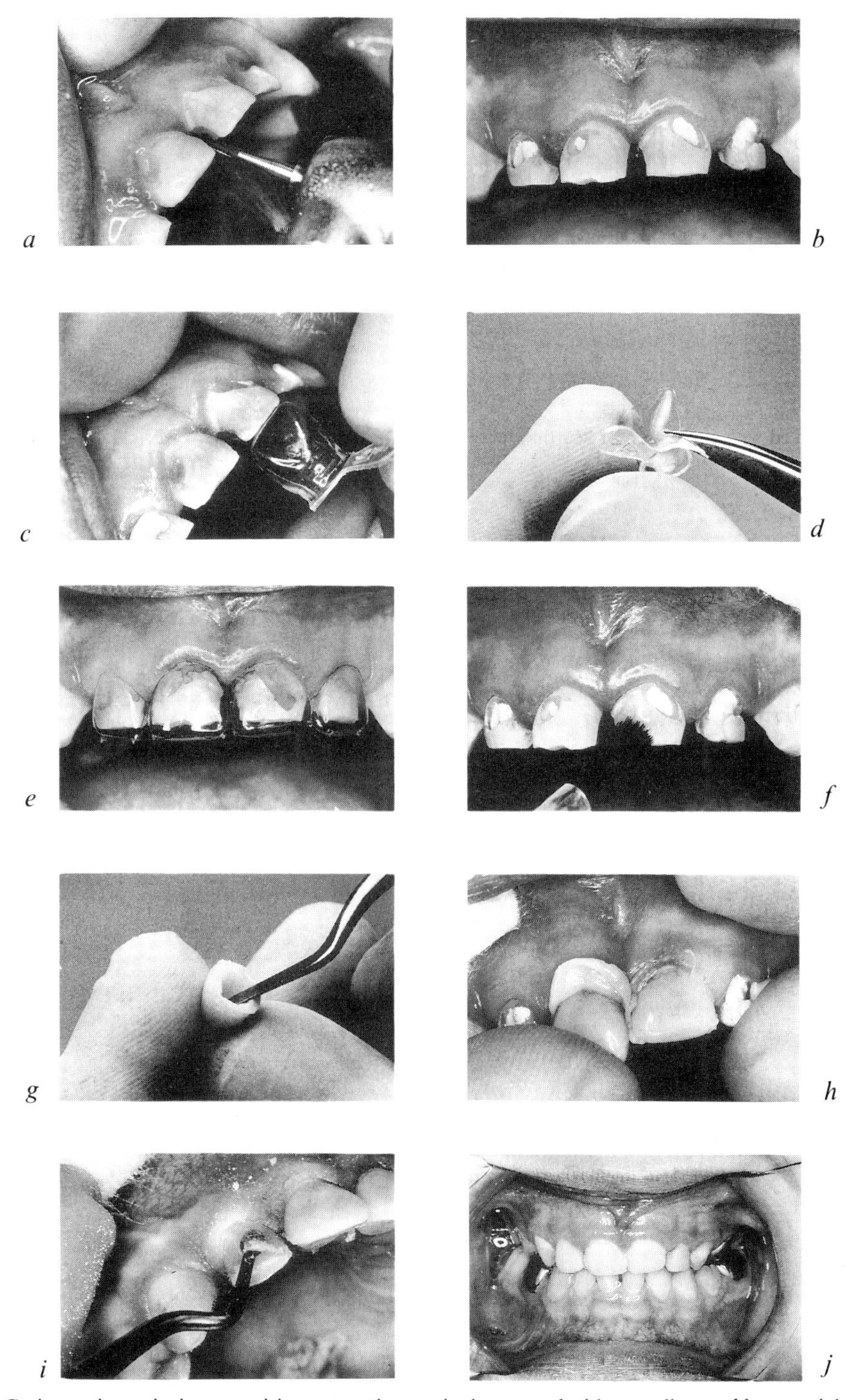

Fig. 11.3. *a*, Carious primary incisors requiring restoration: caries is removed with a small, round bur; mesial and distal slices are then made after reducing the incisal length of the crown. *b*, Pulpal protection with calcium hydroxide linings. *c*, Selection of correct-sized crown form. *d*, Trimming of strip-crown form with fine scissors. *e*, Crown forms trial-fitted. *f*, Tooth crowns etched. *g*, Crown form filled with composite resin. *h*, Filled crown form is seated on prepared tooth. *i*, Removal of crown form with probe or excavator. *j*, Finished crowns on four maxillary incisors. (Courtesy of Dr M. Pollard; reproduced with permission of Martin Dunitz Ltd., London.)

The strip-crown technique is a quick and simple method for the restoration of primary incisors. Parents and children are often delighted with the improvements that can be achieved without resorting to extractions. Experience also shows that restoring these teeth encourages an interest in dental health from both parents and child.

Metal crowns with resin facings

Recently a new type of crown form for anterior primary teeth has become available. Its aim is to combine the ease of fit and strength of the preformed stainless-steel crown with the aesthetics of the strip crown. These crowns, marketed as Kinder Crowns (Mayclin Studio Inc., Minneapolis, MN), may be used in place of the strip crown, but they are much more expensive.

The aims of reducing incisor teeth for resin-faced crowns are to provide sufficient space for the steel crown, remove the caries, and leave sufficient tooth for retention of the crown. Mesial and distal slices are required to clear the interproximal contacts. The gingival margin should have no ledge or shoulder; rather the chamfer should merge with uncut, apically placed tooth structure at the free gingival margin. Incisal reduction is required to prevent unnecessary elongation of the tooth. Tooth reduction should not destroy undercuts for mechanical retention; thus labial and lingual undercuts are left whenever possible.

Lingual reduction is necessary when the overbite is complete, such that the mandibular incisors are in contact with the lingual surfaces of the maxillary incisors; enamel should be removed uniformly with a diamond stone. When an incomplete overbite or open bite exists, and there are indications that it will not close, the lingual surface need not be reduced; the undercut towards the gingival margin is used for retention. For this same reason the only tooth reduction that should occur on the labial surface is that which will remove caries. A No. 169L, plain-cut, tapered fissure bur is compatible with the minimal preparation required. A pulp-protecting base is placed in the deepest areas of the preparation. Crown selection and contouring are done in the same way as for posterior crowns. The finished crowns provide an aesthetic restoration with the strength of the metal crown.

Post crowns in non-vital primary incisor teeth

Sometimes, because of the site of the carious lesion combined with attrition, virtually no tooth structure is left to retain a crown. After caries removal there may be a small supragingival stump remaining; it is not surprising to find that the pulp is cariously exposed. Although it might be thought that an extraction would be indicated, a successful alternative in a co-operative child is pulp treatment and a post crown. A high-standard pulpotomy or pulpectomy should be performed (Chapters 18 and 19). Depending on preoperative pulp status, this is done in one or two visits, the root-filling material is placed, and the pulp chamber up to and just apical to the cementum–enamel junction is used for retention (*Fig.* 11.4). Resin is placed in the pulp chamber and built up to act as a post and core. The strip-crown form is then used, as described above, to build the crown, ensuring that it is trimmed so that its margins are subgingival. Relief holes can be placed at the incisal corners to allow expression of resin during placement.

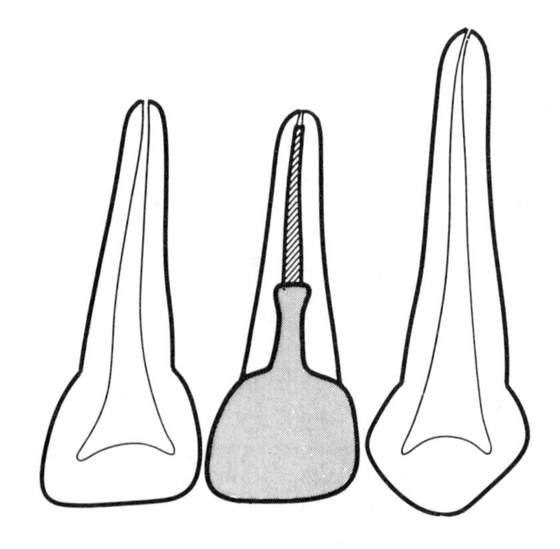

Fig. 11.4. Pulpectomy on a maxillary lateral primary incisor–resin post and crown fitted.

Retention can be enhanced by acid-etching all available enamel. Because of difficulty in retaining primary anterior crowns, the resin should overlap the enamel surface in a feather edge rather than meeting at a butt joint. In this manner more etched enamel is available to the

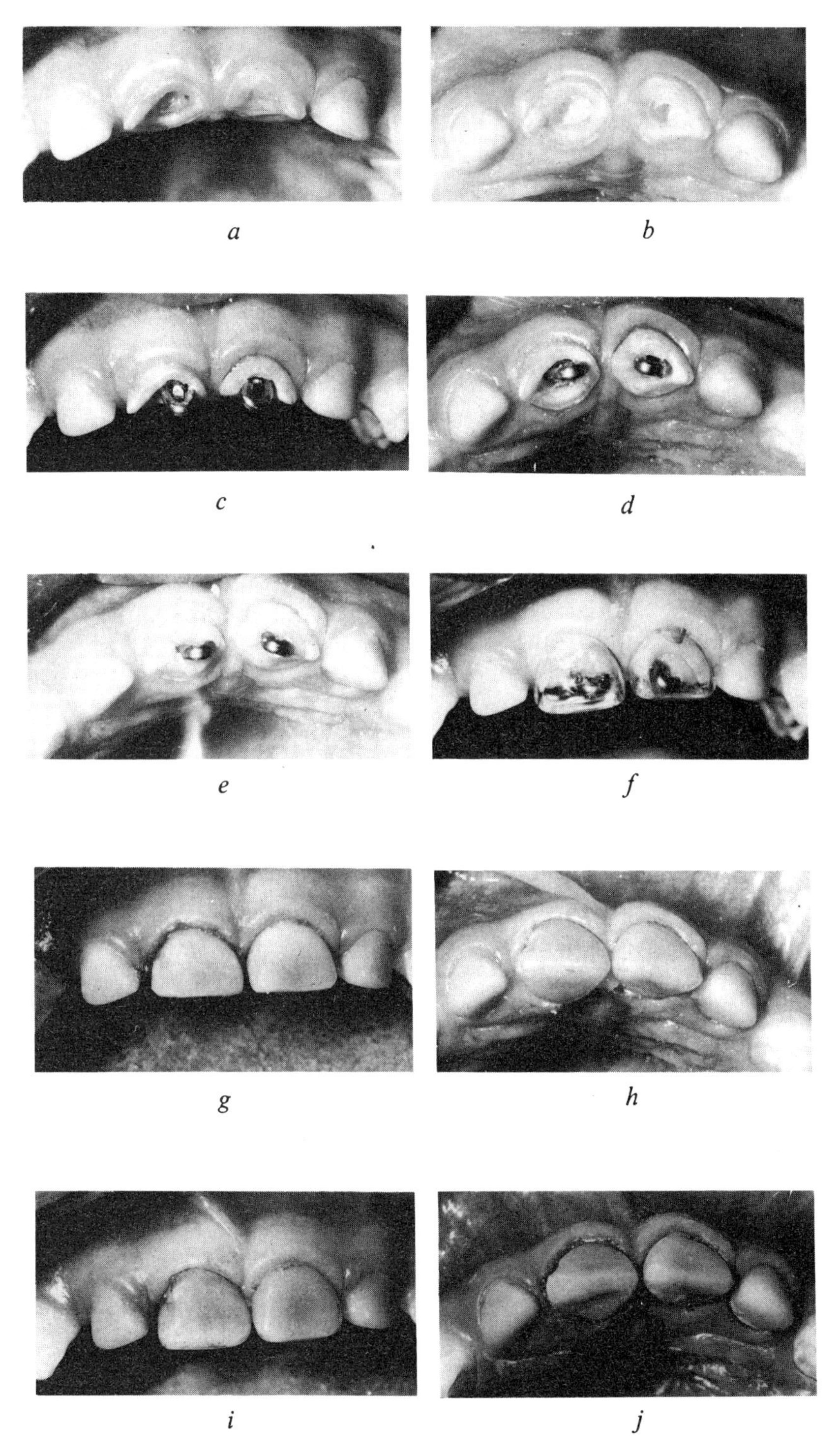

Fig. 11.5. Composite post crowns with wire reinforced post in 51, 61 (A|A), 52, 62 (B|B) have strip crowns placed. *a*, Preoperative. *b*, After pulpectomy. *c*, Wire in canal. *d*, Occlusal view. Wire in canal. *e*, Post cemented in canal with composite. *f*, Strip crown forms. *g*, Composite placed. Buccal view. *h*, Composite placed. Occlusal view. *i*, Finished restoration. Buccal view. *j*, Finished restoration. Occlusal view.

resin. In some instances it will be necessary to accept a subgingival flash of resin in the interest of retention. Once the resin is set, the crown is finished as described before.

Pin reinforcement of the resin post and core can be provided with orthodontic wire (*Fig.* 11.5). Non-vital primary incisors treated in this way may exfoliate prematurely; the problems associated with resorption of primary teeth treated by pulpectomy and root-canal filling are described in Chapter 19. However, it should be emphasized that, because of its relatively coronal position, the post part of the post crown rarely represents a problem in resorption.

Discing

Discing of the interproximal area may be considered only as a temporary measure to remove superficial caries and make the area self-cleansing, or at least more readily cleansed. Sandpaper discs are recommended since they remove tooth surface more slowly and probably generate less heat than 'lightning strips' or metal discs; they are also less traumatic to the soft tissues should the lips and tongue be improperly retracted. The exact angulation of the disc is dictated by the site of the lesion. After discing, the incisal edge must be no wider than the maximum gingival mesiodistal width so that the area is easily cleaned. The end result should be a parallel-sided or tapered tooth, narrowest at the incisal edge. Closed contacts should be opened by the discing in the hope of preventing recurrence of the lesion.

It is seldom possible to remove all decay by discing; to do so may expose the pulp. Therefore the oral environment must be changed so that the remaining caries will arrest. Fluoride varnish should be applied to the disced surfaces, and this may need to be repeated until the child's co-operation has improved to the extent that strip crowns can be fitted.

It should be emphasized that discing is only a temporary expedient to slow down the progress of dental caries in incisors in very young children. It should *never* be considered as a definitive treatment. When discing is used, restoration of the incisors must be planned to take place within 3 months. It is hoped that any remaining caries will arrest, or slow down, until such time as a permanent restoration (strip crowns) may be placed. The size and anatomy of the primary anterior pulp impose limitations on the extent of the discing which should therefore be minimal.

References

Doyle W. A. (1967) Esthetic restoration of deciduous incisors: a new Class IV preparation. *J. Am. Dent. Assoc.* **74**, 82.

Hennon D. K., Stookey G. K. and Muhler J. C. (1969) Prevalence and distribution of dental caries in preschool children. *J. Am. Dent. Assoc.* **79**, 1405.

Kennedy D. B. (1986) The Class 4 Lesion. In: *Paediatric Operative Dentistry*, 3rd edn. Bristol, Wright.

O'Sullivan E. A. and Curzon M. E. J. (1991) The efficacy of comprehensive dental care for children under general anaesthesia. *Br. Dent. J.* **171**, 56.

Pollard M. A. and Fayle S. A. (1994) Strip crowns for primary incisors. In: *Restorative Techniques in Paediatric Dentistry*. ed. Duggal M. S. London, Dunitz.

Chapter 12

The Class 5 lesion

Diagnosis

The Class 5 lesion is considered separately from those lesions that appear in developmental pits, which were discussed in Chapter 8. It occurs on the gingival one-third of the tooth and its aetiology can be directly linked with poor oral hygiene, since this area is accessible to the toothbrush; indeed, it is probably the only lesion that can be prevented by toothbrushing alone. Dietary habits, such as sucking mints and chewing gum, can also be an aetiological factor. The initial decalcification is caused by the breakdown of foods containing fermentable carbohydrates held in close proximity to the buccal surfaces of the posterior teeth for long periods.

Diagnosis of Class 5 lesions should present no problem since they are clinically obvious to exploration. However, if the practitioner examines the patient in too hasty a manner, he or she may fail to diagnose cervical caries in those areas that require retraction of soft tissues to improve access and visibility. Such areas are the buccal surfaces of maxillary molars and the lingual surfaces of mandibular molars.

Class 5 lesions are more prevalent in the more distally positioned teeth. Therefore the first primary molars are affected less than second primary and the first and second permanent molars. The most likely reason for this is the better accessibility to the toothbrush of anterior teeth. Also, food debris from the distobuccal surface of the maxillary first and second permanent molars may be retained due to inactive tongue and cheek muscles. Further, the first permanent molar erupts at a time when parental control of dietary habits is diminished now that the child is of school age.

In the very young, Hennon et al. (1969) found that decay in primary canines was most often located on the buccal surfaces in the 18–39-month age groups. It could be that a neonatal hypoplastic defect commonly seen on the buccal surface of mandibular primary canines acts as an area for plaque retention and subsequent caries development in these young children whose oral hygiene is often neglected. Furthermore, many parents do not realize the need to brush the teeth of infants, which should be as soon as there are teeth to brush.

Considerations in treatment

The treatment of these lesions needs to be discussed in broader terms than a mere description of the design of the Class 5 cavity. This is because the Class 5 lesion, particularly when it occurs in all quadrants of the mouth simultaneously, is almost pathognomonic of a severe dietary and/or oral hygiene problem. The history and any projected changes in patient behaviour must be taken into consideration when operative treatment is performed.

Regular examination and preventive care, including topical fluoride application, should permit the practitioner to diagnose the lesion in its early stages. At this time the initial decalcification may present as a white chalkiness or brown stain limited to the enamel. When the patient is a regular attender with a low past decay experience and there is no other decay in the offending teeth, it is appropriate to scale the decalcified areas, polish the surface smooth, and apply topical fluoride, such as fluoride varnish where available, to arrest the incipient lesion. However, if the lesion extends into the dentine, a Class 5 cavity should be prepared.

At the same time, vigorous attempts should be made to improve the oral home-care. Disclosing tablets and solutions can demonstrate the plaque to both child and parent. Toothbrushing instruction should be given, followed by an assessment of the child's ability to brush that area. With young children, particularly those of preschool age, it is necessary for the parent to perform the brushing (Pinkham, 1975). Children under 7 years do not have the manual dexterity to use a toothbrush correctly; and their parents should be instructed in the scrub-brush method, which is most effective for plaque removal in the primary dentition (Sangnes et al., 1972).

When gingival decalcification is occurring in many areas, a fluoride mouthrinse should be recommended. However, this is appropriate only for children of school age who can rinse effectively. The parent and child should be warned of the severity of the problem. Such multiple decalcified areas should be re-evaluated earlier than at the normal 6-month recall. With small children, parents can be advised to apply fluoride mouthrinse solution on a cotton-tipped applicator (Q-Tip). This conservative approach is justified on the basis that the patient has been and will continue to be a regular attender. In that case the decalcification can be interpreted as the result of a lapse in oral hygiene and dietary habits. Alterations in the child's daily toothbrushing routine can easily be caused by such things as parental illness or breakdown of a marriage, while an increase in the eating of sweets may be attributed to the child's increased access to the sweet shop or corner shop. This occurs particularly in the preteenage period when children gain increasing independence, both social and financial.

The treatment of multiple areas of gingival decalcification in a new patient must also allow for any other caries present. Since access to the Class 5 lesion can be as difficult for the operator as it is for the child's toothbrush, it is more difficult to place an excellent restoration and there is less chance of the restoration being well cleansed. The longevity of a Class 5 restoration is thus put in doubt, and the patient's dental age must be considered to determine if the Class 5 lesion could be better treated by a method other than cavity preparation and restoration.

A preschool child who presents with extensive gingival decalcification may have Class 2 lesions in the same teeth. The operator can place both Class 2 and Class 5 restorations in the primary molars of this child and expect them to last more than 6 years until the premolars erupt. This approach may result in disappointment if the restorations fail, as they often do. Perhaps the child's oral hygiene and diet may not improve or the Class 2 cavity design will have encouraged marginal deterioration (Chapter 9). This is most likely to occur in mandibular first primary molars (Castaldi, 1957; MacRae et al., 1962). Much time would be saved for both patient and practitioner if a stainless-steel crown had been placed at the outset. The success rate of multisurface restorations in primary molars is nowhere near as good as that of the preformed crown (Roberts and Sheriff, 1992).

The orthodontic implications of cervical caries in the first permanent molar must be considered by the practitioner. When extensive lesions are present close to the eruption time of these teeth, their longevity is in question. If a malocclusion would be best treated by extractions, teeth with a poor long-term prognosis should always be considered as possible choices for extraction. Orthodontic extraction of the first permanent molars may be considered for a child with a Class I skeletal base, an Angle's Class I molar relationship, a full complement of permanent teeth, none of which is developing ectopically, and minimal crowding (Houston et al., 1992). Such a serious and far-reaching decision should be made in conjunction with an orthodontist. Treatment planning in relation to the first permanent molar has been well described (Crabb and Rock, 1971). Unfortunately, removing four permanent molars under general anaesthesia is often more attractive to the busy practitioner than managing a difficult child while placing extensive restorations or preformed crowns. However, the apparently easy route may not be in the child's best dental or emotional interests. Every child must be carefully evaluated and treatment must be performed in their best interests and not for the convenience of the dentist.

The Class 5 cavity

Once cavity preparation has been undertaken, every effort should be made to place a restoration which will be long-lasting. Rubber-dam application is essential, mainly because of the improved access afforded. Outline form should be limited to the carious lesion and any adjacent decalcified areas. Decalcified areas and carious defects occurring 2 mm apart should be included in the same cavity outline as extension for prevention, rather than as separate lesions. The Class 5 cavity may be kidney-shaped; a gently curved outline form is as acceptable as a square, sharp outline form at the mesial and distal margins. The No. 330 bur can be used to cut the cavity. Dentinal undercuts for mechanical retention will be placed if the pear-shaped bur is used. Any remaining caries can be removed with a slow-running, round No. 2 bur. A pulp-protecting base should be used in deep areas of the cavity. The gingival enamel margin should follow a regular curve parallel to the gingival attachment unless the lesion extends subgingivally. The margins should be trimmed with hatchets to ensure that no enamel unsupported by dentine remains. This is especially important because of the possible decalcification adjacent to the lesion.

Although the appearance may not be ideal in anterior teeth, amalgam alloy is the material of choice when improvement in oral hygiene and dietary habits is expected. Since that will not always be the case, a fluoride-releasing cement is recommended (Hatibovic-Kofman and Koch, 1991). It will normally last at least 2 years and in many instances considerably longer. An advantage of this semipermanent restoration is the continued fluoride release, which outweighs the dissolution that occurs with time. This fluoride release is most beneficial to margins that are both susceptible to further caries and finished somewhat less than perfectly due to difficult access. With time, age and increased eruption, there may be improvements in the access, oral hygiene and dietary habits, and the restoration can then be placed with amalgam alloy or composite resin.

References

Castaldi C. R. (1957) Analysis of some operative procedures currently being used in paedodontics. *J. Can. Dent. Assoc.* **23**, 377.

Crabb J. J. and Rock Y. P. (1971) Treatment planning in relation to the first permanent molar. *Br. Dent. J.* **131**, 396.

Hatibovic-Kofman D. and Koch G. (1991) Fluoride release from glass ionomer cements *in vivo* and *in vitro*. *Swed. Dent. J.* **15**, 253.

Hennon D. K., Stookey G. K. and Muhler J. C. (1969) Prevalence and distribution of dental caries in preschool children. *J. Am. Dent. Assoc.* **79**, 1405.

Houston W. J. B., Stephen C. D and Tulley W. J. (1992) *A Textbook of Orthodontics*, 2nd edn. London, Wright.

MacRae P. D., Zacherl W. and Castaldi C. R. (1962) Study of defects in Class II dental amalgam restorations in deciduous molars. *J. Can. Dent. Assoc.* **28**, 491.

Pinkham J. R. (1975) Oral hygiene in children: relationship to age and brushing time. *J. Prevent. Dent.* **2**, 28.

Roberts J. F. and Sherriff M. (1992). The fate and survival of amalgam and preformed crown molar restorations placed in a specialist dental practice. *Br. Dent. J.* **169**, 237.

Sangnes G., Zachrisson B. and Gjermo P. (1972) Effectiveness of vertical and horizontal brushing techniques in plaque removal. *J. Dent. Child.* **39**, 94.

Chapter 13

Matrices

Justification for use

Restoration of the primary dentition prevents space loss by maintaining arch length; carious teeth should thus be restored to their original dimensions and contour whenever possible. Restorations should be provided whose contour discourages the retention of food debris, bacteria and plaque so that they will not be detrimental to gingival health or encourage recurrent caries. To fulfil these objectives, a well-adapted and contoured matrix must be used when restoring Class 2 and 3 cavities. This recommendation applies both to permanent and temporary restorations, since the requirements are the same.

Maintaining correct arch length by properly contoured interproximal restorations is especially important in the young child since tooth movement accompanies the transition from primary to permanent dentition. The first permanent molars often erupt into a cusp-to-cusp relationship; this occlusion may then change to an Angle Class I by differential mesial migration, either at the expense of the mandibular primate space, if present, or when the primary molars are lost (Baume, 1950). There is more leeway space in the mandibular than in the maxillary arch since the mandibular second primary molar is larger mesiodistally than its maxillary counterpart. When the primary molars are lost, this small discrepancy allows the mandibular first permanent molar to migrate farther mesially than its maxillary counterpart; hence an Angle Class I relationship is obtained. Undercontoured maxillary Class 2 restorations may permit early mesial migration of the maxillary first permanent molar from a cusp-to-cusp relationship into an Angle Class 2 before any mandibular leeway space has been used. Steep cuspal inclines may then prevent any spontaneous alteration of this iatrogenic malocclusion (Davey, 1967).

Undercontoured interproximal restorations with either flat or open contacts encourage retention of plaque. Also, restorations with overhanging margins may provide an area for plaque retention. Nothing is more discouraging than to see an iatrogenic gingivitis in an otherwise healthy mouth when the cause is related to improper use of matrices.

Matrices for primary molars

The matrix band must be compatible with the size of the primary molar and the child's oral environment. It must have good adaptation to the interproximal margins of the cavity, enough stability to withstand the pressures of condensation, and retention to resist any effort of the child to dislodge it. Although it is impossible to reproduce interproximal contour precisely, the best results are obtained when the matrix is contoured, wedged and supported (Phillips et al., 1956) The ideal interproximal contour is shown in *Figs* 13.1 and 13.2; there should be a smooth contour and a positive contact with the adjacent tooth. Matrices for primary molars should be restricted to small Class 2 restorations. Large restorations, such as mesial–occlusal–distal, are contraindicated, with the use of stainless-steel crowns preferred.

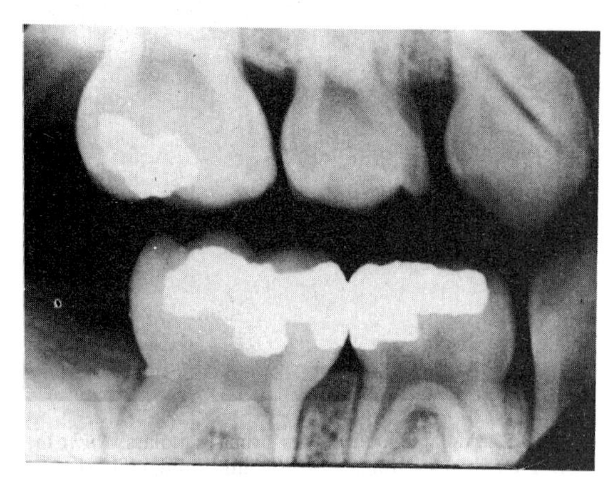

Fig. 13.1. Postoperative bitewing demonstrating correct interproximal contour of Class 2 amalgam restorations.

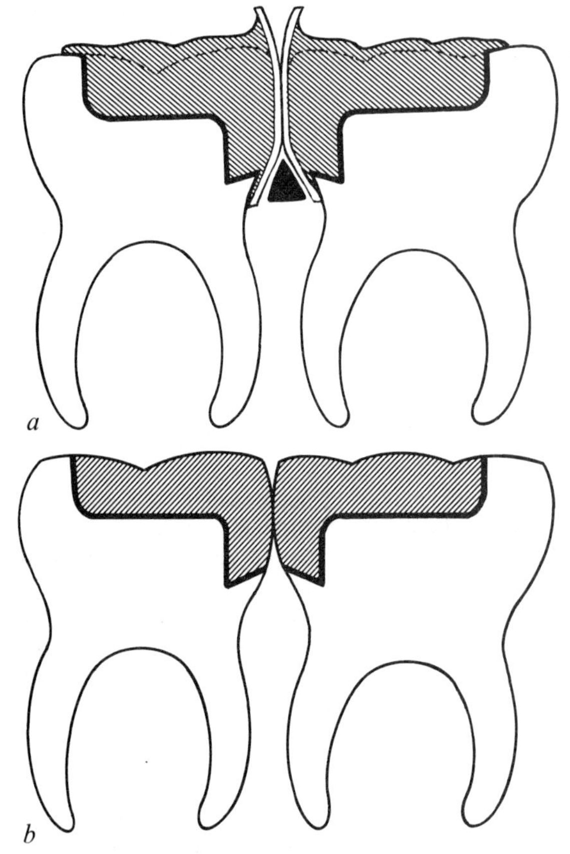

Fig. 13.2. *a*, Correctly wedged matrices for adjacent Class 2 restorations in primary molars. *b*, Correct interproximal contour of adjacent Class 2 restorations in primary molars.

Wedging

A wedge must be used with any of the matrices to be described so that a cervical overhang of restorative material is avoided (Phillips et al., 1956). The correctly placed wedge improves the cervical adaptation of the band to the cavity walls and stabilizes it. The wedge can be inserted from either the lingual or the buccal, depending on ease of access; occasionally both a buccally and lingually placed wedge are necessary to obtain good adaptation. Pressure is recommended to spring the teeth slightly apart and thus help re-establish any pre-existing tight contact following wedge removal. The thickness of band material must be compensated for by using heavy condensation pressures and separation by positive wedge placement. If the wedge is placed too far occlusally, a flat contact may result with an overhang gingivally (*Fig*. 13.3). Failure to use any wedge invariably results in a gingival overhang (*Fig*. 13.4). The use of an orange wooden wedge (Hawes-Neos wedges; Procare Dental, Bradford BD5 9BJ) is compatible with the size and anatomy of primary molars.

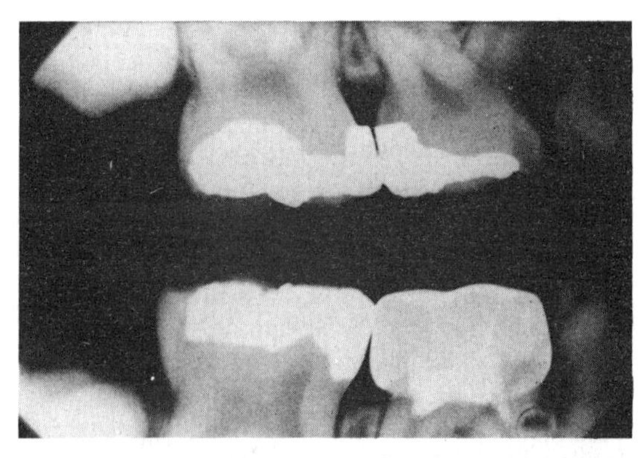

Fig. 13.3. Bitewing demonstrating that incorrect location of wedge for adjacent Class 2 restorations has resulted in a flat contour and gingival overhang. Note also the undercarved marginal-ridge area.

Analgesia

Adequate analgesia is required to place a matrix and wedge effectively and painlessly. Local analgesia will almost certainly have been used for interproximal cavity preparation. When necessary, palatal and long buccal

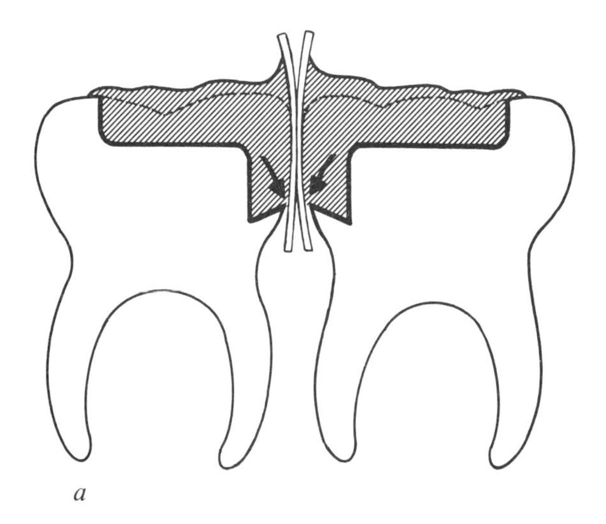

a

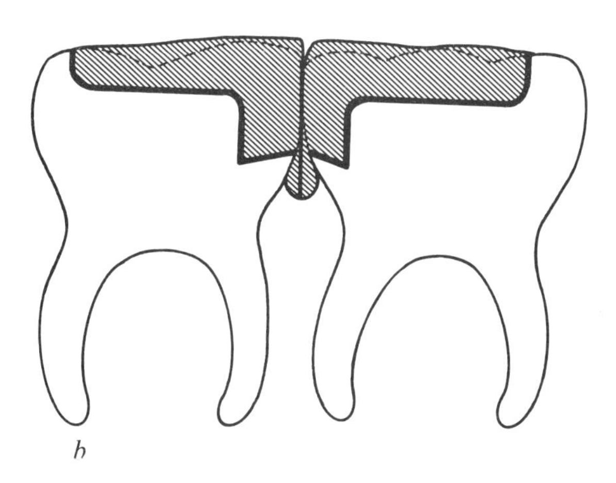

b

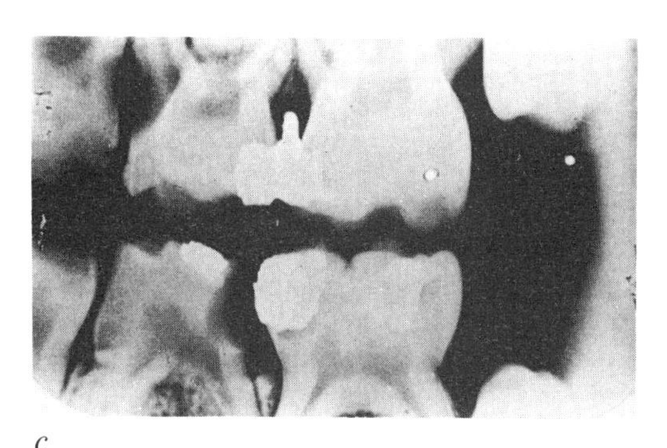

c

Fig. 13.4. *a*, Failure to use a wedge in adjacent Class 2 restorations in primary molars invites the production of an overhang. *b*, Resulting overhang. *c*, Bitewing demonstrates gross overhang from failure to use a wedge or carve the interproximal area between 64 and 65 (|DE).

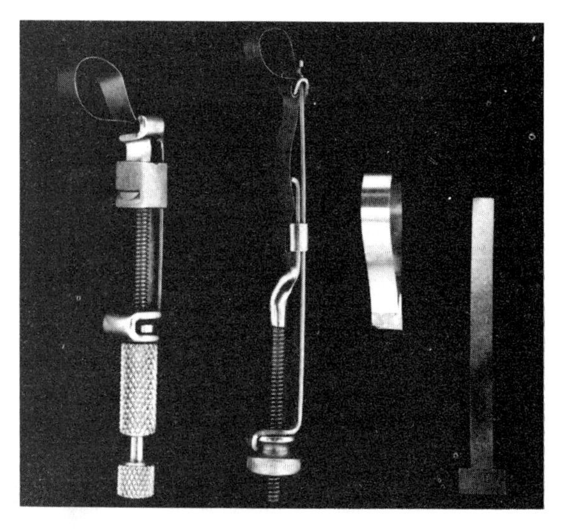

Fig. 13.5. Available matrices for primary molars. *Right to left:* T-band, custom-made orthodontic band, child-size Siqueland, child-size Tofflemire.

analgesia (in upper and lower arches, respectively) assures the operator that all procedures can be performed painlessly. Alternatively, lingual topical anaesthesia may be sufficient.

Posterior matrices

The following posterior matrices are commonly used:

(1) custom-made, spot-welded orthodontic band,
(2) T-band,
(3) Tofflemire or Siqueland (*Fig.* 13.5).

1. Custom-made orthodontic band

This is the best matrix to use on primary molars. It is similar in size and shape to the T-band, but it can be prepared either before or after cavity preparation and fits the bulbous contours of the primary molar. Alternatively the matrix material for the Siqueland can be used instead (*Fig.* 13.6). A $1\frac{1}{2}$ in long strip (approx. 40 mm) of 3/16 by 0.020 in orthodontic steel band material is spot-welded to form a loop larger than the average-sized primary molar. This loop is placed on the tooth; where necessary a tight contact can be sprung open by a wedge to allow the loop to be placed. The Howe 033/110 plier (Procare, Bradford) is used to draw the loop tight buccally (*Fig.* 13.7). It is removed and spot-welded to maintain this

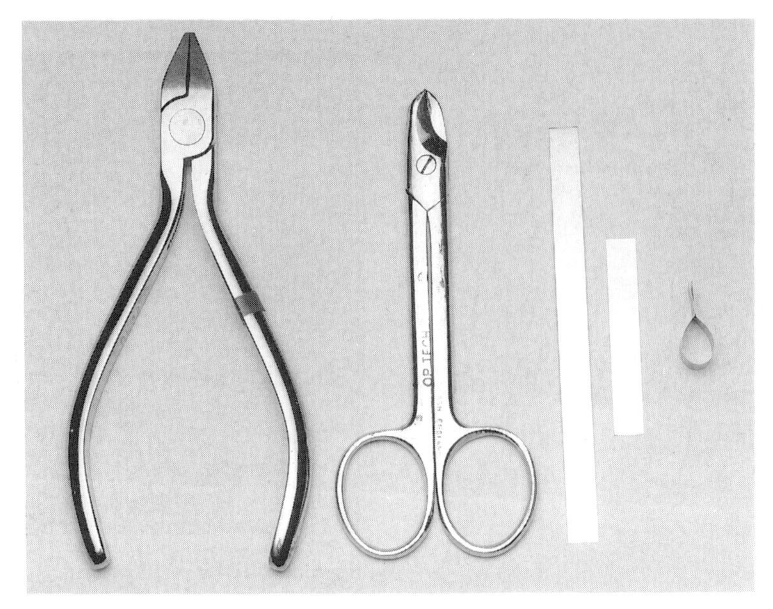

Fig. 13.6. Pliers, crown scissors and band material. Siqueland band has been cut in half, fitted around a primary molar and then spot-welded to size.

accurately adapted contour (*Fig.* 13.8). Excess band material, which may impinge on buccal tissues, is cut with scissors away from the second spot-weld.

Following cavity preparation the band is tried on the tooth and contoured if necessary with a No. 114 or 137 plier, then wedged as previously described (*Fig.* 13.9). To remove the band after placement and preliminary carving of the restoration, a plastic instrument (e.g. Hollenbach carver) is passed between the tooth and band material on the buccal side close to the spot-weld. While the band is stabilized with finger pressure, the spot-weld is broken by drawing the instrument buccally. The importance of using the correct amount of spot-welding to join the band is now evident; this is best achieved on a trial-and-error basis. The wedge is removed and the band is withdrawn in a buccolingual direction. A useful tip is to place the end of a large amalgam plugger on the marginal ridge as any matrix band is removed. This helps to prevent fracture of the ridge (*Fig.* 13.10).

A major disadvantage of the custom-made orthodontic band is the expense of a spot-welder. Those in exclusive paediatric dental practice are encouraged to use this method routinely since the spot-welder may also be employed for appliances used in minor tooth movement.

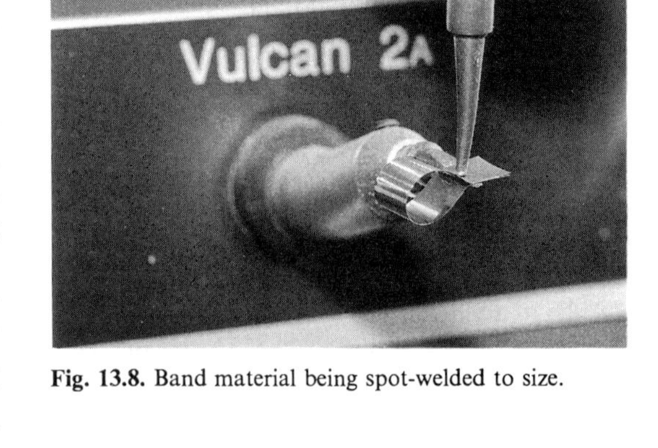

Fig. 13.8. Band material being spot-welded to size.

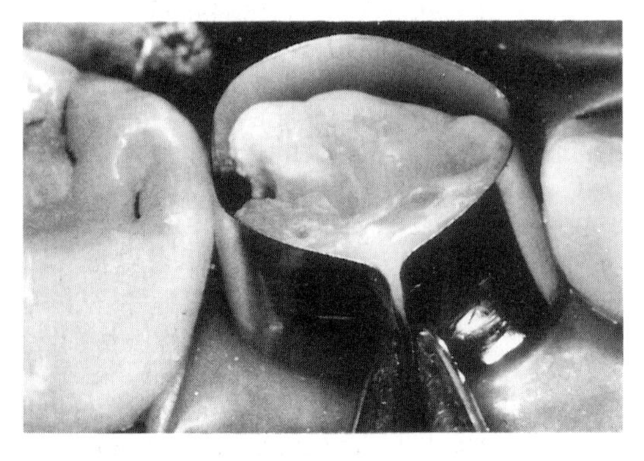

Fig. 13.7. Photograph of band material placed around a primary molar and drawn tight with pliers.

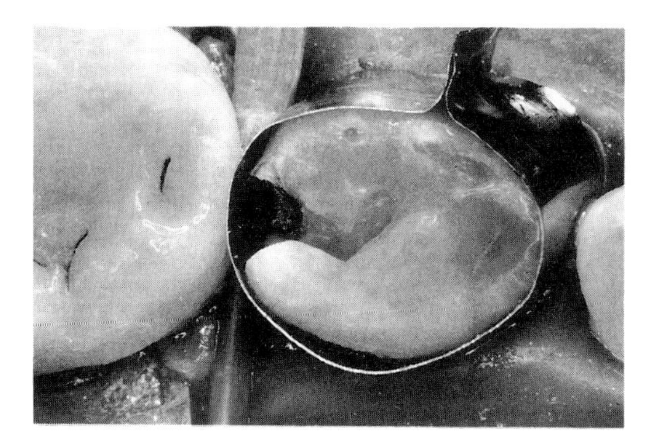

Fig. 13.9. Photograph of spot-welded band placed around primary molars.

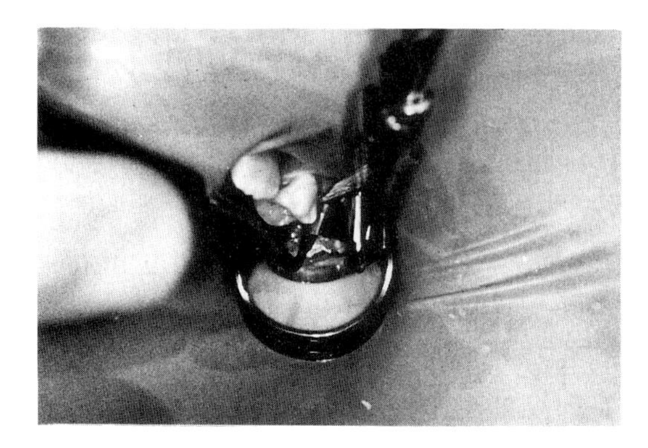

Fig. 13.10. Removal of a matrix band with a plugger used to hold the marginal ridge in place during matrix removal.

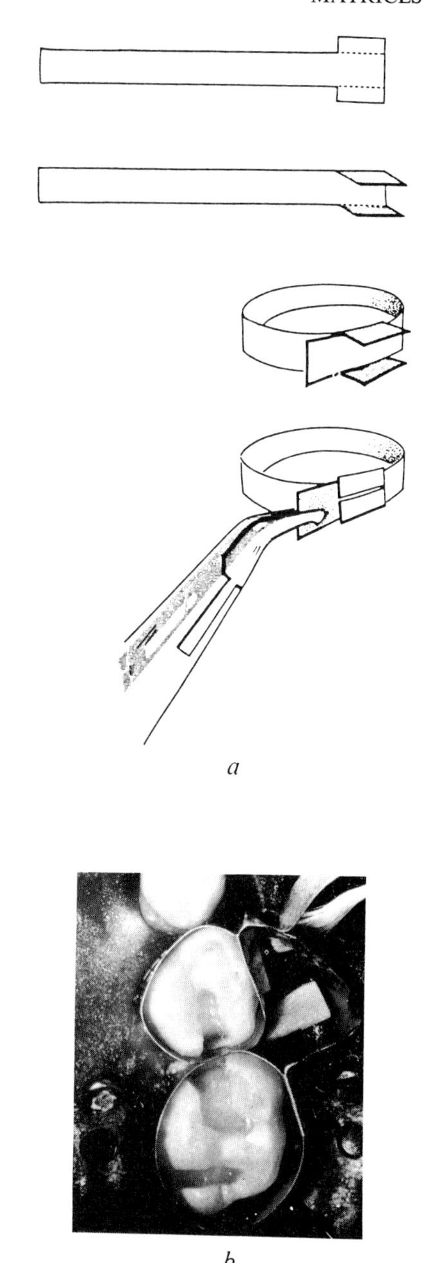

Fig. 13.11. *a*, T-band formation. *b*, T-bands placed on adjacent primary molars.

2. T-band

The T-band can be purchased prepinched in different sizes (Tofflemire narrow-size band material, Wm. Getz Corporation, Chicago; Siqueland narrow retainer, 5 mm band material, Procare, Bradford) or can be custom-made from strips of brass or German silver alloy. The band is fabricated either before or after cavity preparation; a T-shaped metal band is cut, with the proportions shown in *Fig.* 13.11. The short arms of the 'T' are folded over to form a loop; the free end is passed through the loop, ensuring that it is on the buccal side of the band and freely sliding. The band is placed on the tooth so that it passes below the level of the gingival seat of the proximal box. The plier (Howe 033/110) applied to the free arm tightens the band and at the same time finger pressure stabilizes it. Once tightened the band's dimensions are maintained by bending the free sliding arm back on itself. The folded-over short arms of the 'T' act as a fulcrum. This can be done either inside or outside the mouth. Excess band material is cut away with scissors. The band can also be tightened on a trial-and-error basis out of the mouth.

The advantage of both the spot-welded and the T-band is that adjacent mesio- and disto-occlusal restorations can be packed simultaneously as the band material is thin enough not to leave an open contact. When filling adjacent cavities in this way the gingival depths of each restoration should be filled first and alternately.

The band is cut if it impinges on the gingiva; this commonly occurs on the lingual surface of first primary molars. It is then contoured with a No. 114 or 137 plier out of the mouth. After reinsertion, it is wedged and checked for adaptation and retention before placement of the restoration. The T-band is often difficult to use either because of insufficient anaesthesia or inadequate contouring and wedging.

In removing the T-band, the loop is first undone and the wedge removed so that the band is loose. The band is then cut close to the marginal ridge, and the remaining interproximal band material is grasped with the No. 110 plier or locking cotton tweezers and withdrawn in a buccolingual direction, sliding it through the contact area. A condenser/plugger can be used to hold the marginal ridge area lightly as described for the spot-welded band. It will be very difficult to remove the band occlusally if it has been properly contoured, as occlusal withdrawal invites fracture of the marginal ridge.

3. Tofflemire or Siqueland

These can also be used for the primary dentition, although the narrow-sized Tofflemire band material (5 mm compared to 6 mm) is recommended to prevent excessive gingival trauma and to improve retention of the matrix. The main advantage of these bands and retainers is that the clinician may feel proficient with them because they are commonly used for adults. An advantage of the Tofflemire is that, as with the T-band and custom-made orthodontic bands, the band material can be removed in a buccolingual direction. It will also require wedging; not always the case with the Siqueland retainer, although wedging is recommended whenever possible.

These advantages are outweighed on several counts. First, the Siqueland has to be removed occlusally, which invites marginal-ridge fracture, as described earlier. Second, compared to the T-band and custom-made orthodontic band, there is additional bulk in the child's mouth, which may rest against lip, cheek and tongue. The additional tactile stimuli increase salivation; also the retaining arms may annoy the child so that he or she will dislodge the band, often just when the alloy is to be inserted. Both of these disadvantages are eliminated when the rubber dam is in place. Third, the retainer part of these matrices is bulky in the child's small mouth. Lastly, when applying the matrix band to a tooth which is clamped with a rubber-dam clamp, the bulkiness of the band-holder prevents correct positioning of the band. In this situation the custom-made ortho-band is the preferred option.

General considerations

A final selection of matrix band must be left to the individual practitioner. Whichever band he or she selects, they should use a mirror and an explorer to test its marginal adaptation to the cavity walls before inserting the restoration (see *Fig.* 13.9). Any discrepancies should be corrected before the restoration is placed, unless those areas can be adequately contoured post-operatively.

Quadrant dentistry should always be the aim of any dental practitioner, particularly when treating children. Accordingly the placing of adjacent Class 2 restorations may well arise. Some clinicians recommend that this be done at separate visits to obtain the best interproximal contour. However, there is no evidence to contradict placing two adjacent Class 2 restorations in primary teeth at the same appointment, provided each is supported by its own matrix band. In fact, such treatment may remove the need for a second visit by the patient and a second injection for that particular quadrant.

When adjacent interproximal lesions are restored at the same visit, the alloy should be condensed alternately in the interproximal boxes (Hill, 1973). This prevents one restoration from being overcontoured and the other undercontoured. When a wedge is placed before cavity preparation, the adjacent primary molars are sprung apart slightly. This prewedging results in the re-establishment of a tight contact area.

Unfortunately, not all Class 2 lesions lend themselves to ideal cavity preparation; with adjacent deep interproximal lesions that have been untreated for some time space loss may already have occurred. As matrix application is

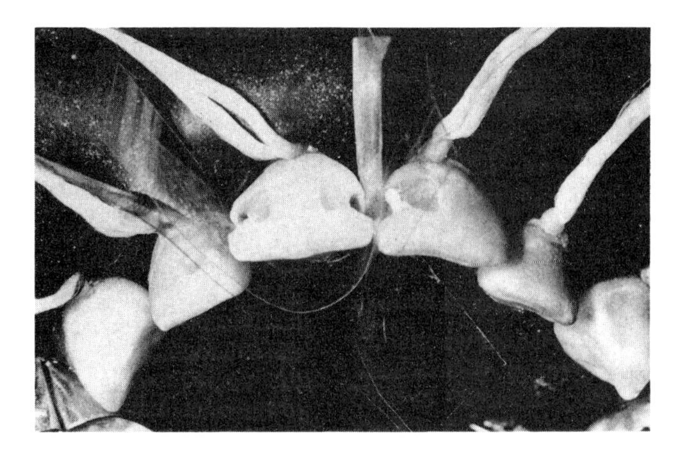

Fig 13.12. Wedged celluloid matrices.

difficult in these instances, floss should be passed between the adjacent bands before the wedge is inserted. After the alloy has been placed and the wedge and band removed, the floss can dispose of any overhanging gingival excess before the alloy is set. Rubber dam will also retract the papillae so that postoperative carving is occasionally possible. Alternatively, a gold knife or curette can be used once the alloy is set.

Anterior matrices

Where alloy is used, as in Class 3 distal cavities in primary canines, a wedged metal matrix is essential to provide strength to resist amalgam condensation. A flat, straight piece of band material (5-mm Dentatus matrix band, A. B. Dentatus, Hagerstein, Sweden or Siqueland matrix band child size, Amalgamated Dental Co., 26 Broadwick St, London) about 20 mm long is recommended. It should be looped around the tooth to be treated and the tooth adjacent to the lesion so that the band appears S-shaped when viewed from the occlusal. In this way, there will be access for condensation of the restorative material and good support of the band to prevent displacement during condensation.

A wedged celluloid matrix is advised for Class 3 cavities when resin is used (*Fig*. 13.12). One advantage is that the operator can see through the translucent matrix to determine whether the resin is adequately condensed and contoured.

Class 4 cavities no longer present a problem as the use of the strip crown now replaces the need for Class 4 restorations (see Chapter 11). Should a Class 4 restoration be completed, then the easiest form of matrix is a celluloid crown cut diagonally across to form a triangular matrix covering the incisal edge to be restored. This is very simple and leaves the composite resin with a finished surface so that all that is needed is trimming of the enamel–composite junction.

References

Baume L. J. (1950) Physiological tooth migration and its significance for the development of occlusion. 1. The biogenetic course of the deciduous dentition. *J. Dent. Res.* **29**, 123.

Davey K. W. (1967) Effect of premature loss of primary molars on the anteroposterior position of maxillary first permanent molars and other maxillary teeth. *J. Dent. Child.* **34**, 383.

Hill C. J. (1973) Approximating Class II amalgam restorations for primary molars. *Dent. Clin. North Am.* **17**, 1, 77.

Phillips R. W. et al. (1956) Proximal contour of Class II amalgam restorations made with various matrix band techniques. *J. Am. Dent. Assoc.* **53**, 391.

Chapter 14

Preformed crowns (the stainless-steel crown)

The stainless-steel crown, developed for use in paediatric dentistry in the early 1950s, has helped to solve the problem of the extensively carious tooth. Because of the alarming rate of failure for extensive Class 2 amalgam restorations in primary molars, particularly the mandibular first primary molar, the paediatric dentist has used the stainless-steel crown as a routine treatment in selected cases. The crown is prefabricated in a variety of sizes for each tooth. Tooth preparation precedes the fitting, contouring if necessary, and cementation, all at one appointment. Unlike the gold or porcelain crown, an impression is unnecessary. Also, the finished tooth preparation may have undercut areas. The elasticity of the metal allows the preformed crown to expand past the position of maximum bulbosity, and then to spring back to form a tight collar into these undercuts at the cervical area. The fit into the residual undercuts does help somewhat in the retention of the cemented crown (Savides et al., 1979). One further difference from cast crowns is that the cement is not a thin lute, rather it acts as a space-filler around the irregularly shaped preparation as well as a cementing medium.

Indications

The stainless-steel crown is indicated in a variety of circumstances. To the general practitioner the thought of placing steel crowns in all these instances (to be described) may be daunting. Inexperience and resulting slow clinical speed with the technique can be deterrents. However, before passing off the stainless-steel crown as an unnecessary luxury treatment performed only by specialists, a dentist should evaluate the results of his or her extensive alloy restorations. There are likely to be several, large, Class 2 alloy restorations that will require replacement before tooth exfoliation. One has to question whether replacement would be necessary if a steel crown had been placed initially (Papanathasiou et al., 1994). Braff (1975) reported that 88.7% of primary molars in his study that had been restored with multisurface amalgams needed subsequent treatment before they exfoliated. In contrast, only 30.3% of his sample of primary molars with stainless-steel crowns needed further treatment. Roberts and Sherriff (1990) showed a replacement rate of only 2.8% for the stainless-steel crowns in their 10-year prospective study. The stainless-steel crown is indicated in the circumstances detailed next in subsections 1–5.

1. Extensive decay in primary teeth

The interpretation of extensive decay is subjective and therefore specific examples must be given. The further the intracoronal preparation progresses beyond the minimal, classical design described in Chapters 8 and 9, the greater is the indication for a stainless-steel crown. Thus a crown is indicated whenever one or more cusps are destroyed or weakened by caries. This commonly occurs in the first primary molar when the distal interproximal lesion is not treated early. When the decay then involves the whole of the broad, flat contact area, the distolingual and distobuccal cusps are both weakened. Attempts at a Class 2 cavity preparation would result in a proximal box whose buccal and lingual walls flare markedly towards the embrasure; this would encourage failure of the amalgam at these margins (Chapter 9). In the primary incisor, interproximal decay occurring both mesially and distally, particularly when there is also a Class 5 lesion present, would be an indication for crown placement (see Chapter 11).

A factor to consider in the preoperative evaluation is the dental age of the patient, which is judged by the stage of resorption of the primary tooth, or the root development of the underlying tooth. When a primary tooth can be expected to exfoliate within a year of restoration, a large intracoronal restoration may last satisfactorily. However, parent, child and operator may all be frustrated by the failure of extensive amalgam restorations in primary teeth, and would each have benefited from the initial placement of the steel crown. The experienced clinician can place a stainless-steel crown faster than a three-surface amalgam alloy restoration, and so the disadvantage of additional time is overcome. If a dentist is working under a capitation system, providing replacement restorations at his or her own expense may be a further reason to place a preformed crown at the outset, given their superior survival rates.

2. Following pulp therapy

In both primary and permanent teeth, pulp therapy leaves the treated tooth more brittle. That the tooth structure might subsequently fracture has led to the accepted wisdom of cuspal coverage after endodontics in permanent teeth. This doctrine should also apply to primary teeth. Should the fracture occur below the epithelial attachment, subsequent repair of the tooth may be impossible. It is therefore recommended that postoperative failure be prevented by placing a stainless-steel crown in the first place (Duggal and Curzon, 1989). A tooth that is a candidate for pulp therapy will probably also be a candidate for a crown for reasons described in the previous section. Berg and Donly (1988) have suggested using a combination of glass-ionomer cement and composite resin to restore primary molars that have had a pulpotomy. Perhaps this would be more suited to those teeth where the access cavity is confined to the occlusal surface, and which do not have the weakened cusps frequently encountered with pulpally involved proximal cavities.

3. As a preventive restoration

It has been implied in the preceding sections that the stainless-steel crown is a preventive restoration because it helps avoid amalgam failure or tooth fracture. It can be used also to prevent caries from developing in other areas of the tooth, while an interproximal amalgam restoration cannot protect the buccal and lingual surfaces. Evidence of a developing Class 5 lesion is a sign of a lapse in dietary and oral hygiene habits (Chapter 12). When this occurs in the preschool child who also has a Class 2 lesion in the same tooth, the stainless-steel crown should be seriously considered. This recommendation is prompted by the failure rate of disto-occlusal amalgam restorations in mandibular first primary molars (Castaldi, 1957) and the length of time in the mouth required of the alloy. It also ensures final treatment and prevents the need for difficult Class 5 restorations. This application should be fully used in the handicapped child whose lack of oral hygiene may encourage further decay.

The anatomy of the first primary molar accounts for the difficulty in placing durable mesial–occlusal–distal (MOD) restorations. The marked convergence of buccal and lingual walls towards the occlusal surface close to the mesial contact explains the difficulty in preparing the mesial box. It is extremely difficult to leave the mesiobuccal wall well supported. Also, Castaldi (1957) and MacRae et al. (1962) report that the distobuccal margin of mandibular first primary molars was most commonly deficient in their analyses of Class 2 primary molar alloys. Therefore many practitioners no longer place MOD restorations in the first primary molars of preschool children; instead they place a stainless-steel crown. We would suggest taking this idea one stage further, by not placing MOD intracoronal restorations in any primary molar.

A further advantage of the stainless-steel crown is that dental plaque is more readily seen than on enamel. This, when pointed out to the child and parent, can stimulate them to improve oral hygiene practices.

4. For teeth with developmental defects

Linear hypoplastic defects can undermine the occlusal surface of first primary molars if the aetiological systemic upset occurred at or around birth (Jaffe et al., 1973). Similarly, amelogenesis and dentinogenesis imperfecta can alter tooth morphology and predispose the dentition to excessive wear and loss of the vertical dimension. Hypoplastic and hypocalcified defects on teeth may be more susceptible to caries if the anatomy encourages plaque retention, although this does not always occur. Often the location and extent of the hypoplastic defects do not lend themselves to amalgam restorations. In all these instances the stainless-steel crown can be considered. The preformed crown on the first permanent molar is frequently used as a semipermanent restoration. If extractions are required for orthodontic crowding the hypoplastic molars should be chosen instead of healthy premolars; with modern fixed-appliance therapy this does not pose a great problem for the orthodontist. If this approach is unnecessary or undesirable, the stainless-steel crown will last through the teenage years before placement of a gold or a porcelain bonded-to-gold crown. Pulp morphology, the length of clinical crown, and considerations of costs may preclude the use of cast crowns in the child under 12 years of age.

Caution is required in placing steel crowns on hypoplastic teeth. As the treatment may well involve the crowning of teeth in all four quadrants (often all posterior teeth) there is a very real danger of altering the vertical dimension by impinging on the freeway space. Therefore, it is recommended that the practitioner fit the crowns in quadrants, proceeding to tooth preparation in the next quadrant only when the previous crowns are cemented. In this way there is less likelihood of opening the bite. On the other hand, it is acceptable to open the bite by less than 2 mm if extensive abrasion has already resulted in loss of the vertical dimension; however, leaving the crown excessively high may result in tenderness of the treated tooth and possibly an adverse pulp response.

Developments in adhesive techniques have offered alternatives to the stainless-steel crown for hypoplastic molars, and in particular the first permanent molar. Consideration can be given to the placement of etch-retained, porcelain or chrome–cobalt alloy occlusal onlays to cover the defective enamel, accepting that these are both more expensive to provide than stainless-steel crowns.

5. As an abutment for a space maintainer or denture

The stainless-steel crown can be used as an abutment for a fixed space maintainer. When the abutment tooth presents an indication in its own right for a steel crown, the space maintainer can be incorporated as a crown and loop; alternatively, a band is fitted over the crown and the space maintainer attached to the band. When the abutment tooth presents none of the other indications, but also does not lend itself to banding or to clasping, a stainless-steel crown can be considered. An example is the first primary molar whose buccal and lingual walls converge occlusally, thereby presenting little or no undercut.

Should the second primary molar need to be lost before the first permanent molar erupts, a distal-shoe appliance can be fabricated with an intragingival extension into the second primary molar socket. This prevents mesial migration of the first permanent molar and guides it into occlusion (Hicks, 1973). Since the first primary molar can seldom be satisfactorily banded, it can be crowned and either the appliance is constructed integrally with the crown, or the shoe can be welded on to a band that has been adapted to the undercuts of the preformed crown.

Tooth preparation

1. Anterior

With the development of the acid-etch retained, composite strip crown (Chapter 11), the indications for anterior stainless-steel crowns have fallen markedly. Although stainless-steel crowns are very functional and long-lasting, their appearances provide a great barrier to their acceptance by both patients and parents. Recently, several companies have offered stainless-steel crowns for primary incisors with a composite resin veneer bonded labially. The brittleness of this veneer limits the amount by which the labial surface of the metal crown can be adapted.

The aims of tooth reduction are to provide sufficient space for the steel crown, remove the caries, and leave sufficient tooth substance for retention of the crown. Mesial and distal reductions are required to clear the interproximal contacts. The gingival margin should have no ledge or shoulder; instead, there should be a feather edge at the free gingival margin. Incisal reduction is required to prevent unnecessary elongation of the tooth. Tooth reduction should not destroy undercuts for mechanical retention; thus labial and lingual undercuts are left whenever possible. Lingual reduction with a diamond stone is necessary when the overbite is complete such that the mandibular incisors are in contact with the lingual surfaces of the maxillary incisors. When an incomplete overbite or open bite exists, and there are indications that it will not close, the lingual surface need not be reduced; the undercut towards the gingival margin is used for retention. The only tooth reduction that should occur on the labial surface is that which will remove caries. A Jet pattern, No. 699, tapered fissure bur is compatible with the minimal preparation required. A pulp-protecting base is placed in the deepest areas of the preparation. Crown selection and contouring are done in the same way as for posterior crowns.

The anterior steel crown can be closed, or open-faced for better aesthetics. In this latter instance, the crown should be fitted up to the point of cementation before its labial surface is finally removed. The small dimensions of the anterior steel crown make it most difficult to manage. The crown must be handled with care to prevent unwanted distortion both while contouring and during preparation of the labial window. The labial window is best prepared out of the mouth with a high-speed bur, leaving at least 1 mm of labial collar at the gingival margin. The open-faced crown is polished and cemented with a non-eugenol cement. The exposed labial enamel is etched, washed and dried, and then a veneer of composite resin applied flush with the steel crown.

2. Posterior (*Figs* 14.1–14.8)

The aims of tooth reduction are the same as those described for anterior crowns and reduction is accomplished using a No. 699, tapered fissure, turbine bur throughout. The case described here is shown in *Fig*. 14.1, where recurrent caries has occurred around a defective two-surface amalgam. Decay has also recurred around the occlusal amalgam. Replacement by further amalgams would seriously weaken the crown of the tooth and almost certainly lead to further failure. A stainless-steel crown is indicated here. The steps in its placement are described in the following subsections.

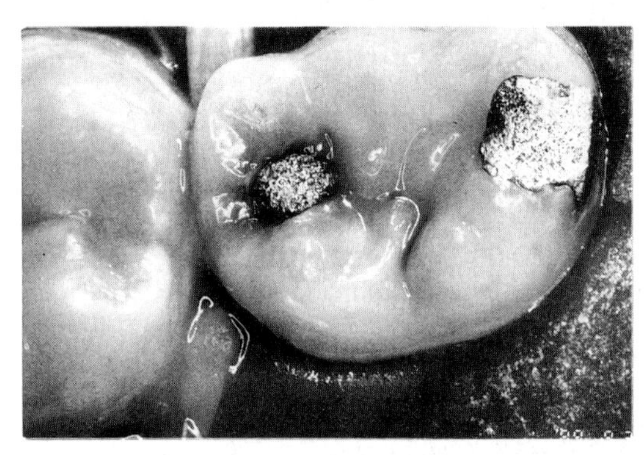

a

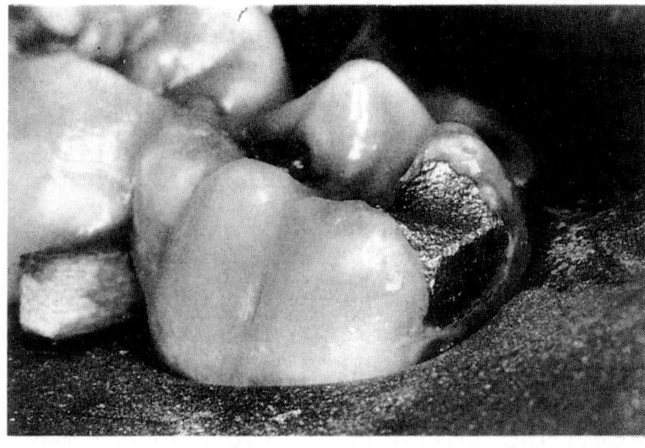

b

Fig. 14.1. Recurrent caries around amalgam restorations in a second primary molar. *a*, Occlusal view. *b*, Buccal view showing deficient gingival margin and recurrent caries.

Caries removal

This is best accomplished before the main preparation for the crown begins. If pulp therapy is subsequently required, it will not be compromised by the gingival bleeding that might result from the crown preparation. Also, if the child's co-operation deteriorates, a temporary dressing is easier to place into a Class 1 or 2 cavity than over a tooth prepared for a crown. The caries and/or old amalgam restorations are removed with the bur as shown in *Fig*. 14.2.

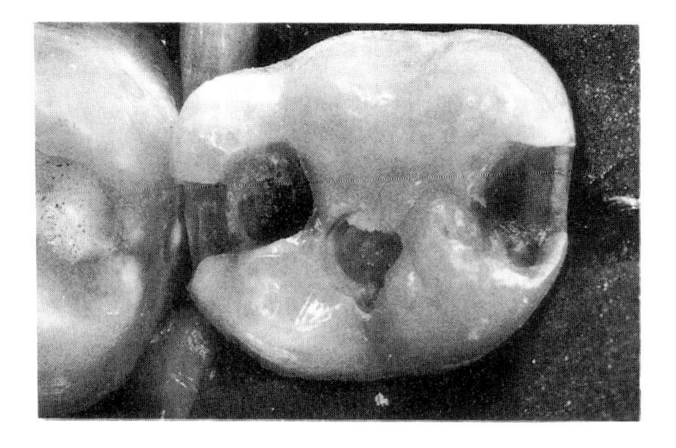

Fig. 14.2. Removal of old amalgam restorations and caries.

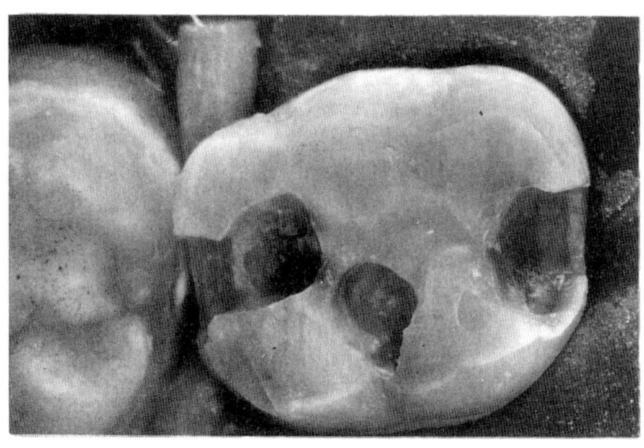

a

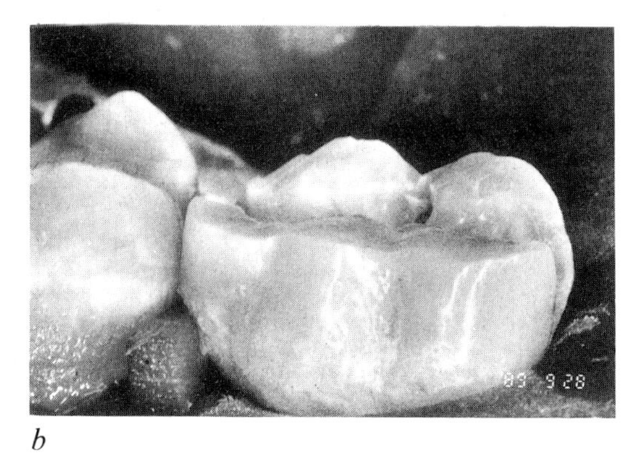

b

Fig. 14.3. Occlusal reduction. *a*, Occlusal view. *b*, Buccal view.

Occlusal reduction

This should approximately follow the anatomy of the tooth to a depth of 1.0–1.5 mm, which allows sufficient space for the metal crown (*Fig*. 14.3). Mink and Bennett (1968) recommended initial placement of 1-mm deep grooves in the occlusal surface to help establish the correct amount of reduction; undoubtedly this is the most accurate approach but it is time-consuming. The cusp height of adjacent teeth gives the operator a good baseline from which to judge the amount of occlusal reduction; similarly, the lingual and buccal developmental pits and grooves in maxillary and mandibular molars are useful reference points. Occasionally, due to hypoplastic wear or gross tooth breakdown, very little clinical height of the natural crown remains. Savides et al. (1979) showed that retention of the cemented metal crown was still relatively high even in teeth grossly decayed to the gingival margin.

Proximal reduction

Mesial and distal reduction takes the form of a ledge- or shoulder-free vertical slice that clears the contact area buccally, lingually and gingivally (*Fig*. 14.4*a*). The contact needs to be cleared for two reasons: first, caries starts at or beneath the contact area; and second, if there is no clearance then the metal crown is unable to slide past the contact area and into the residual undercut. Distal reduction is required even when there is no erupted tooth distally, such as occurs in the preschool child's second primary molar. Failure to follow this recommendation will result in an oversized crown being fitted, which may impede the eruption of the first permanent molar.

The No. 699, plain-cut, tapered fissure bur is preferred to a diamond disc for preparation of the slice because of the unwarranted dangers of soft-tissue trauma that can be caused by discs. However, some operators may prefer to use discs. If so, they should always be safe-sided, used with a guard and then only when the preparation is made under the rubber dam.

An interproximal wedge simplifies the interproximal reduction by slightly springing the teeth apart, thus helping to prevent damage to the adjacent tooth. The tapered fissure bur is positioned buccally or lingually to the contact with the adjacent tooth, at a distance from that tooth which will prevent damage when the bur is taken through the contact-area enamel. Its angulation and depth towards the gingival margin that will allow the contact area to be

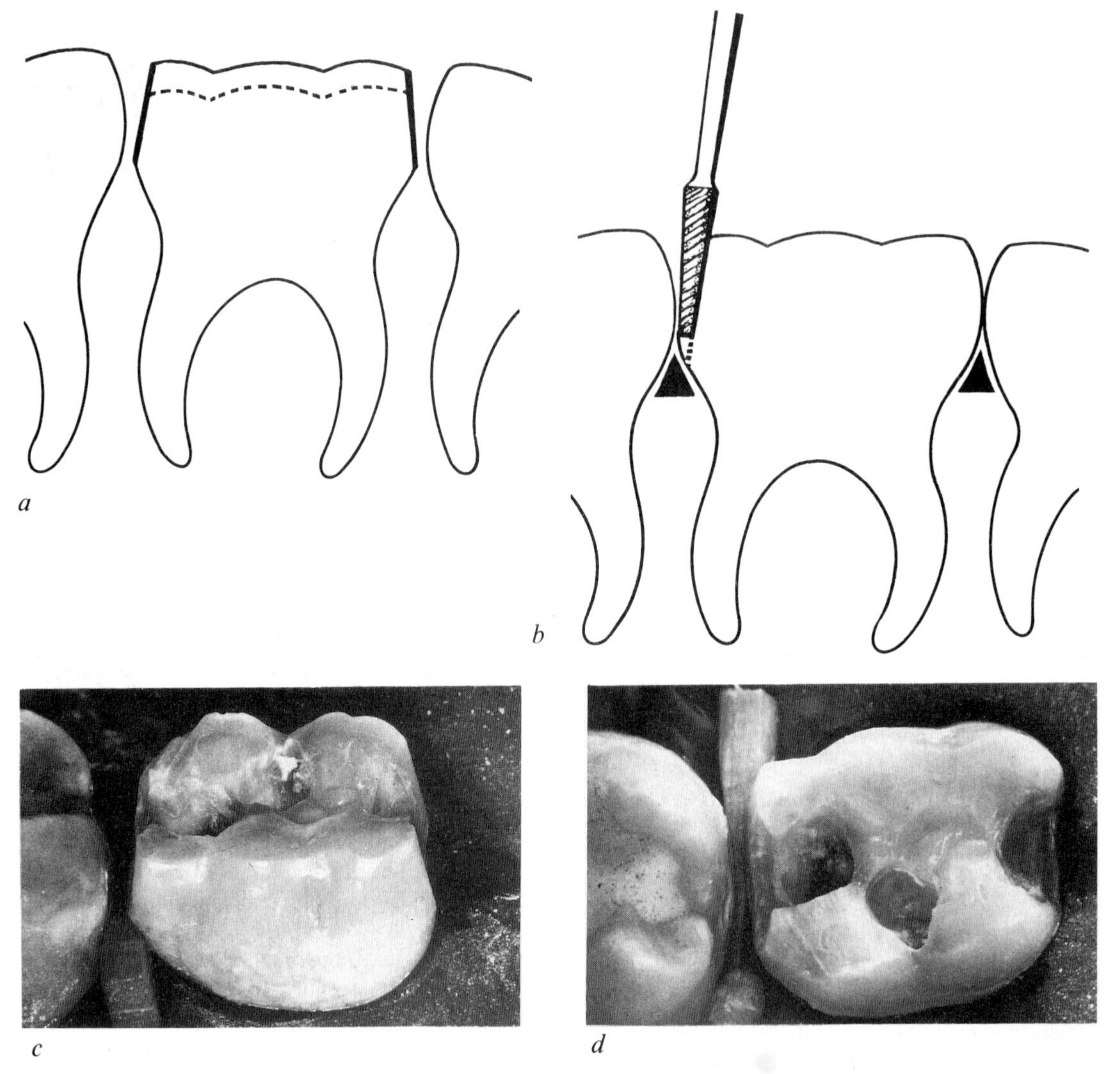

Fig. 14.4. *a*, Mesial and distal reduction; note angulation, clearance of contact point and feather edge. *b*, Positioning of bur, note wedges to protect gingival tissue. *c*, Occlusal view showing mesial and distal reduction. Note the interproximal wedge. *d*, Buccal view.

cleared can be judged before tooth cutting commences. As it is a fissure bur that is being used, and not an end-cutting bur, this approach seems preferable to one where the interproximal reduction is made from the occlusal surface downwards, simply blunting the end of the fissure bur.

Provided the interproximal cut is not started too far into the tooth away from the proximal surface, when the reduction just clears the adjacent contact the desired feather-edge finish line will be established (*Fig.* 14.4). Occasionally this approach results in a shoulder; bearing in mind the bulbosity of primary molars at the cervical aspect of the crown, the shoulder can be converted to a feather edge simply by taking the finish line further gingivally. With the interproximal wedge in position, the rubber dam and interproximal gingival tissues are protected from the bur.

Distal reduction under rubber dam

As preparation of a second primary molar is being carried out under rubber dam it may be that this tooth is also being clamped. Therefore a problem arises when the distal proximal slice needs to be made without snagging the rubber dam in the bur. This can be dealt with by simply pushing the rubber away from the distal tooth surface with a large, flat-plastic instrument, or a Ward's carver. The dam is held away while the enamel slice is made with the tapered fissure bur (Duggal and Curzon, 1994).

Buccal and lingual reduction

Great diversity of opinion exists over this part of the preparation, from no reduction at all to removal of all undercuts to the bottom of the gingival pocket. Mathewson et al. (1974) and Savides (1979) believed that retention depended more upon cement than upon the remaining undercut, but Savides showed that retention was higher with greater buccal and lingual residual undercuts. We should aim, therefore, to remove as little as possible from the buccal and lingual aspects of the tooth crown. However, it becomes more difficult to adapt the margins of the metal crown to the cervical area of the tooth when large undercuts remain, especially when the Ion crowns are used, because they are harder and stiffer than other types. The aim of buccal and lingual preparation should therefore be to reduce the residual undercut to an amount where the metal crown will expand past the position of maximum bulbosity of the tooth and then spring back under its own elasticity to form a tight collar within the gingival pocket. Our clinical experience leads us to suggest that if the supragingival bulbosities are removed (*Fig.* 14.5), sufficient undercut will remain within the gingival pocket for the Ion crown to click firmly into position. It will form a tight collar around the tooth, yet be easy to remove prior to cementation.

Finishing

Any remaining caries should be removed with a slow-running round bur. The preparation is completed by bevelling the external line angles around the occlusal part and where the proximal reduction meets the buccal and lingual surfaces (*Fig.* 14.6). This will ensure proper seating of the stainless-steel crown whose internal contour is free from sharp angles.

Retention of the crown will be obtained by encompassing the normal gingival bulbosity of the primary molars leaving the crown margins in the gingival sulcus. This is why, in our

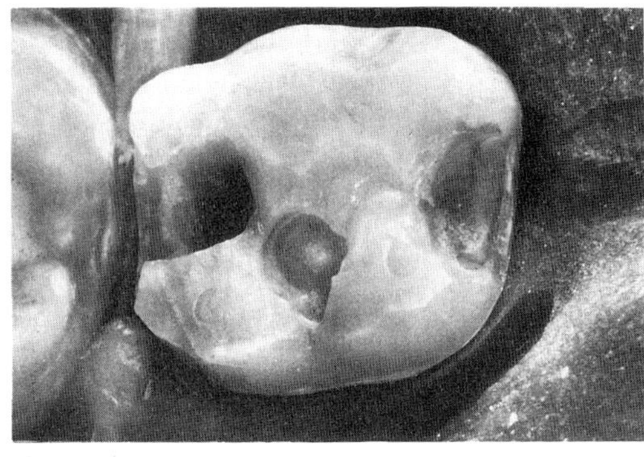

a

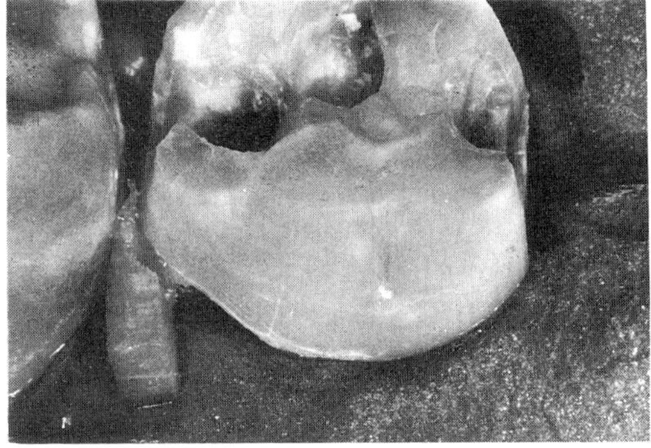

b

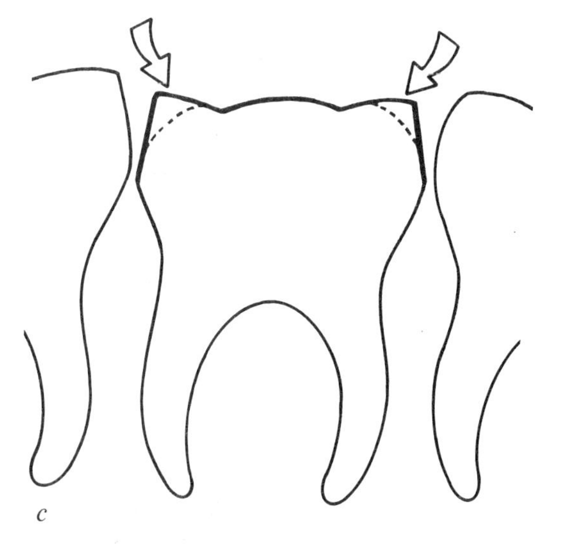

c

Fig. 14.5. Buccal and lingual reduction of bulbosities to the gingival margin. *a*, Occlusal view. *b*, Buccal view. *c*, Rounding of mesial and distal external line angles if necessary. This was not required in the preparation shown in (*a*) because of the removal of caries and old amalgam restoration.

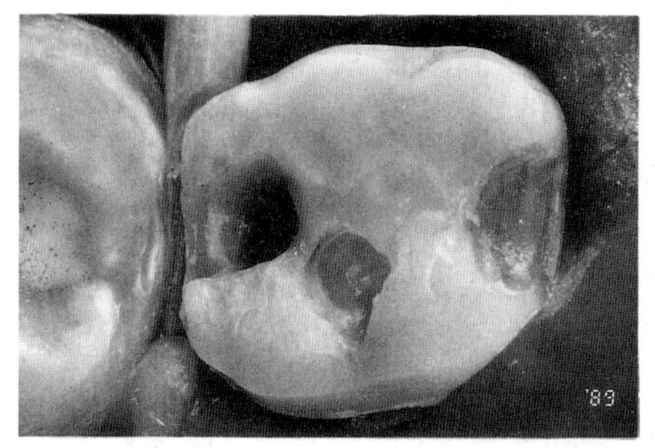

a

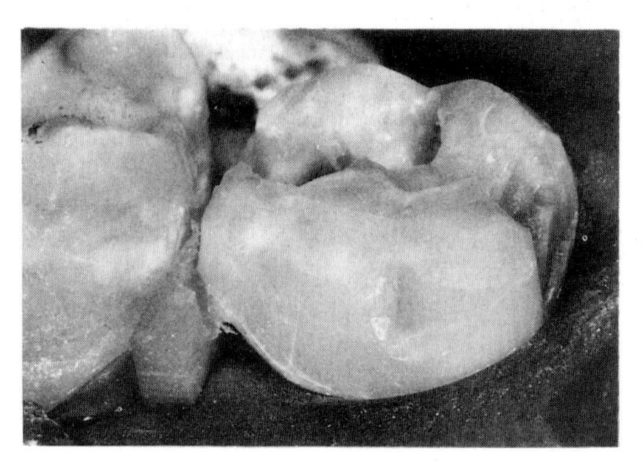

b

Fig. 14.6. Bevelling of external line angles. *a*. Occlusal view. *b*, Buccal view.

opinion, it is undesirable to remove these undercuts (*Figs* 14.5 and 14.6).

Where caries has been removed and a pulpotomy or pulpectomy has *not* been completed, then pulp protection is required. Therefore, after final caries removal, a suitable protective base should be placed (*Fig.* 14.7). The tooth is now ready for trial fitting of the crown.

Crown selection

Several makes of stainless-steel crowns (Unitek Corporation, Monrovia, CA) are available, and practitioners will make their choice on the basis of experience. A correctly selected crown, prior to trimming and contouring, should cover all the tooth preparation and provide resistance to removal. Some crowns can be purchased either festooned (partially trimmed) or non-festooned (untrimmed); the latter require more reduction to prevent the margins from impinging on the gingiva, but are useful when the preparation extends subgingivally. Handling properties of the various crowns differ markedly; some work-harden very quickly while others are almost too readily distorted by contouring pliers. The festooned Unitek or Ion (3M Co., St. Paul, MN) stainless-steel crown is superior to the others mentioned because it most accurately reproduces the tooth morphology and requires the least trimming and contouring, thereby reducing clinical time. This crown will be suitable for the majority of primary and young permanent teeth.

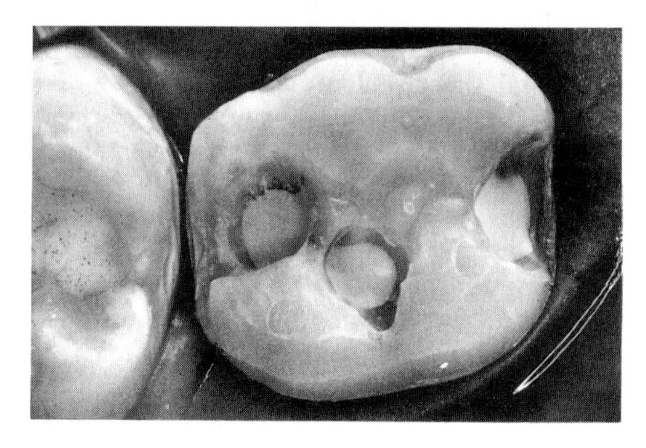

Fig. 14.7. Placement of Dycal to cover all deep, exposed dentine surfaces.

Primary molars with deep interproximal caries extending subgingivally may warrant a non-festooned crown (Rocky Mountain, Metal Products Co., Denver, CO) to encompass the margins of the preparation. However, in an alternative approach, any required pulp treatment can be performed before the tooth is temporarily restored with a glass-ionomer cement or amalgam alloy. The crown margins can be left on this restoration. This latter approach reduces the need to use non-festooned crowns, which usually require more trimming and contouring than their festooned counterpart.

The correct size of preformed crown will seat into the residual undercut with a degree of pressure from a finger or thumb. One that does not form a close collar at the amelocemental junction will lead to plaque retention and poor gingival health. Preoperative assessment should consider the presence or absence of primate

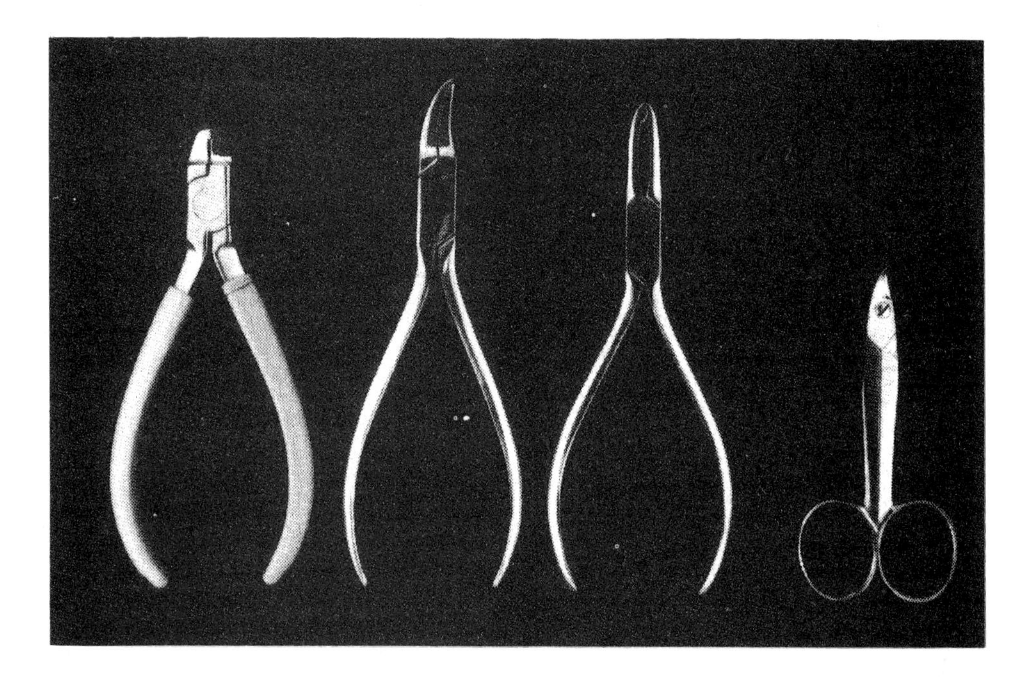

Fig. 14.8. Crown-trimming scissors and contouring pliers. *From right to left:* scissors, 114, 137, 800–412.

spaces when first primary molars are being crowned. Impingement upon the primate space by an oversized crown may prevent early mesial migration of the mandibular first permanent molar from a cusp-to-cusp occlusion into an Angle Class I relationship (Baume, 1950). Similarly, overcontoured and oversized steel crowns on second primary molars can prevent the normal eruption of the first permanent molars.

Crown trimming and contouring

The purposes of crown trimming and contouring are, respectively, to leave the crown margins in the gingival sulcus and to reproduce the tooth's morphology. The festooned, precontoured crowns such as NiChro will seldom require this time-consuming procedure. The amount of gingival reduction can be accurately assessed by scratching on the crown a mark at the level of the free marginal gingiva and reducing the crown with small, curved crown-and-bridge scissors (in the UK, crowns and pliers are available from Procare Ltd., Queens House, Queens Road, Bradford) (*Fig.* 14.8). This should be done away from the child's face to minimize the danger of slivers of metal lodging in the eye. Crown contouring subsequently will reduce the effective occlusogingival crown height, and so the crown should be left slightly long at this stage. Final gingival trimming is done after crown contouring and is most accurately accomplished with a stone wheel. The whole preparation should be covered by the crown, whose margins fit in the free gingival sulcus. There should be no blanching of the gingiva, which indicates overextension. However, when caries requires a subgingival preparation, it is both desirable and necessary to extend the margins apically.

Initial crown contouring is performed with the No. 114 plier in the middle one-third of the crown to produce a belling effect. This will give the crown a more even curvature than one which is contoured only in the gingival one-third (*Fig.* 14.9). During contouring and trimming, the crown is trial-fitted, and the margins and adaptation are checked both visually and

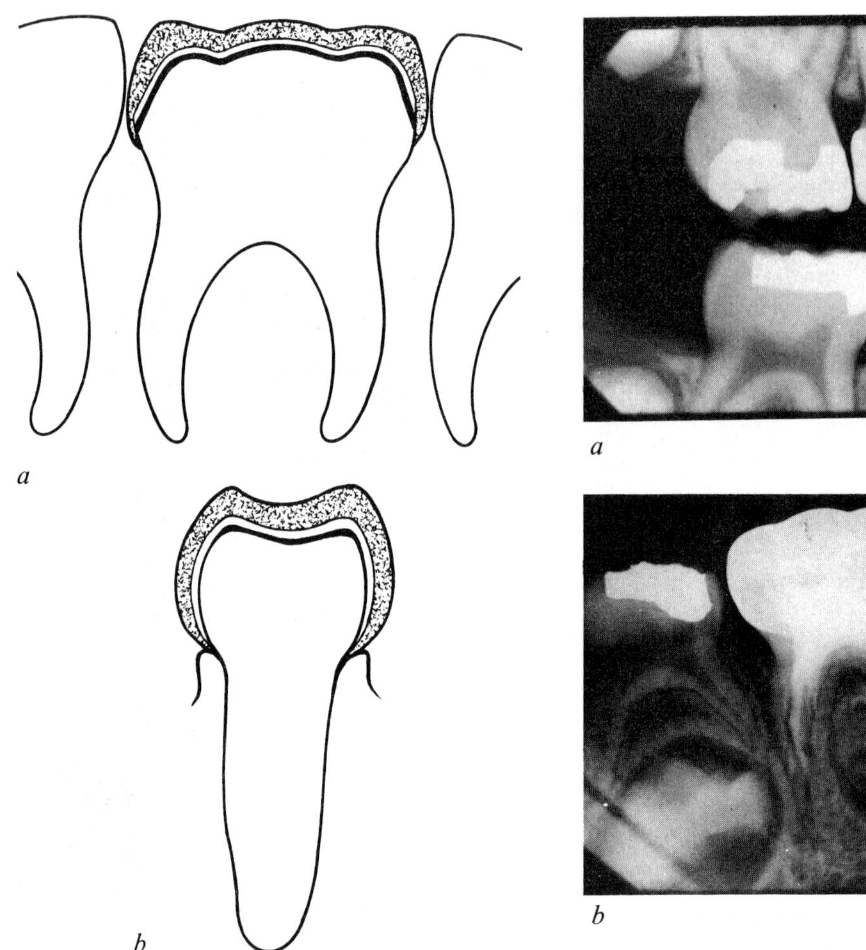

Fig. 14.9. Correct fitting of crown. *a*, Buccal view; note that the gingival margins of the crown have been crimped in to engage the undercuts of the crown bulbosity. *b*, Mesial view.

Fig. 14.10. *a*, Bitewing radiograph demonstrates properly contoured mandibular crown. Note the even curvature, positive contact and absence of overhang. The maxillary crown is undercontoured and exhibits an open contact distally. This crown has only been contoured in the gingival one-third and not in the middle one-third. *b*, Mandibular periapical radiograph of a 3-year-old child demonstrating well-adapted and contoured stainless-steel crown. The tooth has been treated by partial pulpectomy.

with an explorer. Adaptation of the gingival one-third of the crown is done with the No. 137 plier. Any marked gingival crimping of the crown can also be accomplished with a Unitek 800 412 plier (*Fig*. 14.8).

As it is impossible to burnish the margins of the crown in the mouth, all contouring and trimming must be performed out of the mouth. The finally trimmed and contoured crown should be evenly and smoothly shaped with no marked changes in contour. Corectly fitted stainless-steel crowns are shown in the radiographs illustrated in *Fig*. 14.10.

The buccal and lingual margins are more readily evaluated than the interproximal fit. The ability of the crown to fray waxed dental floss indicates an unsatisfactory inaccuracy in interproximal adaptation. The floss also checks the presence or absence of a sound contact (alterations in contact areas will be discussed later).

Trial fitting and also cementation are best accomplished if the crown is placed lingually and then rolled towards the buccal aspect of the tooth. In this way, as the crown is being rolled from lingual to buccal, the interproximal adaptation can be assessed by looking at right angles to the preparation and comparing the depth of the preparation to the depth and contour of the crown. A degree of pressure from a finger or thumb will be necessary to seat the crown. When the crown margins pass over the cervical bulbosity on the buccal surface, a definite snap or click is often heard; this assures the operator of the crown's retention and a good fit. The occlusion should be checked to see that the crown is not interfering. Insufficient occlusal tooth reduction, or sharp external line angles result in inability to seat the crown. The thickness of the metal of the preformed crown does not permit reduction without danger of perforation; therefore occlusal adjustment must involve further tooth preparation, or further crown trimming.

Polishing and cementation

If the stainless-steel crown has been trimmed or contoured, then it should be polished to remove all scratches prior to cementation (Durr et al., 1982). The crown margin should be blunt since a knife-edge finish merely produces sharp slivers of stainless steel, which act as areas for plaque retention. A broad stone wheel should be run slowly across the margins towards the centre of the crown; this improves the adaptation of the crown by drawing the metal closer to the tooth without reducing crown height (Roche, 1970). Final lustre can be achieved with Shofu points or wheels.

Pulp-protecting bases should be placed over the deep areas of the preparation (*Fig.* 14.7). The cementing medium can be zinc phosphate, polycarboxylate cement, zinc oxide cement or glass-ionomer luting cement. Although it has been reported that zinc oxide has reduced retentive powers compared with zinc phosphate or polycarboxylate cements when used for cementing stainless-steel crowns (Myers et al., 1981), Roberts and Sherriff (1992) reported that only 0.3% of the stainless-steel crowns in their study, all cemented with a reinforced zinc oxide cement, were lost. A consistency similar to that used for cementing gold inlays is recommended, although a thicker mix can be used when only one crown is being cemented. When the assistant hands the filled crown to the dentist, its orientation is made easy by the fact that the tooth notation and crown size are stamped on the buccal aspect of the crown. The tooth should be clean and dry before cementation. Knotted floss can be passed interproximally before the cement has set to assist in the later removal of set subgingival cement. Excess cement in the gingival sulcus should be removed thoroughly with an explorer prior to final polishing of the crown with pumice and a rubber cup (*Fig.* 14.11).

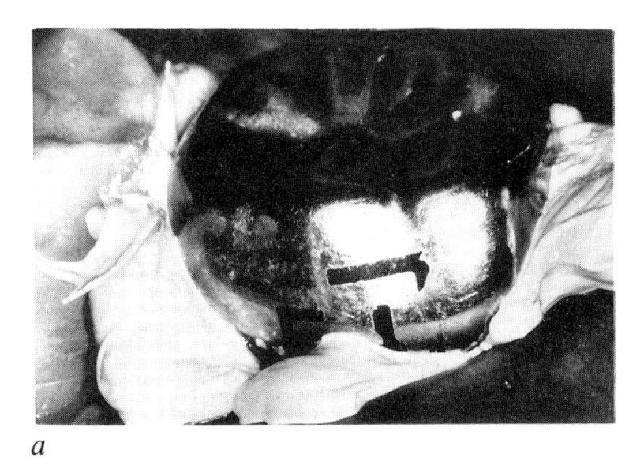

a

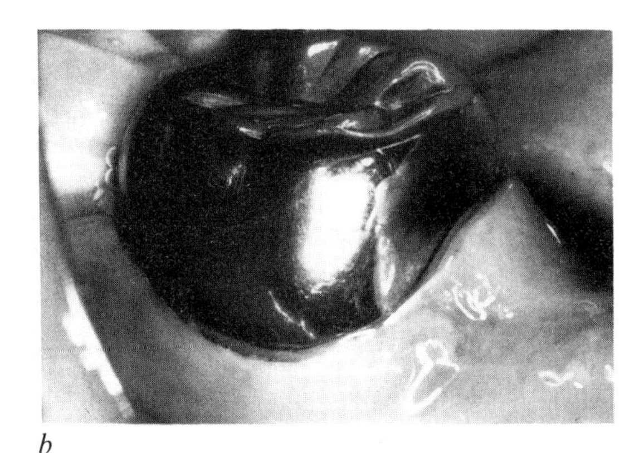

b

Fig. 14.11. *a*, Stainless-steel crown filled with cement and seated on to prepared tooth. Excess cement exudes around the gingival margins and can be removed once set. *b*, The same crown as in (*a*) 1 week later. Note small amount of cement on mesial gingival margin, which will need removal.

The use of crowns in quadrant dentistry

The child who presents with extensive decay may require pulp therapy and stainless-steel crowns in adjacent primary molars. A note of the crown size should be made on the patient's records; since tooth size is fairly constant for each individual, this will be of value when selecting appropriate crowns for teeth in other quadrants. As noted in Chapter 4, treatment planning should minimize the number of appointments and re-administration of local analgesia; therefore it may be desirable to place steel crowns on adjacent primary molars that are also candidates for pulp therapy. This can be performed in one visit, very little additional time being required if the pulps are vital. Confidence in preoperative assessment of pulp status (Chapter 17) may encourage the operator to perform the crown preparation before embarking on pulp therapy. This approach is efficient since the high-speed cutting instruments and water coolant are used only once. However, an error in diagnosing pulp status may necessitate a two-visit pulp procedure, which is unfortunate once the crown preparation has been completed. The alternative operative sequence is to perform the pulp therapy first and then prepare the tooth for crowning. Although this method requires a second use of high-speed cutting instruments for the crown preparation, it does make temporary dressing, if required, much easier, and any possible gingival bleeding from crown preparation does not complicate pulp therapy.

Crown preparation for adjacent primary molars must provide sufficient interproximal clearance to allow for the bulk of two stainless-steel crowns. Completing one restoration before beginning the second usually prevents insufficient interproximal reduction. Although each crown will be trial-fitted individually, both crowns must be tried on together prior to cementation. Occasionally one of the crowns has a path of insertion which is hindered if the other is already seated; in these cases the insertion sequence must be reversed.

Adjacent stainless-steel crowns are considerably more difficult when there has been long-standing interproximal caries that requires subgingival reduction to encompass the depth of the decay. Furthermore, space loss from interproximal caries leaves little interproximal clearance for both crowns. It is impossible to regain lost space from crowning alone; rather, the crowns have to be adapted to the altered space. During selection it may be necessary to reduce the mesiodistal width of the crown by squeezing it with a No. 110 plier, which will flatten the interproximal contour and provide more bulk of metal buccally and lingually (McEvoy, 1977).

The stainless-steel crown is also placed adjacent to Class 2 amalgam restorations; in this type of quadrant dentistry the sequence of operative procedures is most important. A typical example of one-visit quadrant dentistry is the mesio-occlusal alloy on the second primary molar, the stainless-steel crown on the first primary molar, and the distal restoration on the primary canine (*Fig.* 14.12). If the alloys are completed first, there is danger of amalgam fracture and inadequate contact areas when the crown is trial-fitted and cemented. If all cavity and crown preparations are made first and the crown is then cemented, the excess cement from the crown will flow into the cavity

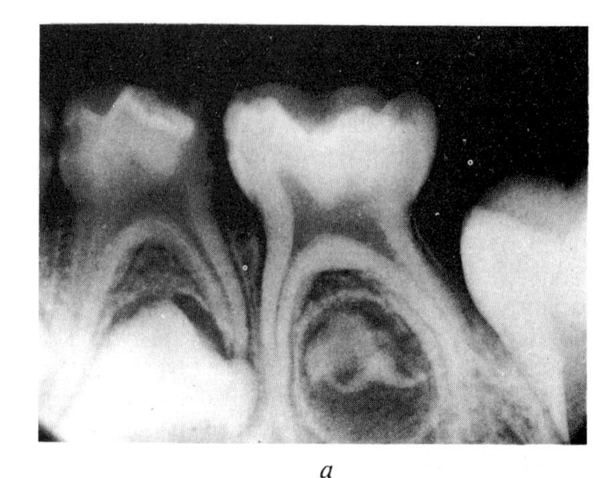

a

b

Fig 14.12. *a*, Preoperative mandibular periapical radiograph of a $4\frac{1}{2}$-year-old. *b*, Postoperative mandibular radiograph shows the treated quadrant. The canine has been restored with a composite, the first molar by pulpotomy and crown and the second molar with amalgam. Note the good reproduction of contour.

preparations and need to be removed. Also, it is easier to overcontour the crown so that its dimensions impinge on the space for the alloy. Furthermore, the Class 2 cavity preparation may require further modification after the adjacent crown has been cemented, in order to make the interproximal margins cleansable. Therefore the crown should be prepared and cemented prior to any adjacent preparations. In this way all the above disadvantages are avoided.

Stainless-steel crown modifications

There are several ways of modifying the stainless-steel crown (Mink and Hill, 1971; McDonald and Avery, 1994). These can be summarized as follows:

- *The undersized tooth or the oversized crown.* This commonly occurs when there has been space loss as a result of long-standing interproximal caries. The crown is cut vertically along the buccal wall. The free crown margins are approximated and spot-welded to reduce the crown's dimensions. After contouring, the cut and relocated area is soldered and polished.
- *The oversized tooth or the undersized crown.* A vertical cut is made on the buccal surface of the crown. The margins are pulled apart and an additional piece of stainless-steel band material is spot-welded to the buccal surface, increasing the dimensions of the crown. After contouring, solder is applied to fill any microscopic deficiency in seal. The crown is polished and cemented.
- *Deep subgingival caries.* If this occurs interproximally, the unfestooned Rocky Mountain crown will normally be deep enough to encompass the preparation. Failing to stock such crowns or making an error in crown trimming can be compensated for by lengthening the crown with a spot-welded and soldered piece of band material, as described in the previous item.
- *The open contact.* Inability to establish a closed contact area (except for the primate space) will result in food packing, increased plaque retention and subsequently gingivitis. Selection of a larger crown may solve this problem. Alternatively, exaggerated interproximal contour can be obtained with a No. 112 (ball-and-socket) plier to establish a closed contact. Localized addition of solder can also build out the interproximal contour.

Complications

The stainless-steel crown is by no means a panacea for the treatment of extensive caries or a means of avoiding amalgam failure. Handled improperly, these crowns can do as much damage as a poorly finished amalgam alloy. Some of the common complications that arise are mentioned next, together with appropriate treatments.

Interproximal ledge

Incorrect angulation of the tapered fissure bur can produce a ledge instead of a shoulder-free interproximal slice. Further tooth reduction to remove this ledge should be attempted cautiously, because of the possibility of an iatrogenic pulpal exposure. Failure to remove the ledge will result in inability to seat the crown, whose margins will bind on the ledge (*Fig.* 14.13).

When the adjacent tooth is partially erupted and the contact area is poorly established, the interproximal slice is difficult to prepare. Extensive subgingival tooth reduction is re-

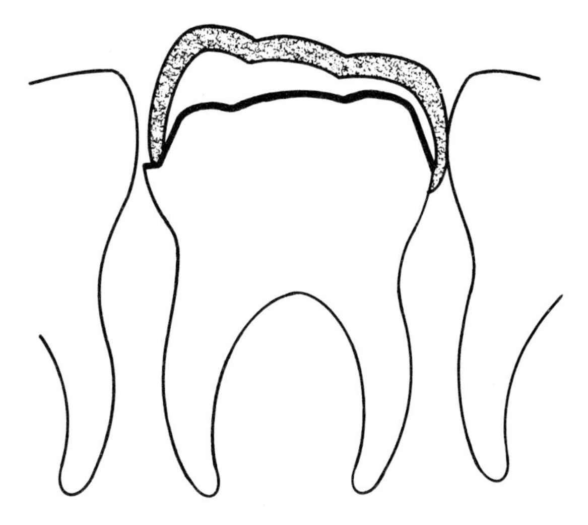

Fig. 14.13. Inability to seat the crown results from a ledge on the preparation. This must be removed, taking care not to expose the pulp.

quired to clear the contact area; difficulty in access increases the likelihood of establishing a ledge or damaging the erupting tooth, which would be unfortunate if it were the first permanent molar. In such instances it may be wise to delay crowning until the contact areas are properly established, which may occur in as little as 3 months.

Crown tilt

Destruction of a complete lingual or buccal wall by caries or overzealous use of cutting instruments may result in the finished crown tilting towards the deficient side. Lack of tooth support encourages this tilting which is commonly seen on the lingual aspect of mandibular primary molars. Placement of an amalgam alloy, or glass-ionomer cement, restoration prior to crowning provides support to prevent crown tilt, the restoration acting as a core. The clinical significance of crown tilting is minimal unless it occurs on young permanent molars where unfavourable supra-eruption of the opponent tooth may occur.

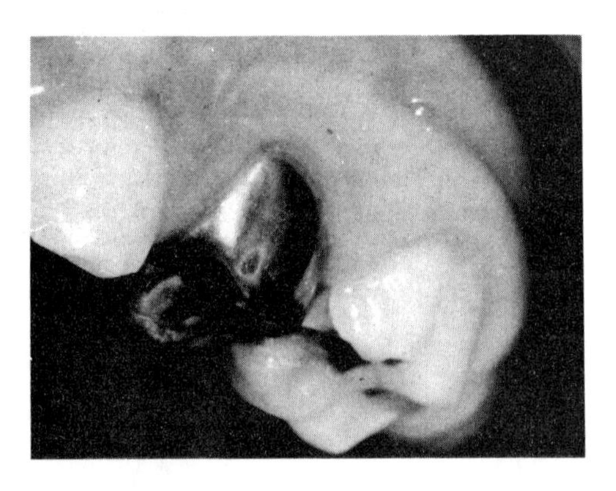

Fig. 14.14. Good gingival response to well-adapted stainless-steel crown.

Poor margins

The marginal integrity of the crown is reduced when it is imperfectly adapted. Recurrent caries seldom appears around open margins. However, as the marginal discrepancy increases, so does the chance of plaque retention and subsequent gingivitis (Henderson, 1973; Myers, 1975) (*Fig.* 14.14). It is speculated that any chronic inflammation of the supporting tissues which is caused by open or overextended margins may result in premature exfoliation of that tooth; however, this speculation awaits clinical verification.

Aesthetics

Sometimes parents complain about the appearance of metal crowns as being ugly. Usually the crowns involved are first primary molars. In these cases a mesiobuccal facing can be placed after the crown has been cemented into place. The technique has been described by Roberts (1983).

Inhalation or ingestion of the crown

Fortunately these accidents are rare, particularly when rubber dam is used as we advocate for all dentistry for children. Sudden, unpredictable movement may result in inhalation or ingestion of the crown if the rubber dam is not in place. Should this occur, an attempt at removal can be made by holding the child upside down as soon as possible; if this is unsuccessful, referral for an immediate chest X-ray is mandatory. If the crown is in the bronchi or lung, medical consultation and referral will probably result in an attempt to remove it by bronchoscopy. The presence of a cough reflex in the conscious child fortunately reduces the chances of inhalation, ingestion of the crown being more likely. Ingestion is of less consequence, but none the less must be diagnosed by the absence of the crown on a chest radiograph. The stainless-steel crown will usually pass uneventfully through the alimentary tract within 5–10 days. The parent should assume the unpleasant task of locating the expelled crown.

Anguish and stress to child, parent and clinician are reduced by taking all possible precautions to prevent crown ingestion or inhalation. Therefore, crown preparation, trimming and trial fitting should be performed with the rubber dam in place (see *Figs* 14.4–14.13). When a crown is being fitted adjacent to the clamped tooth, the interproximal rubber can be cut and the ligature removed so that the gingival margins are visible. Experience with crowns will encourage the operator to cement on the crown with the rubber dam in place; while the cement is setting, the cut rubber dam is removed and the occlusion checked.

Occlusal wear

Children with tooth-grinding habits may exhibit wear through existing stainless-steel crowns. When this wear occurs the crown should be replaced. If the wear is confined to a small area on the tip of a cusp then a small amalgam restoration can be placed in the hole in the wear facet so as to preclude the cement dissolving away and leaving a defect.

References

Baume L. J. (1950) Physiological tooth migration and its significance for the development of occlusion. *J. Dent. Res.* **29**, 123; 331; 440.

Berg J. H. and Donly K. J. (1988) Comparative approach for restoring primary molars after pulpotomy technique. *J. Dent. Child.* **55**, 463.

Braff M. A. (1975) A comparison between stainless steel crowns and multisurface amalgams in primary molars. *J. Dent. Child.* **42**, 474.

Castaldi C. R. (1957) Analysis of some operative procedures currently being used in paedodontics. *J. Can. Dent. Assoc.* **23**, 377.

Duggal M. S. and Curzon M. E. J. (1989) Restoration of the broken down primary molar: 2. stainless-steel crowns. *Dent. Update.* **16**, 71

Duggal M. S. and Curzon M. E. J. (1994) Stainless steel crowns for primary molars. In: *Restorative Techniques in Paediatric Dentistry*. London, Dunitz.

Durr D. P., Ashrafi M. H. and Duncan W. K. (1982) A study of plaque accumulation and gingival health surrounding stainless steel crowns. *J. Dent. Child.* **49**, 343.

Henderson H. Z. (1973) Evaluation of the preformed stainless steel crown. *J. Dent. Child.* **40**, 353.

Hicks P. E. (1973) Treatment planning for the distal shoe space maintainer. *Dent. Clin. North Am.* **17**, 1, 135.

Jaffe E. C., Stimmler L. and Osborne J. A. (1973) Enamel defects associated with neonatal symptomatic hypocalcaemia. *Proc. Br. Paedodont. Soc.* **3**, 25.

McDonald R. E. and Avery D. R. (1994) Restorative dentistry. In: *Dentistry for the Child and Adolescent.* 6th edn. St Louis, Mosby.

McEvoy S. A. (1977) Approximating stainless steel crowns in space-loss quadrants. *J. Dent. Child.* **44**, 105.

MacRae P. D., Zacherl W. and Castaldi C. R. (1962) Study of defects in Class II dental amalgam restorations in deciduous molars. *J. Can. Dent. Assoc.* **28**, 491.

Mathewson R. J., Lu K. H. and Talebi R. (1974) Dental cement retentive force comparison on stainless steel crowns. *J. Calif. Dent. Assoc.* **2**, 42.

Mink J. R. and Bennett J. C. (1968) The stainless steel crown. *J. Dent. Child.* **35**, 186.

Mink J. R. and Hill C. J. (1971) Modification of the stainless steel crown for primary teeth. *J. Dent. Child.* **38**, 61.

Myers D. R. (1975) A clinical study of the response of the gingival tissue surrounding stainless steel crowns. *J. Dent. Child.* **42**, 281.

Myers D. R., Bell R. A. and Barenie J. T. (1981) The effect of cement type and tooth preparation on the retention of stainless steel crowns. *J. Pedodont.* **5**, 275.

Papanathasiou A. G., Curzon M. E. J. and Fairpo C. G. (1994) The influence of restorative material on the survival rate of restorations in primary molars. *Pediatr. Dent.* **16**, 282.

Roberts J. F. (1983) The open faced stainless steel crown for primary molars. *J. Dent. Child.* **15**, 262.

Roberts J. F. and Sherriff M. (1992). The fate and survival of amalgam and preformed crown molar restorations placed in a specialist dental practice. *Br. Dent. J.* **169**, 237.

Roche J. R. (1970) In: *Current Therapy in Dentistry*, Vol.4, p. 540. St Louis, Mosby.

Savides N. L., Caputo A. A. and Luke L. S. (1979) The effect of tooth preparation on the retention of stainless steel crowns. *J. Dent. Child.* **46**, 385

Chapter 15

Dental materials

This chapter supplements previous chapters on cavity preparation and matrices. It is by no means complete in its description of dental materials. No attempt will be made to discuss in detail their physical and chemical properties; rather, their use will be justified and described as they relate to paediatric operative dentistry.

Fluoride

Teeth or quadrants of teeth isolated during operative dentistry should be polished with a fluoride prophylaxis paste and should also receive a topical fluoride application as part of the operative procedures. The fluoride solution is best applied as soon as cavity preparations are complete, so that adjacent interproximal surfaces are protected. The margins of the restoration also require protection, and fluoride, either in solution or in the form of a varnish, should be applied to the completed restorations. This is supplementary to the normal applications every 6 months, when used. Fluoride varnishes are particularly useful in that they act as a slow-release system so that fluoride is available on surfaces adjacent to the restorations for days if not weeks (Hatibovic-Kofman and Koch, 1991).

Another possible means of increasing topical fluoride exposure is to use a fluoride rinse as the mouthwash in place of the usual pink mouthrinse solution, although care must be taken that it is not swallowed. This mouthrinse can be followed up by home use on a daily basis. Because of the dangers of fluoride overdosage, this should be used only in those children who are old enough to spit out the fluid, over 5 years of age. One potential advantage of using the fluoride rinse is based on the fact that those children who require the most visits for operative dentistry are the ones who require the most preventive care; and they will be receiving the additional fluoride exposure.

Pulp-protecting bases

A base is recommended in those cavities where removal of caries leaves the pulpal floor and/or axial wall in close proximity to the pulp. The main purpose of the base is to minimize thermal insult to the pulp through the restorative material. Such a base may help stimulate the formation of secondary dentine as in indirect pulp treatment (Chapter 16). These recommendations on pulp protection apply both to primary and permanent teeth. Contrary to previously accepted teaching, there is evidence to indicate that deep lesions in primary teeth benefit from pulp-protecting bases (Geller et al., 1971).

The small dimensions of cavity preparations in primary molars require that a thin layer of base be used which can not only withstand the condensation pressures of amalgam but also leave sufficient room for the restorative material. A hard-setting calcium hydroxide base (e.g.

Dycal, Procare, Bradford) fulfils these requirements; pure calcium hydroxide powder mixed with water or saline is not recommended as it does not adequately withstand condensation. This also applies to zinc oxide, even though it is effective in stimulating secondary dentine formation (Kerkhove et al., 1967). On the other hand, resin-bonded zinc oxides (e.g. Kalzinol, Procare; Timurex, Interstate Dental Co. Inc., New York) can be recommended, although the handling properties of Dycal are, in our opinion, superior. Zinc phosphate cements are contraindicated because of their acidity, which may adversely affect the pulp.

The decision to place a pulp-protecting base must lie with the individual practitioner. Although the pulp may have already responded to the carious lesion by laying down secondary dentine, this should not discourage the placement of a base, which may stimulate further pulp protection. As a rule, whenever the pink outline of the pulp shows through the cavity walls a base is mandatory; this applies also to dark-stained dentine left in the depths of the cavity. However, it is unnecessary to line out the cavity to ideal dimensions; a minimum of 0.5 mm of Dycal is recommended. Enamel walls must be free from the base. Additional bulk of restorative material is provided by the deeper cavities and this is advantageous in Class 2 cavities.

Varnishes

Varnishes are synthetic or natural resins in a chloroform solvent (e.g. Copalite).

The purposes of the varnish are (in order of importance):

(1) to reduce marginal microleakage;
(2) to minimize ion diffusion;
(3) to protect the pulp by sealing dentinal tubules against acid penetration.

The dye penetration study of Going (1964) demonstrated that Copalite reduces marginal microleakage around amalgam alloy restorations. This is especially important in the immediate postinsertion period, before any amalgam breakdown products fill the marginal discrepancy that always exists between enamel wall and restorative material. The staining within the enamel which occurs close to the margins of amalgam alloy restorations is caused by ion diffusion (particularly of silver and tin) from amalgam to tooth; this is minimized by varnish. The pulp-protecting properties of a varnish are negligible when compared with Dycal; certainly they are no substitute for pulp-protecting bases. Varnishes are applied to the floor and walls of the cavity by a fine cotton pellet or a camel-hair paintbrush. As the chloroform evaporates, the resin contracts and leaves small voids. Re-application after a 20-s period for evaporation is indicated to fill these voids. It is impossible to avoid coating the enamel walls with varnish. However, this is of no clinical significance as the varnish thickness is 4 μm and one purpose is to reduce marginal microleakage around amalgam restorations. Varnishes are recommended prior to amalgam restorations and cementation of crowns on vital teeth. They should not be used prior to any resin restoration (either simple or composite) since polymerization is altered and the resin is softened. Some commercially available products incorporate fluoride within the varnish. In the absence of any clinical studies known to us, the incorporation of fluoride into the varnish must be considered as empirical. Presumably it is hoped that the fluoride will prevent or minimize recurrent decay.

Cements

Cement bases can be used to:

(1) line out large cavities in young permanent teeth;
(2) cover pulp dressings prior to amalgam placement;
(3) cement crowns.

In cavity preparations [indications (1) and (2)] the zinc phosphate cement is used to provide resistance to condensation of amalgam alloy. It can be used to partially fill very large cavities in young permanent teeth where a calcium hydroxide, pulp-protecting base has already been placed. The dimensions of the cavity may require so much amalgam alloy to be placed that it would be impossible to fill it before the alloy had set. A thick mix of zinc phosphate, or polycarboxylate, cement is recommended for such cavity preparations since this reduces the amount of free acid.

Zinc phosphate and polycarboxylate cements, resin-bonded zinc oxides or glass-ionomer cements are recommended for cementing stainless-steel crowns. When the pulp is vital the deep areas of the preparation should be covered with Dycal.

Intermediate restorative materials

These materials are required to hold medications adjacent to the pulp between appointments. They are also needed in the indirect pulp treatment of deep carious lesions in young permanent teeth (Chapter 20). Their capacity to seal the tooth and prevent leakage is most important in avoiding contamination of the pulp; since the material must withstand occlusal forces, and whenever possible restore the tooth to correct contour and function, a matrix band is often essential. If necessary, the material should be supported by an orthodontic band to ensure retention. The notion that a temporary restoration need not be as meticulously placed as a permanent one is dangerous as the ability of the temporary restoration to prevent leakage is most important.

Of these materials, the most commonly used are reinforced cements and zinc oxides (resin-bonded or not). In clinical evaluations of indirect pulp treatment in primary and young permanent teeth (Weaver ct al., 1972), reinforced resin-bonded zinc oxides [(IRM; intermediate restorative material) D. Caulk Co., Milwaukee, available from Procare, Bradford] have produced the best results for periods up to 2 years.

Reinforced cements

In addition to routine use as cement bases, these can be used as satisfactory intermediate materials in teeth receiving indirect pulp treatment (Weaver et al., 1972); of course a calcium hydroxide, protecting base is required initially. The glass-ionomer cements, although not strictly speaking reinforced cements, function very well as intermediate materials and can be used until pulp recovery has occurred, when a final restoration can be placed. These cements are also useful to restore primary teeth which are within 6–12 months of exfoliation. Fluoride-impregnated cements (Hatibovic-Kofman and Koch, 1991) can also be used as a temporary dressing or intermediate restorative material. Fluoride release from these materials may be useful in remineralization of the immediately adjacent enamel. This may be of immense value in patients who have multiple lesions and poor oral hygiene, and who are candidates for indirect pulp treatment. This material is also useful in treating Class 5 lesions (Chapter 12).

Resin-bonded zinc oxides

Of the various commercially available products, IRM has been clinically proven to be superior. Ninety-five per cent of teeth treated by IRM were satisfactory after 18 months (Weaver et al., 1972). One advantage of IRM is its colour (white, blue or pink); the parents can be instructed to check periodically for the material's presence in those teeth where retention is in doubt. Other resin-bonded zinc oxides (e.g. Kalzinol, Timurex) can also be used.

Zinc oxides

These are ideal short-term temporary restorations as they are non-injurious to the vital, unexposed pulp and have good marginal seal initially. However, their crushing strength is low and this, in conjunction with a tendency to dissolve in the mouth, makes them unsuitable for periods exceeding 2 weeks. Furthermore, the smell and taste of the eugenol are distressing to some children. Their routine use cannot be recommended in view of the improved properties of resin-bonded zinc oxides.

Resins

Research over the past 20 years has revolutionized the use of resins in dentistry. Acrylic resins can be termed generation 1 (simple, unfilled resins), generation 2 (filled, composite resins), or generation 3 (microfil, macrofil or hybrid). While simple, unfilled resins and composites are usually self-polymerized, the generation 3 resins can either be self- or light-polymerized. Improved retention and reduced microleakage can be obtained by the routine use of acid-etching. With the superior qualities of the generation-2 and -3 resins, it is inappropriate to discuss the use of simple, unfilled resins. The following is a very simplified review and should be supplemented by reference to comprehensive texts on the subject of dental materials.

Generation-2 resins (filled composites)

The composites are similar in composition to simple resins, but exhibit improved qualities, particularly of increased hardness, reduced coefficient of thermal expansion, and improved abrasion resistance, which are partly attributable to the quartz or glass filler. These tooth-coloured restorative materials are indicated in the anterior region for aesthetic reasons.

The main clinical problems with composite resins are owing to the large filler particles, which result in difficulty in finishing due to differential wear of the filler and resin particles. Furthermore, with increasing abrasion with time, the phenomenon of 'plucking' occurs, resulting in discoloration of the resin restorations. There is progressive and cumulative loss of filler particles, which become plucked out of the restoration surface resulting in stain and uneven colour.

Generation-3 resins

The generation-3 resins are either self- or light-polymerized. They are further subclassified according to their make-up as microfils, macrofils and hybrids (blended macrofil and microfil). In general terms, the *microfils* have a smaller particle size and greater smoothness and polishability. They also have a lower percentage of inorganic filler by weight; this makes them suitable for stress-bearing situations. Therefore the microfils are best suited to non-stress-bearing areas where polishability and aesthetics are of prime importance, such as Class 3 and 5 preparations. By contrast, the *macrofils* have larger particle size and greater percentage of inorganic filler by weight. These are less polishable than the microfils, but better suited for stress-bearing areas such as Class 1 and 2 restorations.

Hybrid resins have two types of filler. They are slightly less polishable than microfils, but definitely more abrasion resistant making them suitable for the strip-crown restoration (Chapter 11).

Light curing

The light-cured, generation-3 resins require a visible light source, which has a longer, more penetrating wavelength than the ultraviolet light previously used with generation-1 materials. The depth of curing is 2.5–3.0 mm per 20 s, which requires curing to be done from both the lingual and labial surfaces in the case of anterior restorations. As the material does not harden until exposed to the light source, the clinician is afforded ample manipulation time; this can significantly reduce the finishing procedures. Light-activated types usually have better colour stability, because of absence of residual chemical activators. By contrast, the chemically polymerized composites suffer the disadvantage of intrinsic discoloration.

Application

There are now too many different types of resins for a detailed description of their individual properties, advantages or methods of application to be included here. The use of calcium hydroxide pulp-protecting bases is recommended in all teeth. Cavity varnishes and zinc oxides are not recommended as they may alter resin polymerization. The materials should be manipulated according to the manufacturer's instructions. Frequently the materials supplied include an etching kit, a bonding agent consisting of an unfilled resin, and the resin material. After etching, the bonding agent is placed with a brush followed by the resin. Elimination of air bubbles from the mix and insertion of the materials before polymerization requires a well-organized approach by the dental team. Generally the resins are bulk-packed. Class 3 restorations require support with a celluloid matrix strip, while the strip crown is self-supported. The use of specially designed, commercially available plastic or Teflon-coated instruments is helpful to condense the material into the depths of the preparation; a pressure syringe can be used to inject the material into the cavity. Metal instruments are not recommended as the resin may be stained by loose metal fragments. The material should be left undisturbed during polymerization and, as with all restorative materials, the best results can be expected when the material is placed free from contamination using the rubber dam. This is particularly true of the resins, as well as the glass-ionomer cements, which are sensitive to moisture and require a completely dry field.

Finishing

Composite resins can usually be finished immediately after polymerization. Because the matrix (polymer) and filler of the composite resin have different hardness and abrasion resistance, any finishing will tend to produce a matt finish because of differential wear. Therefore every effort should be made during placement of the restoration to reproduce tooth contour accurately so that finishing is minimized. Gross excess can be reduced with 12-bladed tungsten-carbide finishing burs run under water coolant at high speed, Soflex discs (3M Company, MN) or Baker–Curson burs. Small, thin flashes of material can be fractured off using sharp, tungsten-carbide-tipped hand instruments (e.g. gold knife, hatchets). The use of petroleum jelly is not advised, as the surface impregnation will prevent addition to defects uncovered during polishing. Polishing with pumice or dark rubber cups is not recommended because of potential staining of the matt surface. Undoubtedly the best surface is produced when finishing is kept to a minimum. Soflex discs and strips are ideal for finishing generation-3 resins. Their size and grade of roughness distribution lend themselves to progressive polishing. A smear layer is formed which results in excellent colour match and stability.

Use in Class 2 restorations

The use of resins in multisurface restorations in primary molars depends very much on the size of the restorations to be used. Recent research comparing various restorative procedures in primary molars has shown that composite resins have a poorer survival rate than amalgam and stainless-steel crowns (Papanathassiou et al., 1994). The main reason for the failures was the use of resins in large cavities, particularly in Class 2 lesions, where the material is insufficiently strong to withstand the stresses applied. The recommendation is that, for primary molars, resins are excellent for small to medium-sized Class 1 restorations and minimal Class 2 restorations. The composite resins can be recommended for restoration of Class 2 primary and permanent tooth preparations in those areas where appearance is a primary consideration and lack of occlusal form is of minimal clinical significance. Others have indicated that the use of resins can be encouraged in paediatric dentistry (Croll et al., 1993) provided that they are placed in low load-bearing areas, where rubber dam has been used and close attention is paid to optimum conditions. These materials are very technique-sensitive and hence require total moisture control.

Compomers

Recently a new group of materials known as 'compomers' has been tested for use in primary teeth. These contain either or both of the essential components of a glass-ionomer cement but at levels insufficient to promote acid–base cure reactions in the dark and are referred to as polyacid-modified composite resins (McLean et al., 1994). It has been claimed that these compomers are ideal for the restoration of primary molars (Croll, 1993). However, there has been little in the way of clinical trials on these materials.

Recently, Frankenmolen et al. (1994) reported in an abstract on a clinical trial of a new compomer restorative material in Class 1 and 2 restorations in primary molars. In 55 children there were placed 92 restorations, mostly Class 2. Results after 1 year showed two cases of failure, but a high rate of wear. The investigators felt that the high rate of wear was less of a problem in primary molars, bearing in mind the limited life required for such restorations. It was suggested that a combination of excellent handling characteristics with the reported high survival rate merited further investigation.

The compomers show potential and would appear to be superior for restoring primary molars than the older glass-ionomer cements. However, until long-term trials have been reported the use of these materials should be viewed with caution.

Use of resins compared with amalgam

A 2-year clinical study (Tonn and Ryge, 1978) of a carvable composite and a fine-cut amalgam alloy in Class 2 cavity preparations in primary molars indicated the superiority of amalgam. As with the permanent teeth, the failures of composite were loss of anatomical form and marginal staining. Similarly, a composite (Profile) was successful only 46% of the time when used in primary and young permanent posterior restorations, compared with 80% success with Dispersalloy over a 3-year study period (Derkson et al., 1984). These poor results with composite may partly be attributed to the dental student operators, but not totally. Only one study has reported favourable results with composite resins in Class 2 preparations in primary molars. Nelson et al. (1980) published the results of a 3-year clinical study of Dispersalloy and Adaptic (either radiopaque or non-radiopaque) in Class 2 preparations in primary teeth. The materials performed comparably and they concluded that an acid-etch-bonded Adaptic restoration is an acceptable restoration in the late mixed dentition where the projected tooth lifespan was 3 years or less.

Success with acid-etching prompted the testing of a modified Class 2 preparation in primary teeth (Paquette et al., 1984). In this technique, only the decay is removed and the area filled with resin after acid-etching. One-year clinical assessment revealed a sufficiently high failure rate to eliminate this technique from the clinician's armamentarium.

Before resins can be recommended for posterior primary tooth restorations, the following areas need to be resolved satisfactorily:

- pulp protection,
- matrix application,
- wedge placement,
- control of insertion,
- finishing.

Amalgam is a very forgiving material in that it is pliable and thus both condensable and carvable. This permits the clinician consistently to produce excellent interproximal adaptation and contour. Its ability to 'self-seal' areas of marginal breakdown, and its inertness to the dental pulp make it an ideal material. By contrast, resin is exceedingly difficult to manipulate, and is less forgiving. It is much harder to produce a tight-fitting, well-adapted and well-contoured interproximal area with resin than with amalgam.

Clinical technique

As in all Class 2 restorations, the resin material must be supported by a wedged matrix (Chapter 13). Ribbons et al. (1971) describe a modification of this which facilitates finishing. A preoperative acrylic splint is made by adapting a thin roll of acrylic dough to the occlusal surfaces of the teeth to be restored and the adjacent teeth. When the lesion is large, contour is established by inlay wax; a lubricant on the occlusal surfaces prevents sticking. This acrylic occlusal splint is used after the composite has been inserted into the wedged, matrixed cavity to reproduce correct contour and hence minimize finishing.

Great care must be taken to ensure correct interproximal contour of the restoration since radiographic evaluation is impossible because of the material's radiolucency. Only minor alterations can be made in the gingival areas of the completed restoration; small flashes can be removed with a gold knife. Furthermore, unlike amalgam, composite cannot be condensed to ensure a tight, positive contact postoperatively. Positive pressure from the wedge is therefore essential to spring the teeth apart and compensate for the thickness of matrix band. During application of the composite it is imperative that no voids be incorporated between cavity and restoration. This is especially important in the interproximal box where access is most difficult. This is difficult to ensure since the sticky texture of the composite tends to let it pull away from the cavity walls. Finishing of the set restoration is the same as that described for anterior teeth. Interproximal adaptation and contour of the set restoration are checked with unwaxed dental floss; any fraying indicates an overhang, which must be removed.

Amalgam

Amalgam alloy is the most commonly used restorative material. Its coefficient of expansion, thermal conductivity, compressive and tensile strengths, biological compatibility, failure to dissolve, ease of manipulation and low cost are some of its advantages. Its significant disadvantages are the metallic appearance when used in the anterior part of the mouth and its seemingly inevitable marginal deterioration. However, the byproducts of the amalgam breakdown are beneficial because they fill the alloy–tooth interface. This may account for the material's longevity in many teeth. Its time-proven qualities make it the material of choice for restoring all posterior cavities (unless a crown is indicated) and for anterior teeth where aesthetic appearance is of secondary importance.

Amalgam has come under close scrutiny of late for two reasons. First, the cost and potentially limited availability of mercury have increased the manufacturer's cost. Second, mercury hazards (real or imagined) have caused investigation and concern. Two hazards exist. The first and more significant is lack of mercury hygiene in the dental office. Failure to use preformed amalgam capsules, lack of adequate air circulation and ventilation, unnecessary handling of the amalgam or mercury, mercury or amalgam spillage, and failure to store waste amalgam under water in a sealed container all contribute to increased mercury levels. The second potential hazard is that of mercury leakage from completed amalgam restorations. Despite emotional oratory to the contrary, this hazard is insignificant. The role of amalgam and its use have been reviewed by Mandel (1991), who has indicated its continued safe use. There continues to be controversy over the use of amalgam, although recent reports have not indicated a health problem (Hansen et al., 1993), and where the use of mercury, in amalgam, has been restricted, as in Sweden, this has been because of environmental problems rather than anything specifically dental. The alternatives to amalgam, reviewed above, are still not sufficiently reliable and long-lasting to be viable (Welbury et al., 1991) for certain restorations. In primary teeth with less than 3 years to go before exfoliation, a case can be made for the use of resin alternatives. In young permanent posterior teeth we would still advocate the use of amalgam.

Selection of alloy

The practitioner is well aware of the variety of commercially available alloys and the claims of improved qualities made by their manufacturers. However, while most of these claims are well documented in laboratory research, few have been subjected to rigorous clinical testing *in vivo*. Although the practitioner will develop a personal preference for a particular material, care should be taken to select one that has been approved by a national testing body, e.g. British Standards Institute or American Dental Association Council on Dental Materials.

Three basic amalgam compositions have been used: fine-cut alloys, spherical alloys, and high copper-content alloys.

Fine-cut alloy

Small, fine-cut alloy particles have the advantage of higher strength, a smoother finished surface and easier manipulation than those prepared from large-grained alloy filings. Because of the smaller surface area it is easier to obtain a homogeneous mix. Zinc-free alloys are preferred since moisture contamination with zinc results in excessive expansion; this in turn leads to marginal deterioration, corrosion and secondary caries. Irrespective of the zinc content, the best properties of the material are obtained when it is condensed in a moisture-free environment.

Spherical alloys

These alloys are prepared from spherical particles; logically there is more complete amalgamation around all of the particles. The initial strength after 1 h is 25% higher than with conventional alloys (Basker and Wilson, 1971); this is important because in the immediate postoperative period the child patient is less likely to be able to follow the recommendation to avoid biting on the new filling. Also, spherical alloys are superior to lathe-cut alloys in marginal strength (Koran and Asgar, 1967). Further advantages of spherical alloy are the improved adaptation into line angles and the reduced expansion on setting.

Undoubtedly the major advantage of spherical alloy is its insensitivity to alterations in manipulation. While this property, which is attributed to the microstructure of the material, can hide inconsistencies and imperfections in clinical technique, it is dangerous because it discourages the clinician from paying sufficient attention to detail in material handling. Compared with lathe-cut alloys, it feels wet and offers little resistance to condensation pressure. This is significant in Class 2 preparations where the establishment of a positive contact point postoperatively is partially dependent upon condensation pressure. Therefore, greater care must be used when preparing the matrix band in teeth restored with spherical alloy (Phillips, 1994).

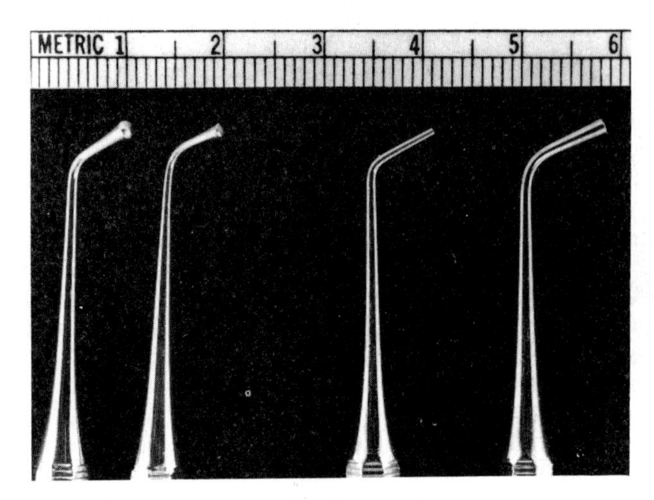

Fig. 15.1 Appropriately sized and shaped condensers for conservative preparations in primary and young permanent teeth.

Despite these properties, the final test is in the mouth over an extended time period. Since a minimum of 2 years is required to demonstrate clinical variations in alloy performance (Mahler et al., 1973), studies covering shorter periods are less meaningful. Weaver et al. (1970) reported that after 3 years, restorations of spherical and conventional filling alloy were identical in clinical performance.

High copper-content alloys

These are characterized by a low creep value (laboratory test) and improved clinical performance as shown by reduced marginal breakdown and gross fracture. Clinical studies correlate with laboratory data in that those amalgam alloys which show improved marginal integrity also exhibit low creep values. These alloys are designed to reduce or eliminate the gamma-2 phase of the amalgam alloy setting reaction, which is shown here as:

$$\underset{\text{(gamma)}}{Ag_3Sn} + Hg \rightarrow \underset{\text{(gamma)}}{Ag_3Sn} + \underset{\text{(gamma-1)}}{Ag_2Hg_3} + \underset{\text{(gamma-2)}}{Sn_8Hg}$$

from Phillips (1973).

The gamma-2 phase is the weakest portion of the hardened amalgam. The oxidation occurs mainly at the gamma-2 phase, which in turn leads to corrosion and subsequent marginal failure. Therefore, reducing or eliminating this phase may minimize marginal deterioration. The gamma-2 phase can be reduced by the addition of copper to the alloy. Dispersalloy, a high copper-content alloy, has been shown clinically to have less marginal failure in both primary (Mathewson et al., 1974) and permanent teeth (Mahler et al., 1973) than the fine-cut alloys. Nelson et al. (1980) found that two different high copper-content alloys (Dispersalloy and Tytin) performed similarly to one another after 3 years of clinical service. They were superior to two other high copper-content alloys (Aristalloy CR and Optaloy II). This study involved over 300 restorations performed in private practice on primary-molar Class 2 preparations. These studies spanned 2 years and therefore are clinically very significant.

For maximum strength, the completed restoration should contain as little mercury as possible. There is a serious loss of strength when the mercury content exceeds 56%; ideally it should be 50% or less (Eames, 1959).

Trituration

This is the mixing of mercury and alloy. The significant variation is the trituration time, which determines:

- the thoroughness of the mix,
- the strength,
- the expansion.

Undertrituration decreases the thoroughness of the mix and its strength, and increases expansion on setting. Overtrituration increases amalgam contraction. It should be remembered that

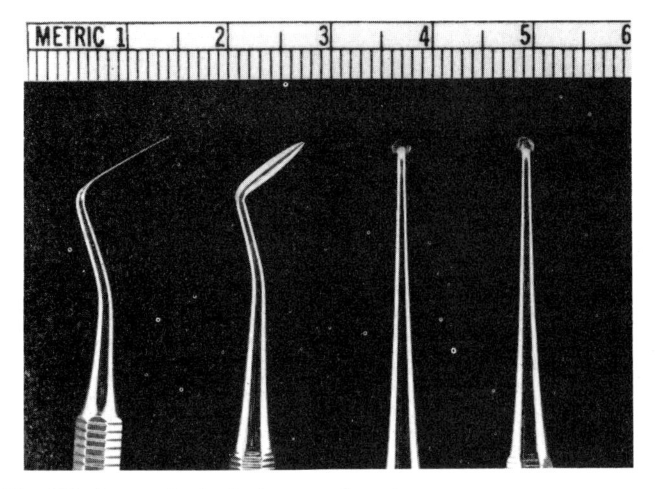

Fig. 15.2. Appropriately sized carvers for primary and young permanent teeth. *From left to right:* Hollenbach 3 half-size (two views), discoid, cleoid. (Available from Procare, Bradford.)

the use of mechanical condensers run at high speed will effectively lengthen the trituration time and therefore adjustments to the manufacturers' recommendations to the times will be necessary.

Condensation

The aims of condensation are to adapt the amalgam as closely as possible to the walls of the cavity, at the same time bringing any excess mercury to the surface. The cavity is deliberately overfilled so that the mercury-rich superficial layer can be removed by carving. The least accessible parts of the preparation should be filled first so that condensation in these areas can be carried out thoroughly. As each increment of material is added, it should be thoroughly condensed before adding further increments.

With small restorations there is little need for mechanical condensers and simple hand condensation of amalgam is sufficient. Small-diameter condensers suitable for very small Class 1 restorations in primary teeth are now available and should be used (*Fig.* 15.1).

The condensation should be completed as quickly as possible. Once amalgam has started to set for 3 min, it should be discarded. If partially set alloy is used, excess mercury cannot be expressed from it. This means that the residual mercury content is too high, resulting in reduced strength and a greater tendency to corrosion, breakdown and secondary caries (Philips, 1994).

Carving

The purpose of carving is to reproduce anatomical features and eliminate flashes or overhanging margins of amalgam. Reproduction of anatomy restores the tooth to correct contour and function. Flashes of amalgam are liable to

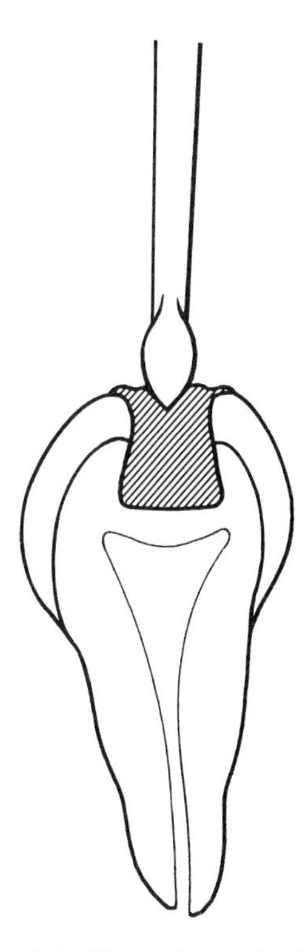

Fig. 15.3. Use of cleoid to define occlusal grooves. This is the first step in the carving sequence.

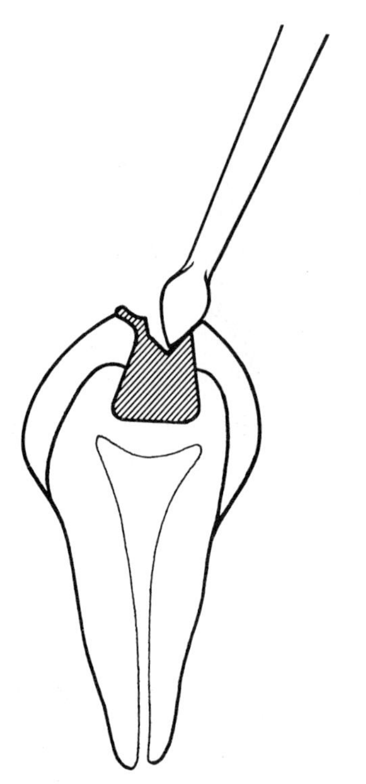

Fig. 15.4. The margin is carved with a more horizontal inclination of the cleoid: the second step.

fracture leading subsequently to marginal deterioration and secondary caries. Although it is often said that the carving of restorations in primary teeth should not be too elaborate, this attitude is dangerous as failure accurately to carve all accessory grooves in the occlusal surface will result in overhanging flashes of amalgam in these grooves.

Knowledge of tooth morphology and selection of appropriately sized instruments (*Fig.* 15.2) greatly facilitate carving. Because of the shallowness of preparations in primary molars, carving should not be too deep since this would impinge on bulk of alloy. Initially the Hollenbach size 3, half-size, which has very small blades, is used for carving anatomy into restorations in primary molars.

A cleoid–discoid instrument is recommended for carving the details into the occlusal surface (Kennedy, 1986). The carving sequence is shown diagrammatically in *Figs* 15.3–15.4. The depth of the fissure is emphasized initially using a vertical inclination and because the instrument is small, there is no danger of exposing the margins. The same instrument is used with a more horizontal inclination to refine the margins of the restoration. The instrument should always be drawn from enamel to alloy in this procedure. Finally, any accessory grooves are refined to eliminate flashes.

The Hollenbach (half-size) is recommended for carving Class 3 and 5 restorations and the interproximal part of Class 2 restorations. The instrument is laid flush with the appropriate enamel surface to smooth Class 3 and 5 restorations. These restorations are easily overcarved, leaving a depression. This should be avoided; rather, the carved restoration should be left slightly proud to allow for further removal during the polishing procedure.

Class 2 restorations should be carved as thoroughly as possible before the matrix is removed. A common error is failure to carve the marginal ridge area, which is essential so that a smooth interproximal contour is maintained. Failure to carve this area will also result in fracture of the ridge when the matrix is removed. The rounded discoid end of the cleoid–discoid carver can be used to obtain a smooth, rounded marginal ridge area after the matrix is removed.

The carvability of amalgam alloy is partially dependent on its stage of setting. For convenience, the busy practitioner may start to carve as soon as condensation is complete. At this time the alloy is often too 'wet' to carve, resulting in the smearing of the alloy into accessory grooves and the production of flashes. Waiting for a couple of minutes allows the material to set a little more so that its carvability improves.

Burnishing and polishing

Burnishing the margins of partially set amalgam has been a controversial topic. It can be done by running hand instruments over the interface or by lightly polishing the carved, partially set material to produce a smooth, scratch-free surface. Clinical evaluation, supported by laboratory data, indicates that this does not predispose the restoration to breakdown. Rather, it reveals discrepancies in carving technique and flashes of amalgam that require removal. Provided excess heat is avoided, which would result in bringing mercury to the surface, burnishing can be recommended.

It was suggested (Phillips, 1994) that polishing be postponed until at least 24 h or longer after initial amalgam placement. This supposedly avoided a mercury-rich outer layer. When

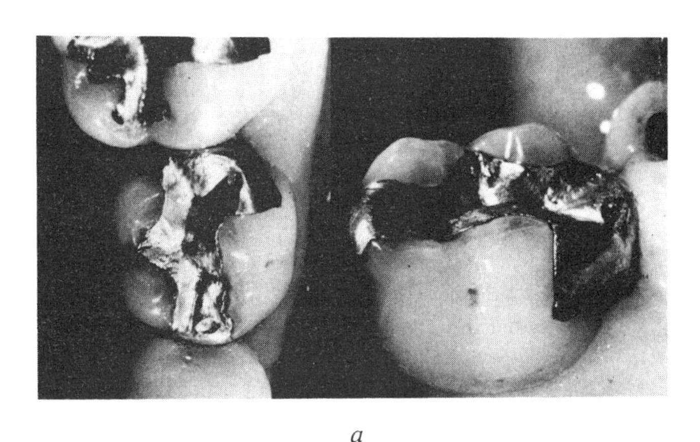

a

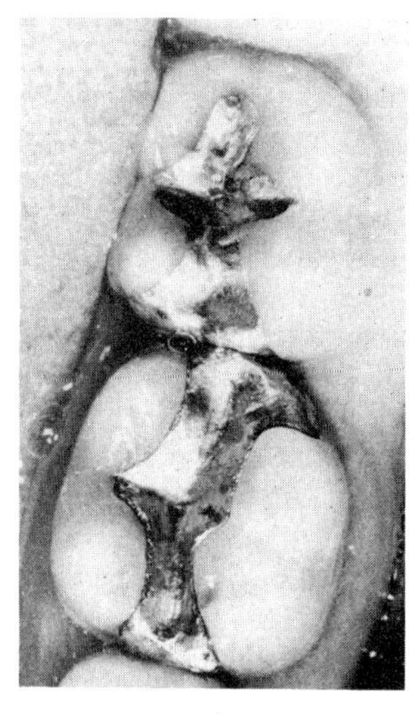

b

Fig. 15.5. *a*, 3-year cut with overlay of distobuccal cusp 75. Note wear facets. *b*, 4-year fine cut on 36, 4-year Dispersalloy on 37 placed same day. Note improved margins with Dispersalloy.

this approach is used, the following technique is appropriate. Finishing burs, which are used to smooth over the surface, should be run at slow speed and always from enamel to amalgam. What is required is a bur that will simultaneously apply equal pressure to both enamel and alloy. Barrel- or pear-shaped finishing burs fulfil this requirement. Flame-shaped burs are not recommended since they produce deep grooves in the restoration. Round burs are contraindicated since their shape tends to cause a depression at the margin. Overzealous use of finishing burs can undo meticulous carving and ruin accurately finished margins.

The depths of the grooves are polished by burnishing with a cleoid, or small-ended burnisher, into them. The accessible interproximal surfaces are refined by plane burs. Scratches are removed from the surface with green or brown Sofu points. Commercially available rubber cups of varying abrasiveness can also be used. Heat should be avoided since this brings mercury to the surface. A smooth, scratch-free, polished restoration is less likely to retain food debris and resists tarnishing and corrosion better.

The necessity to polish restorations has been challenged by the outcome of a 3-year study of Class 1 restorations in permanent molars using a high copper-content, spherical alloy (Tytin) (Straffron et al., 1984). There was no difference in marginal integrity between the carved only and the carved and polished groups, indicating that polishing did not improve the margins. Some of the non-polished (carved only) restorations appeared to undergo a self-polishing process as their surface texture improved with time.

This same group of researchers (Corpron et al., 1983) also compared conventional polishing to polishing with rubber cup and Silex slurry immediately after carving. After 3 years of study, no differences were noted in marginal integrity. The 8-min polished group (polished after carving) demonstrated a more granular surface initially. However, at 3 years, the surface texture was equal for both groups. This supports the use of an unwebbed rubber cup with a slurry of XXX Silex to polish Class 1 restorations in permanent molars immediately after carving, as the only polishing necessary.

Marginal deterioration

Several causes of marginal deterioration in amalgam have been described in Chapter 9. Other causes have been described in this chapter. The causes can be summarized as poor cavity design, faulty manipulation of the alloy and improper selection of the restorative material (*Fig.* 15.5). Although it takes at least 2 years to reveal amalgam failures (Mahler et al., 1973), marginal deterioration may occur well before this time, if only at a microscopic level. A defect of 50 μm will encourage the development of secondary caries (Jorgensen and Wakumoto, 1968). Horwitz et al. (1967) evaluated minimal-extension Class 2 amalgam restorations in primary molars which were prepared and restored under the rubber dam. Refined telemicroscopic apparatus evaluated the margins. In the first 12 weeks the gingival margins exhibited rapid breakdown, which was then superseded by a more rapid occlusal breakdown, presumably due to occlusal forces. This study brought into sharp focus the need to finish accurately the restoration to prevent flashes of amalgam which subsequently break down.

The primary dentition is subject to extensive wear (Nelson et al., 1980). Once abrasion destroys the enamel adjacent to a restoration, there is inadequate support for that restoration unless the restorative material abrades at the same rate. Since amalgam does not abrade well, this may be one reason why primary molar amalgam restorations are subject to marginal fracture. Nelson et al. (1980) feel that the ability of resin to wear at the same rate as the tooth may be a positive sign, as it leaves both restoration and enamel supported.

References

Basker R. M. and Wilson H. J. (1971) Spherical particle amalgam. *Br. Dent. J.* **130**, 338.

Corpron R. E. et al. (1983) A clinical evaluation of polishing amalgams immediately after insertion: 36-month results. *Pediatr. Dent.* **5**, 126.

Croll T. P. (1993) Glass ionomer resin restoration of primary molars with adjacent Class II carious lesions. *Quintessence Int.* **24**, 723.

Croll T. P., Killian C. M. and Helpin M. L. (1993) Restorative dentistry renaissance for children: light hardened glass ionomer/resin cement. *J. Dent. Child.* **60**, 89

Derkson G. D., Richardson A. S. and Waldman R. (1984) Clinical evaluation of composite resin and amalgam posterior restorations: three year results. *J. Can. Dent. Assoc.* **50**, 478.

Eames W. B. (1959) Preparation and condensation of amalgam with a low-mercury alloy. *J. Am. Dent. Assoc.* **58**, 78.

Frankenmolen F. W. A., Peters M. C. R. B. and Roeters F. J. M. (1994) Clinical performance of a new compomer restorative pediatric dentistry. Abstract 90, 2nd European Congress of Paediatric Dentistry, Athens.

Geller J. S., Klein A. J. and McDonald R. E. (1971) Association between dentinal sclerosis and pulpal floor thickness: television radiographic evaluation. *J. Am. Dent. Assoc.* **83**, 118.

Going R. E. (1964) Cavity linings and dentin treatment. *J. Am. Dent. Assoc.* **69**, 415.

Hatibovic-Kofman D. and Koch G. (1991) Fluoride release from glass ionomer cements *in vivo* and *in vitro*. *Swed. Dent. J.* **15**, 253.

Hansen D. J., Horsted-Bidslev P. and Tarp P. (1993) Dental amalgam: a toxicological evaluation. *Ugeskr. for Laeger* **155**, 2990.

Horwitz B. A., Wein A. I. and McDonald R. E. (1967) Intra-oral television micromeasurement of cavity margin deterioration. *J. Dent. Res.* **46**, 700.

Jorgensen K. D. and Wakumoto S. (1968) Occlusal amalgam fillings: marginal defects and secondary caries. *Odont. Tidsskr.* **76**, 43.

Kennedy D. A. (1986) *Paediatric operative dentistry*, 3rd edn, Ch. 12. Bristol, Wright.

Kerkhove B. C. et al. (1967) A clinical and television densitometric evaluation of the indirect pulp capping technique. *J. Dent. Child.* **34**, 19.

Koran A. and Asgar K. (1967) A comparison of dental amalgams made from a spherical alloy and from a comminuted alloy. *J. Am. Dent. Assoc.* **75**, 912.

McDonald R. E. (1974) *Dentistry for the Child and Adolescent*. 2nd edn. St Louis, Mosby.

McLean J. W., Nicholson J. W. and Wilson A. D. (1994) Proposed nomenclature for glass-ionomer dental cements and related materials. *Quintessence Int.* **25**, 58.

Mahler D. B., Terkla L. G. and van Eysden J. (1973) Marginal fracture of amalgam restorations. *J. Dent. Res.* **52**, 823.

Mandel I. D. (1991) Amalgam hazard. *J. Am. Dent. Assoc.* **122**, 62.

Mathewson R. J., Retzlaff A. E. and Porter D. R. (1974) Marginal failure of amalgam in deciduous teeth: a two-year report. *J. Am. Dent. Assoc.* **88**, 134.

Nelson G. V. et al. (1980) A three-year clinical evaluation of composite resin and a high copper amalgam in posterior primary teeth. *J. Dent. Child.* **47**, 414.

Papanathasiou A. G., Curzon, M. E. J. and Fairpo C. G. (1994) The influence of restorative material on the survival rate of restorations in primary molars. *Pediatr. Dent.* **16**, 282.

Paquette D. E. et al. (1984) Modified cavity preparations for composites in primary molars. *Pediatr. Dent.* **5**, 246.

Phillips R. W. (1973) Selection of amalgam alloys: particle form, new formulas. *J. Dent. Child.* **40**, 106.

Phillips R. W. (1994) Restorative materials. In: *Dentistry for the Child and Adolescent*. 6th edn, ed. McDonald R. E. and Avery D. R. St Louis, Mosby.

Ribbons J. W. and Pearson G. J. (1971) A composite filling material. *Br. Dent. J.* **134**, 389.

Straffron L. H. et al. (1984) A clinical evaluation of polished and unpolished amalgams: 36-month results. *Pediatr. Dent.* **6**, 220.

Tonn E. and Ryge G. (1978) Comparison of composite and amalgam in primary molar Class 2 preparations. American Academy of Pedodontics meeting, San Diego, June 1978.

Weaver R. G., Johnson B. E., Cvar J. F. and McCune R. J. (1970) IADR Programme and Abstracts, Abst. 267.

Weaver R. G., Johnson B. E., Cvar J. F. and McCune R. J. (1972) Clinical evaluation of intermediate restorative materials. *J. Dent. Child.* **39**, 189.

Welbury R. R., Walls A. W. G., Murray J. J. and McCabe J. F. (1991) The 5-year results of a clinical trial comparing glass polyalkenoate (ionomer) cement restoration with amalgam restoration. *Br. Dent. J.* **170**, 177.

PART IV

Pulp therapy

Chapter 16

Principles of pulp therapy

This and Chapters 17–20 will deal with pulp treatment of primary and young permanent teeth. Principles of pulp therapy will be discussed in the present chapter; Chapter 17 will deal with diagnosis of pulp pathology; treatment techniques will be described in Chapters 18–20.

Outline of procedures

Indirect pulp treatment

The technique is to remove all decay, except that which, in the clinician's experience, would expose the pulp if it were removed. A pulp-protecting base, such as zinc oxide or calcium hydroxide, is placed over the deep aspects of the cavity, whose margins are well supported and finished. An intermediate or permanent restoration is placed depending on whether a two- or one-visit procedure is being used. Elimination of the majority of the bacteria from the lesion and the substrate by an efficient seal of the restoration will hopefully diminish the rate of progression of the lesion. Since the pulp is no longer insulted by the carious lesion, it is also hoped that it will respond physiologically to this protective layer by depositing secondary dentine, rather than pathologically, were the lesion left untreated. For this treatment to be successful, the pulp must be vital and free of inflammation; at least, if any inflammation is present, it must be reversible so that the secondary dentine can act as a barrier to further insult.

Direct pulp capping

Pulp capping is the placement of material over an exposed, vital pulp. It is hoped that the pulp will respond by remaining free from pathosis and preferably will lay down secondary dentine. For this to be successful the pulp adjacent to the exposure site must be vital and capable of repair. If the inflammation extends throughout the pulp chamber, the chances of success obviously diminish. Therefore the technique is most applicable to small carious or traumatic, vital exposures.

Pulpotomy

Pulpotomy is the partial removal of vital pulp. This is followed by placing some medicament over the radicular pulp stumps that stimulates repair in, fixes, or mummifies the remaining vital radicular pulp. When the pulp is vital and local analgesia is used, the treatment can be performed in one visit; this pulpotomy technique is referred to as vital amputation.

Pulpectomy

In pulpectomy, vital tissue is removed from the coronal pulp chamber and root canals. Following mechanical and chemical preparation of the root canals, they are filled. As with pulpotomy, through common usage, pulpectomy refers to debridement and subsequent filling of the root canals, irrespective of preoperative vitality. Pulpectomy can either be partial or complete depending on the extent of instrumentation of the root canals. The thin, tortuous and branching path of the pulp filaments in the primary molar (Hibbard and Ireland, 1957) precludes the possibility of complete removal of all radicular pulp. Therefore, theoretically any pulpectomy in a primary molar is partial. Through common usage, complete pulpectomy refers to those instances when successful biomechanical preparation and obliteration result in an effective apical seal. Partial pulpectomy is removal of pulp and debris and subsequent filling of the canals short of the apex. The pulpectomy for primary and permanent teeth can be performed in one or many visits. Pulpectomy techniques are applicable to those teeth with inflamed vital radicular pulps or to non-vital teeth.

Comment

Successful pulp therapy for primary teeth is one of the most valuable services a child patient can receive, since there is no better space maintainer than the retained primary tooth. The practitioner must be aware of the dangers of retaining untreated, carious primary molars. A carious primary molar that is left untreated merely invites chronic infection, which may at any time become an acute alveolar abscess. The underlying permanent tooth is put at unnecessary risk during its development by the surrounding inflammation; the possibilities of hypoplasia and hypocalcification are increased, as is that of deflection of the eruption pathway. In addition, the tooth and surrounding periodontium are a focus of chronic inflammation, which is of serious consequence in children with congenital and acquired heart conditions because of the risk of developing subacute bacterial endocarditis. Space loss can also occur as a result of untreated interproximal caries.

The orthodontic implications of premature loss of primary teeth have been outlined in Chapter 1.

Assessment

Thorough preoperative assessment is essential to determine whether pulp therapy or extraction is indicated. If conservation is indicated, the assessment will indicate which type of pulp therapy (e.g. pulpotomy) is applicable. The following should be considered:

(1) medical conditions,
(2) space management decisions and parental attitudes toward dental health,
(3) assessment of the individual tooth.

1. Medical conditions

A full medical history may reveal a systemic problem or disease that will influence treatment. For example, every effort should be made to conserve teeth in haemophiliacs to prevent the hospitalization that may be required if extractions were to become necessary. Another systemic abnormality that influences pulp treatment and operative dentistry is congenital and acquired heart disease. Failure to eliminate any infected pulp or periapical tissue poses a serious health hazard in these children by increasing their chances of developing subacute bacterial endocarditis. Also, the trauma of operative dentistry results in a transient bacteraemia from the gingiva, which places the cardiac patient at further risk. From 75% to 90% of bacterial endocarditis cases are caused by the α-haemolytic streptococcus of the viridans group, an organism commonly found in the gingival sulcus (Sorensen, 1973). For the same reasons a pulpotomy is also contraindicated in immunocompromised children, such as those with acute leukaemia.

There will never be unanimity on the advisability of endodontic therapy in patients with congenital or acquired heart conditions. Each child, each mouth, and each individual tooth must be evaluated. For example, a child may present with three out of four carious primary molars in one arch already committed to removal. Attempts to save the fourth tooth may be unwarranted if its loss can be incorporated into any early orthodontic or space management plan involving the loss of the other three teeth.

The ideal pulp treatment for cardiac patients is indirect since this avoids pulp exposure. Direct pulp therapy should be avoided whenever possible in such patients. The treatment of non-vital primary teeth does not carry a high enough success rate to justify its use in cardiac patients; these teeth should be extracted. Whenever pulp treatment is performed, the clinician must be convinced that the chances of success are high and postoperative results must be carefully monitored. If there is any suspicion that the pulp treatment might fail, the tooth should be extracted.

Although it is generally accepted that patients with cardiac anomalies must receive a course of antibiotics prior to dental treatment, opinions differ on the exact dosage, its timing, and the route and duration of administration. The objective of an antibiotic regimen is to obtain a high blood level at the time of any dental procedure that will result in a transient bacteraemia above the physiological limit. The most effective and certain means of ensuring a high blood level is by an oral dose of amoxycillin 1 h before the dental procedure (BNF, 1994). Where penicillin has been given within the previous month, or the child is penicillin-allergic, oral clindamycin should be given 1 h before the dental treatment. However, the regimen for antibiotic cover is constantly under review and any dentist should always consult the latest guidelines in this regard. Tetracycline should not be used since it is only bacteriostatic and not bactericidal; also there is the unnecessary danger of intrinsic staining in developing permanent teeth.

The latest American Heart Association guidelines for the prevention of bacterial endocarditis have been accepted by the American Academy of Pediatric Dentistry (1993). These are as follows:

- *Children under 60 lb/28 kg:* 50 mg/kg amoxycillin orally 1 h before the procedure, and 25 mg/kg 6 h after the initial dose

  OR

  1 g orally penicillin V 1 h before the procedure and 500 mg 6 h after the initial dose.
- *Children allergic to amoxycillin/penicillin:* Erythromycin 20 mg/kg orally 1 h before the procedure and 10 mg/kg 6 h after the initial dose

  OR

  Clindamycin 10 mg/kg orally 1 h before the procedure and 500 mg 6 h after the initial dose.

Research in the United Kingdom supports the use of amoxycillin rather than penicillin for prophylactic coverage. Oakley and Somerville (1981) report that amoxycillin is better absorbed than penicillin from the stomach and stays in the bloodstream longer after a single dose. The Working Party of the British Society for Antimicrobial Therapy (BNF, 1994) recommended the following doses for prophylactic antibiotic coverage for dental procedures:

- *Adult:* 3 g amoxycillin orally 1 h before the procedure.
- *Children under 10 years:* 1.5 g amoxycillin orally 1 h before the procedure.
- *Children under 5 years:* 0.75 g amoxycillin orally 1 h before the procedure.

Recent animal research supports the use of a second dose of amoxycillin, one-half of the initial dose given orally 6 h later (McGowan et al., 1983). For those patients allergic to penicillin the Working Party of the British Society for Antimicrobial Therapy (BNF, 1994) recommend the following regimen:

- *Adult:* Clindamycin 600 mg orally 1 h before the procedure.
- *Children under 10 years:* one-half of the adult dose (6 mg/kg body wt).
- *Children under 5 years:* one-quarter of the adult dose.

It is both courteous and wise to consult with the child's physician, paediatrician and cardiologist when contemplating treatment for any child with a congenital or acquired heart anomaly. Collaboration can only result in improved care.

An interval of 4–6 weeks between appointments is usually sufficient to prevent sensitization to the antibiotic. Every effort should be made to reduce the number of visits and obtain maximum usage from the antibiotic by performing quadrant dentistry at least, and complete-arch dentistry whenever possible. In some instances, consideration must be given to performing the work under general anaesthesia. If so, a hospital is the only place adequately equipped to deal with any emergency that might arise during anaesthesia.

2. Space management decisions and parental attitudes to dental health

Before each tooth is individually evaluated as to its suitability for pulp therapy, an overall assessment of the mouth must be made. The practitioner must assess why the child has so many untreated carious teeth, all of which may be possible candidates for pulp therapy. It may be that the parent has been unable, despite every effort, to locate a dentist who is prepared to treat the child. Perhaps the child has been examined on various occasions by a visiting school dentist but the parent has ignored the recommendations for dental care, finally being driven to seek an appointment by the child's pain. The latter parent, unlike the former, will probably not be receptive to extensive appointments for pulp therapy and conservative dentistry. The practitioner must attempt to evaluate each parent's attitude towards dental health. If it is negative, an attempt should be made to improve it by motivation and education. However, it may be fruitless to attempt extensive work because of parental apathy manifested by poor appointment keeping and poor response to preventive recommendations. In these cases, the treatment plan may have to be more radical and include extractions.

As the effects of space loss are most extreme prior to the completed eruption of the first permanent molar, every effort should be made to conserve the primary molars in a child under 7 years old. However, when a child presents with primary molars that are candidates for extraction the effects of premature loss on the developing occlusion must be considered (see Chapter 1).

Orthodontic evaluation can be made only with adequate radiographs to permit observation of the developing succedaneous teeth. Well-taken, intraoral, periapical radiographs will permit the most accurate evaluation of the tooth's suitability for pulp therapy, as well as the presence or absence of the developing permanent teeth, the dental age of the child, the possibility of ectopically erupting teeth, the eruption sequence, and the presence of crowding. The alternative radiographic survey is extraoral and can take the form of bimolar, lateral jaw or panoral films, such as the panorex or orthopantomograph. These techniques take less time and are generally easier to perform on an anxious child than an intraoral survey. Also, gonadal radiation dosage is reduced with extraoral films. The bimolar and lateral oblique films require no additional X-ray equipment. Extraoral films, particularly the bimolar and lateral oblique film, can also demonstrate the presence or absence of 'stacking' in the permanent molar region, which is indicative of potential crowding. However, the practitioner must realize that the detail of the pulp and periodontal tissues is of superior quality in intraoral films.

When extractions are unavoidable, compensating and balancing extractions of other primary molars must also be considered. Compensating extractions are those performed in the opposing arch but on the same side of the mouth. The objective is to obtain equal mesial movement of the first permanent molars on that side and good cuspal interdigitation of the permanent dentition. Balancing extractions are those performed within the same arch but on the opposite side. The objective is to maintain symmetry in space loss within the affected arch; the subsequent localization of crowding may later necessitate bilateral loss of permanent teeth. The location of other carious primary molars, the extent of tooth destruction and the tooth's suitability for pulp therapy must be taken into account when considering the use of compensating and balancing extractions. These extractions may also be indicated in children whose parents are negative towards dental health. It should be remembered though, that wholesale compensating and balancing extractions do little to improve the parents' attitude; rather, they are likely to become more convinced that primary teeth are not worthy of restoration.

The use of space-maintainers should also be considered when primary molar extraction is necessary (McDonald et al., 1994). They have the same ability to maintain symmetry in an arch as have balancing extractions. While there will never be uniform agreement on the value of space-maintainers, they do have a definite place in paediatric dentistry. The problems they pose can be minimized by correct planning, construction and supervision of the appliance. Those who are experienced with their use tend to advocate them while those who are skilled in correcting the malocclusions that develop from early loss of primary molars tend to deprecate them (Holloway and Swallow, 1975). It is hoped that the final decision on their use is made with the best interests of the child at heart and not the ability or whims of the dentist.

3. Assessment of the individual tooth

Three considerations must be kept in mind:

(1) Can the tooth be restored if pulp therapy can be performed?
(2) Does the dental age of the child warrant retention of the particular tooth?

(3) Is the pulp status such as to be amenable to pulp therapy? (This third question will be discussed in Chapter 17.)

The use of the stainless-steel crown has increased the number of primary teeth that can be restored after pulp therapy. A minimum of supragingival tooth structure may be all that is necessary to retain a stainless-steel crown. However, caries extending on to the root surface may be untreatable. Similarly, extension of caries to the furcation defies all attempts at conservation and necessitates extraction.

The dental age, judged by root development, also influences the decision to perform pulp therapy or extract the tooth. When the roots of primary molars have been more than half resorbed by the erupting succedaneous teeth, extraction should be seriously considered. However, the effects of an unfavourable eruption sequence on the occlusion of the first permanent molar must also be analysed critically.

References

American Academy of Pediatric Dentistry (1993) *Guidelines for the Care of Children*. Chicago, AAPD.

BNF (*British National Formulary*) (1994) Vol. 27, Section 5.1: Antibacterial drugs. London, BMA.

Council on Dental Therapeutics (1985) Prevention of bacterial endocarditis. Committee report of the American Heart Association. *J. Am. Dent. Assoc.* **110**.

Hibbard E. D. and Ireland R. L. (1957) Morphology of the root canals of the primary molar teeth. *J. Dent. Child.* **26**, 250.

Holloway P. J. and Swallow J. N. (1975) *Child Dental Health*, 2nd edn. Bristol, Wright.

McDonald R. E., Hennon D. K and Avery D. R. (1994) In: *Dentistry for the Child and Adolescent*. 6th edn. Ch. 26. St Louis, Mosby.

McGowan D. A. et al. (1983) Prophylaxis of experimental endocarditis in rabbits using one or two doses of amoxycillin. *Br. Dent. J.* **155**, 88.

Oakley C. M. and Sommerville W. (1981) Prevention of infective endocarditis. *Br. Heart J.* **45**, 23.

Sorenson H. W. (1973) The pedodontic patient with heart disease. *Dent. Clin. North Am.* **17**, 1, 173.

Chapter 17

Diagnosis of pulp pathology

General considerations

No single type of pulp therapy will be uniformly applicable or successful. The success of the treatment used depends mainly upon an accurate preoperative assessment of pulp status. Once this has been established, a treatment procedure can be selected which will eliminate the pathology believed to be present. For example, a non-vital primary tooth with premature root resorption (over two-thirds resorbed) should be extracted. Attempts to pulp cap that non-vital primary molar will fail because any drainage that may have occurred previously through an open lesion will be prevented. On the other hand, a complete pulpectomy may be unnecessary on a primary molar that has a minute, traumatic exposure. In these last two examples, the treatment performed in no way relates to the pulp status.

The clinician is faced with emergency patients who require a prompt, accurate diagnosis of pulpal pain so that a palliative service can be rendered. Unfortunately, the most accurate diagnosis of pulp status is by microscopic evaluation of the extracted tooth. As this is obviously impractical, the clinician must use a variety of diagnostic aids, including an accurate history, to determine the true extent of the microscopic pathosis of the pulp. Various diagnostic aids have been evaluated by correlating clinical data with the histological diagnoses in primary and permanent teeth. These individual aids will be discussed and related to the preoperative decision regarding suitability for treatment and to the postoperative evaluation of success.

Diagnostic features

Pain

An accurate history must be obtained of the type of pain experienced, including its duration, frequency, location and spread, as well as aggravating and relieving factors. As pain is subjective, the clinician must be aware of the varying responses given by the child and parents. A fearful child may have been kept awake the previous night with a toothache only to report that he or she has no pain when faced with the immediate dental experience. On the other hand, a parent who has neglected seeking dental care for the child may describe agonizing pain of 3 weeks' duration in the hope that comprehensive care will be performed immediately for the child. Indeed, it is often difficult to elicit an accurate history from the parent, who is effectively the third party and who is eventually responsible for, and feeling guilty about, the child's oral condition.

The absence of toothache does not preclude a histological pulpitis, either in primary (Hobson, 1970) or permanent teeth (Hasler and Mitchell, 1970). For example, children are seen who have non-vital primary molars with fistulae, although their parents will truthfully deny any history of toothache. The active lives of children, together with their short attention spans, may mean that minor discomfort passes without comment in a whirlwind of activities. However, the clinician should be sensitive to the extreme pain that some patients report. Its severity can probably be attributed to increased pressure within the enclosed hard tissue confines of the tooth and supporting structures.

A positive history of toothache suggests definite pulp pathology. However, it is difficult to correlate the type of pain with the degree of pathosis. Sensitivity to thermal stimuli indicates that the pulp is vital. The immediate response to hot or cold that disappears on removal of the stimulus (momentary pain) indicates that the pathosis is limited to the coronal pulp; in such cases, pulpotomy would be appropriate treatment. Momentary pain in response to thermal stimuli may also be due to the exposure of dentine from a leaking restoration or an open lesion; sealing the exposed dentine may relieve this type of pain. Persistent pain from thermal stimuli would indicate widespread inflammation of the pulp, extending into the radicular filaments to contraindicate single-visit pulpotomy (Koch and Nyborg, 1970).

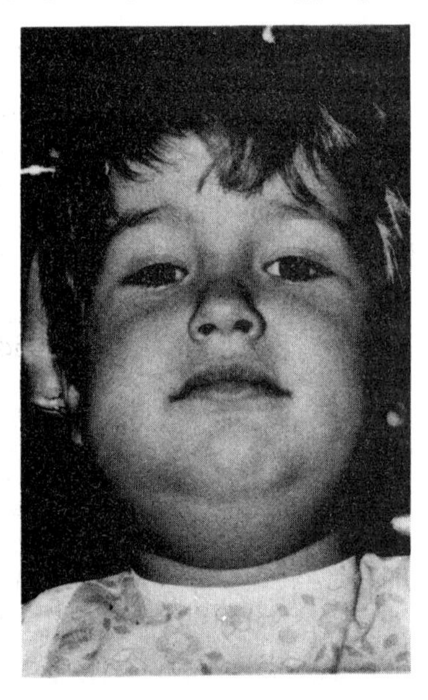

Fig. 17.1. Extraoral swelling (cellulitis). The mandibular right second molar is non-vital.

Spontaneous pain in primary teeth has been linked with extensive inflammation extending throughout the radicular filaments and microscopic internal resorption in the root canals (Guthrie et al., 1965). Spontaneous pain refers to that pain which is not elicited by any direct stimulus, such as thermal changes; it occurs well away from meal times and frequently at night. Single-visit pulpotomy techniques are contraindicated in such teeth, since inflamed tissue within the root canals would not be removed or mummified. Pain on chewing or biting will be discussed later.

Swelling

Swelling may present intraorally, localized to the infected tooth, or extraorally in the form of cellulitis (*Figs* 17.1 and 17.2). It is caused by the inflammatory exudate associated with a non-vital tooth. Since swelling may not exist at the time of examination the clinician must thoroughly question both child and parent to uncover any history of swelling. The relationship of muscle attachments, particularly that of the buccinator, to the inter-radicular and periapical areas determines whether the swelling has an intraoral or extraoral location. The presence of swelling does not necessarily indicate that an extraction is needed, as with

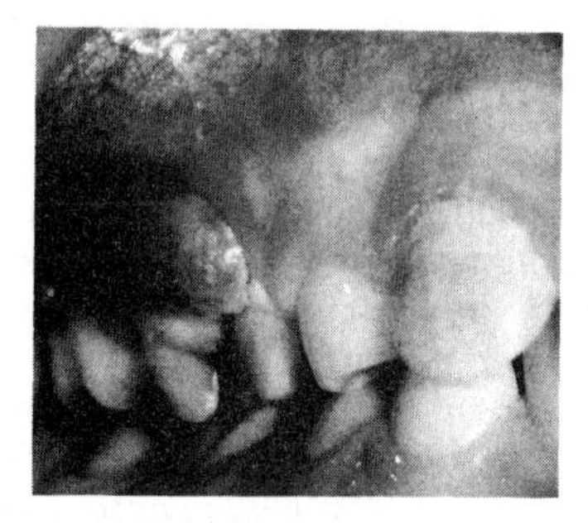

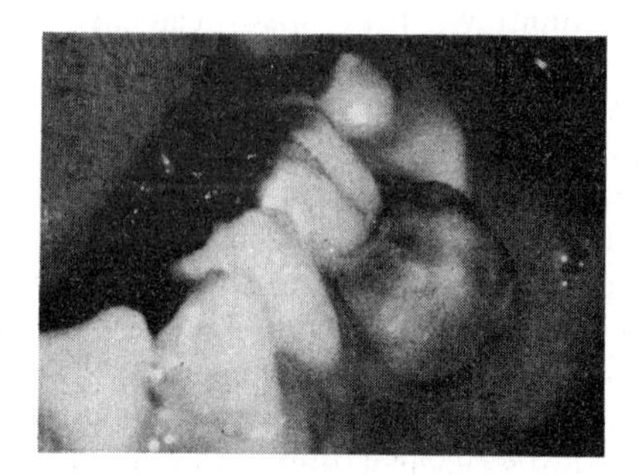

Fig. 17.2 *a*, Fistula adjacent to a non-vital tooth. *b*, Abscess is draining through the gingival margin.

modern antibiotic therapy the swelling can be resolved and pulp therapy initiated, often within 72 hours (Paterson and Curzon, 1992).

Diagnosis of pulp pathology

Swelling

Intraoral swelling is usually apparent on the buccal aspect, although it may in rare instances present lingually or palatally. There is less buccal than lingual or palatal bone through which the inflammatory products from the periapical or inter-radicular regions penetrate, taking the path of least resistance. The pressure of the swelling will eventually result in spontaneous drainage if treatment is not rendered. Drainage may occur through an open lesion in the tooth, although the fine apical foramina of primary molars usually preclude this possibility. Most commonly, drainage occurs intraorally either via the gingival margin or by the establishment of a fistula. The fistula is a small, elevated nodule of tissue which is patent to permit drainage. It is generally seen at or near the junction of the attached gingiva and alveolar mucosa, as that site is adjacent to the inter-radicular region where the inflammatory products are normally located in non-vital primary molars.

The tissue adjacent to a fistula is frequently inflamed to give the appearance of a white nodule surrounded by an crythematous base. The fistula's patency may be tested by the ability to milk serous exudate or pus from it. Once a fistula is present, the infection is seldom acute since drainage has already occurred. Therefore, radical decisions (which may include surgery) regarding treatment of an asymptomatic tooth with a fistula should be delayed until a treatment plan has been formulated.

Extraoral swelling presents as a cellulitis, the location of which is dependent on the spread of infection along fascial planes. In the mandibular arch, the submandibular region is commonly involved as a result of non-vital second primary or first permanent molars. In the maxillary arch, the swelling from non-vital primary canines and first primary molars can be so severe as to close the child's eye. Drainage of the extraoral swelling would eventually occur through the path of least resistance, which may unfortunately be the skin. The pyrexia associated with such swellings, together with the obvious abnormality, usually stimulates parents to seek care before extraoral drainage occurs.

The pulp of a tooth having either an intra- or extraoral swelling or a fistula will be non-vital. However, it is possible for vital tissue, although inflamed, to be present in one canal while an adjacent canal will be non-vital; the fistula will be adjacent to the non-vital canal. For treatment purposes, the whole pulp must be considered non-vital. However, because there may still be some vital tissue left, this means that local analgesia should be used during treatment.

Mobility

Mobility in a primary tooth may result from physiological or pathological causes. Radiographic evaluation of the remaining root of a primary tooth, the crown position, and the amount of root formation of the underlying permanent successor will determine whether any mobility is physiological or pathological. Physiological root resorption of more than one-half the root length contraindicates pulp therapy and extraction should be considered.

Pathological mobility is due to root or bone resorption or both, and it is associated with a non-vital pulp. Bone resorption is identified radiographically by a periapical or inter-radicular radiolucency or both, most commonly the radiolucency appears in the furca. The degree of pathological mobility is of no particular value in ascertaining the degree of microscopic pathosis (Guthrie et al., 1965).

Percussion

Pain from pressure on a tooth indicates that supporting periodontal structures are inflamed. Depression of the tooth into this inflamed tissue results in this type of pain. Occasionally the radiograph will demonstrate that the tooth has been slightly extruded from its socket and is in premature occlusion. As the teeth occlude, the inflamed tissue around the apex is irritated by trauma. As with pathological mobility, pain from percussion indicates that the tooth is most likely non-vital and that the surrounding periodontium is inflamed. It is possible, however, to have an inflamed, vital pulp associated with apical periodontitis in permanent teeth (Seltzer et al., 1963).

It is not necessary to perform a percussion test by hitting a tooth with a mirror handle; indeed this may be overly traumatic, especially if the child reports that the tooth is sensitive to pressure. Rather, a definite history will often reveal the diagnosis. A useful clinical test is to apply finger pressure to the tooth and observe the child's response by watching the eyes.

Constricted pupils are indicative of pain.

Vitality tests

Vitality tests, either thermal or electrical, are of little value in primary teeth. While they may sometimes give an indication of pulp vitality, the response does not identify the degree of pathosis present. Fear of the unknown may make the child patient apprehensive of the electric vitalometer; he or she may then give the response they feel is correct rather than an accurate one. Also, normal healthy primary teeth may not respond to vitality tests.

The real value of vitality tests, either thermal or electrical, is in permanent teeth when comparison can be made with normal antimeres over a time period. The obvious example involves traumatized incisors, when serial testing may reveal that a fractured tooth requires additional current to effect a response compared with its untraumatized antimere. If identical responses have been obtained with the same current at a previous appointment, a trend is developing which would indicate that the fractured tooth may become non-vital. However, since no single diagnostic aid is pathognomonic of the true histological status of the diseased pulp, the clinician should be wary of relying solely on this one particular aid.

It is important that the results of vitality tests be compared with those for normal antimere teeth. Even so, the thickness of tooth structure separating the pulp chamber from the vitality tester influences the possible degree of response. Also, recently erupted permanent teeth, particularly lateral incisors, have failed to produce responses to vitality tests up to 3 years after eruption, even though they were clinically and radiographically normal. Furthermore, the liquid contents of a necrotic tooth's pulp chamber may account for a positive electric vitality test response from some non-vital permanent teeth (Reynolds, 1966).

Radiographs

Recent preoperative radiographs are prerequisites to pulp therapy in primary and young permanent teeth. Besides providing information on the child's dental development (see also Chapter 5), they may demonstrate pathological entities which contraindicate some forms of pulp therapy or indicate failed treatment. As noted earlier, the position of the succedaneous permanent tooth will dictate the decision on performing pulp therapy for primary tooth retention. Let it be emphasized again (as in Chapter 16) that intraoral radiographs of the periapical type provide the best detail of the pulp and the supporting structures. Extraoral radiographs, though excellent for demonstrating the developing dentition, are inadequate for diagnosis of pathology in the pulp and supporting tissues.

Despite its immense diagnostic value, the radiograph can deceive the clinician into thinking that periapical or inter-radicular pathosis is absent when in fact it may be histologically present. This is because the microscopic lesion must be of certain dimensions before it is manifested radiographically. Furthermore, superimposition of permanent successors masks the true appearance, particularly in maxillary primary teeth. A bitewing radiograph should be used to supplement the maxillary periapical primary-molar film, since less superimposition of the developing premolars occurs in the critical trifurcation region.

Experimentally produced lesions in exarticulated bones become radiolucent only when the cortical plate is perforated (Ramadan and Mitchell, 1962). The observation of histologically present but radiographically absent periapical pathosis was also confirmed in permanent teeth by Bender et al. (1966).

The following abnormalities are sometimes observed in conjunction with carious primary teeth.

Pulp calcifications occasionally occur in the horn area of extensively carious primary molars. They represent the pulp's response to a long-standing lesion by the laying down of very irregular dentine. These calcifications are associated with advanced pulpal degeneration extending into the root canals, contraindicating single-visit pulpotomy.

Internal resorption will be radiographically

apparent only when the resorption occurs on the mesial or distal aspects of the root canal; buccal or lingual resorption may pass undetected due to the angulation of the radiograph. Microscopic internal resorption is associated with spontaneous pain at night and inflammation extending throughout both vital coronal and radicular pulp to contraindicate single-visit pulpotomy procedures. The radiographic postoperative presence of internal resorption after pulp capping or pulpotomy would indicate failure (*Figs* 17.3 and 17.4); it is likely that the resorption was present preoperatively but was not radiographically apparent.

External root resorption can occur physiologically or pathologically (see section on Mobility above). The clinician should be familiar with the normal appearance of primary molar roots and their physiological resorptive pattern. It is not uncommon, however, for the distal root of a mandibular first primary molar to be foreshortened to almost one-half the length of the mesial root. This should not be interpreted as pathological if a normal periodontal membrane space is seen, with no radiolucency. Pathological root resorption is invariably associated with periapical radiolucency (*Figs* 17.5 and 17.6). It is indicative of a non-vital pulp

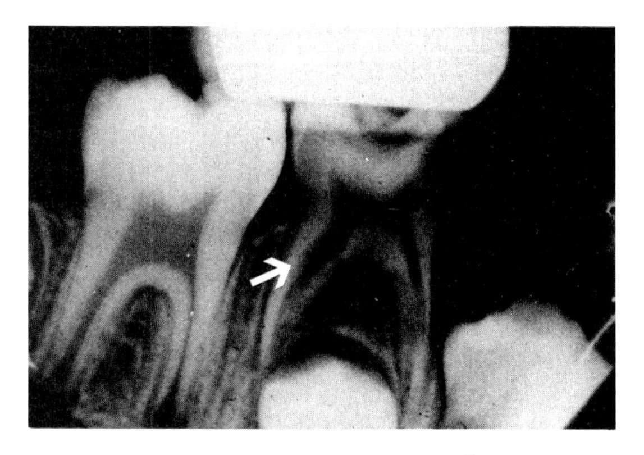

Fig. 17.3. Internal resorption in distal root of mandibular second primary molar: this was undiagnosed and a pulpotomy was performed.

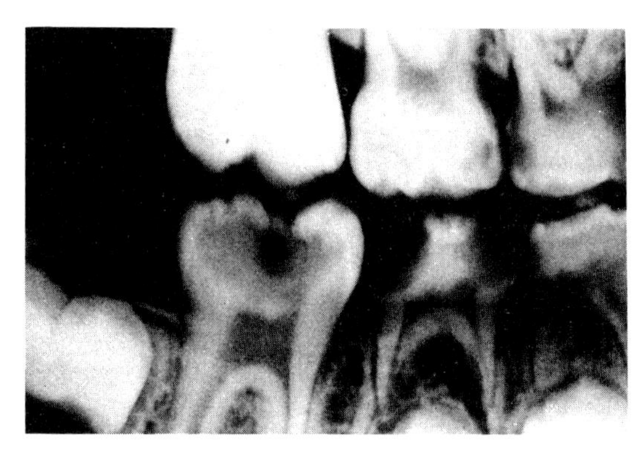

Fig. 17.5. Early resorption of the mesial root of a mandibular second primary molar. This tooth was considered for pulpectomy, see *Fig.* 17.6.

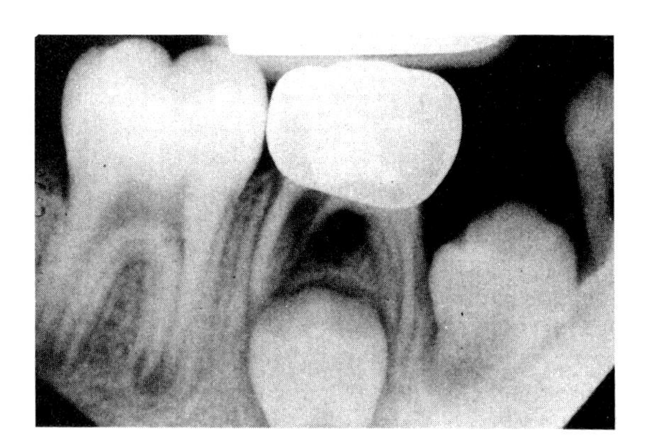

Fig. 17.4. Three-month postoperative radiograph of *Fig.* 17.3 demonstrates progression of internal resorption despite pulpotomy. The pulp treatment failed and a pulpectomy or an extraction was originally indicated.

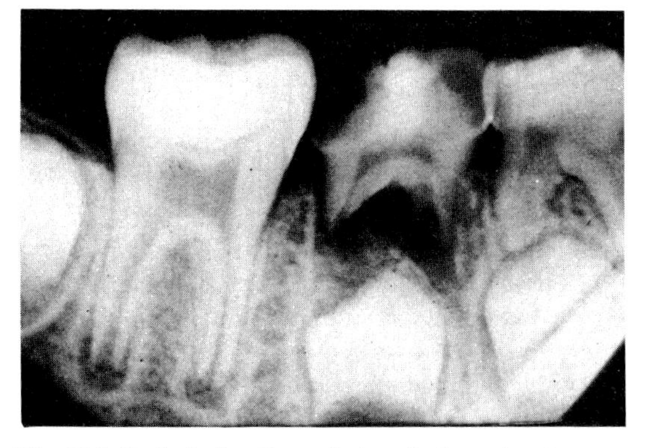

Fig. 17.6. Periapical radiograph 4 weeks later than in *Fig.* 17.5, at the time the first permanent molar was subjected to indirect pulp treatment, demonstrates marked progression of external root resorption of the second primary molar. This tooth had to be extracted. Note the speed at which resorption occurred and therefore the need for radiographs at appropriate intervals.

and extensive inflammation in the supporting tissues; the only viable treatment is pulpectomy or extraction.

Bone resorption will present as a radiolucency if the cortical plate has been penetrated. It indicates that there is inflammation extending beyond the tooth and into the supporting periodontium. The pulp will probably be non-vital, although it is also possible that the canals contain vital, inflamed pulp. In either circumstance, a pulpectomy procedure would carry the highest chance of success. When bone loss is extensive, extraction is indicated.

Radiolucency in primary molars is usually seen at the furcation and not at the periapex. It is possible that the inflammatory exudate cannot penetrate the fine, branching ramifications of the primary molar root canals. This is not the case in the young permanent molar where it is more common to see periapical than inter-radicular radiolucency. The high incidence of furcation radiolucency in primary molars has been attributed to the presence of accessory canals in the bifurcation region of human primary molars (Winter, 1962). Also, the pulpal floor in infected primary molars may be more porous and permeable (Moss et al., 1965). The accessory canals and porous pulpal floor, which is thinner in primary than in permanent teeth, may permit the diffusion of inflammatory exudate more readily; this would explain the high incidence of inter-radicular rather than periapical pathology in necrotic primary teeth.

Depth of the lesion The proximity of the lesion to the pulp can be estimated preoperatively by a radiograph. If the lesion is radiographically very close to the pulp, there is a 75% chance of an exposure when all the caries is removed (DiMaggio and Hawes, 1963). A broken-down marginal ridge is indicative of probable pulp exposure in Class 2 lesions in primary molars (Stoner, 1967; Hobson, 1970) (*Fig.* 17.7). The clinician should therefore plan on some form of pulp therapy when the clinical and radiographic appearances indicate a deep lesion. Correct preoperative assessment will permit accurate scheduling of appointment times and reduced stress during the clinical technique.

The clinician should also be aware of the possibility of an undetected avascular, microscopic pulp exposure. Whenever the pulpal floor of the cavity is so thin that the pulp outline is shown by pink colouration, there may well be a microscopic pulp exposure. This phenomenon should encourage the clinician to err to the radical and to proceed to a pulpotomy rather than risk pulp capping these teeth. The more conservative method of stopping short of exposure is not recommended, as in the authors' experience these teeth become non-vital and then a pulpectomy is required, often as an emergency procedure (Paterson and Curzon, 1992). The success rate of the vital pulpotomy is so high (Morawa et al., 1975) that it is better to proceed directly to use this technique.

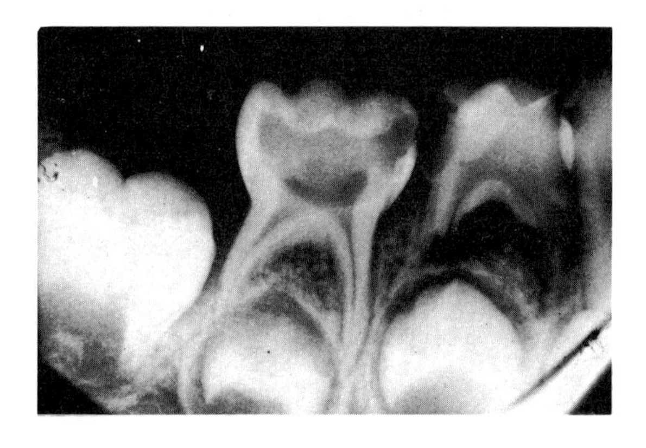

Fig. 17.7. Periapical radiograph of a 3-year-old child. Note that when the marginal ridge of a primary molar is broken down the lesion is close to the pulp. Note also the premature root resorption.

The exposure site

Both the size of the exposure site and the nature of exudate expressed from it are useful diagnostic aids (Koch and Nyborg, 1970). Exposure sites in excess of 1 mm^2 do not lend themselves to direct pulp capping. Indeed, only traumatically induced exposure sites and those whose surrounding dentine is bacteria-free in asymptomatic teeth are suitable for pulp capping. The colour and amount of blood at the exposure site have been shown to be a reliable guide to the extent of pulpal inflammation in primary teeth. Light-red blood and haemorrhage that can be arrested easily are associated with inflammation that is limited to the coronal pulp in primary teeth. Profuse haemorrhage from the exposure site, with deep-red blood, is histologically associated with inflammation extending into the root canals of primary molars. The former instance would be compatible with pulpotomy procedures while the latter would not and would require a pulpectomy.

The amputated pulp stumps

In pulpotomy procedures, the coronal pulp is removed and amputated from the radicular filaments at the entrance to the root canals. Uncontrollable haemorrhage from these pulp stumps will occur if the blood vessels are dilated, as seen in the inflamed pulp. It is therefore imperative that no astringent or vasoconstrictor be placed over these pulp stumps since observing the ability to arrest this haemorrhage is useful to the clinician in assessing radicular pulp status and the extent of inflammation.

References

Bender I. B., Seltzer S. and Soltanoff W. (1966) Endodontic success – a reappraisal of criteria. *Oral Surg.* **22**, 780.

DiMaggio J. J. and Hawes R. R. (1963) Continued evaluation of direct and indirect pulp capping. *J. Dent. Res.* **41**, 38.

Guthrie T. J., McDonald R. E. and Mitchell D. F. (1965) Dental pulp hemogram. *J. Dent. Res.* **44**, 678.

Hasler J. E. and Mitchell D. F. (1970) Painless pulpitis. *J. Am. Dent. Assoc.* **81**, 71.

Hobson P. (1970) Pulp treatment of deciduous teeth. *Br. Dent. J.* **128**, 232.

Koch G. and Nyborg M. (1970) Correlation between clinical and histological indications for pulpotomy of deciduous teeth. *J. Int. Assoc. Dent. Child.* **1**, 3.

Morawa A. P., Straffon L. H. and Han S. S. (1975) Clinical evaluation of pulpotomies using dilute formocresol. *J. Dent. Child.* **42**, 360.

Moss S., Addelston H. and Goldsmith E. D. (1965) Histologic studies of pulpal floor of deciduous molars. *J. Am. Dent. Assoc.* **70**, 372.

Paterson S. A. and Curzon M. E. J. (1992) Amoxycillin versus penicillin V in the treatment of acutely abscessed primary teeth. *Br. Dent. J.* **174**, 443

Ramadan A. E. and Mitchell D. F. (1962) A roentgenographic study of experimental bone destruction. *Oral Surg.* **15**, 934.

Reynolds R. L. (1966) The determination of pulp vitality by means of thermal and electrical stimuli. *Oral Surg.* **22**, 331.

Seltzer S., Bender I. B. and Zionitz M. (1963) The dynamics of pulp inflammation: Correlations between diagnostic data and actual histologic findings in the pulp. *Oral Surg.* **16**, 846.

Stoner J. E. (1967) Dental caries in deciduous molars. *Br. Dent. J.* **123**, 130.

Winter G. B. (1962) Abscess formation in connection with deciduous molar teeth. *Arch. Oral Biol.* **7**, 373.

Chapter 18

Pulp therapy techniques – emergencies and one-visit pulpotomy

The emergency patient

The child with a toothache, who presents as an emergency patient, manifests special problems. Unless time has been allotted in the appointment book for emergencies, such patients will disrupt the daily schedule. This problem is compounded by the fact that both parent and child may be upset from a sleepless night. These factors contribute to the possibility of a negative experience for the child.

The principles of management for the child with a toothache can be listed as follows:

(1) identify the *urgency* of the problem;
(2) take a history and make a *diagnosis*;
(3) be aware of both parental and child *anxiety*;
(4) *relieve the pain* (without extraction if possible).

1. Urgency

The receptionist should screen all incoming telephone calls to determine the urgency of the problem. The dental surgery or office should have firmly established instructions for the receptionist who handles these calls. The following set of guidelines has withstood the test of time: emergency patients are asked a series of questions with regard to their toothache. The response to the questions determines whether the emergency is classified as 'same day' or 'next day'.

The following formula has been successfully used in clinical practice.

- Crying child
- Child awake at night
- Swelling
- Fractured teeth

} same-day emergency

- Intermittent pain of long duration
- Fistula

} next-day emergency

2. Diagnosis

A diagnosis of the pulpal condition must be made prior to initiating any treatment. A history must be taken, followed by a clinical examination and the taking of appropriate radiographs. Many of the above procedures can be accomplished by properly trained auxiliaries if laws permit. In this manner the disruption to the daily schedule is minimal and children receiving routine care do not have their treatment compromised.

3. Anxiety

Parents and child may all have had sleepless nights as a result of toothache. Unnecessary waiting can seem an endless time for those with a true emergency problem. During both the initial telephone call and the history taking, the dental staff must be sensitive to the parents' feeling regarding the dental emergency. Apart from the guilt felt by parents because of their child's toothache, the emergency dental appointment may constitute a severe upset to the family routine. Sometimes parents may express their concerns for immediate care in a hostile manner; they are often unable to realize the disruption they cause to the dental office and act as though theirs was the only child who required treatment. This aggressive behaviour must not be misinterpreted by the staff; rather, the staff should have empathy towards the parents' problem associated with the dental emergency.

4. Relief of pain

The main purpose of the emergency visit is the relief of pain. If definitive treatment can be provided in a manner that will not endanger either the child's future co-operative behaviour or the developing occlusion, this is also advantageous. Personal experience reflects an opinion that too frequently the dentist tries to accomplish too much at an emergency visit, only to realize the error several visits later. Because of the child's apprehension associated with an awareness of an existing dental problem (Wright and Alpern, 1971), a minimum of operative dentistry should be attempted.

Relief of pain from non-vital teeth with associated swelling is achieved by establishing drainage and the use of antibiotics, if the temperature is elevated by 2° or more and if lymphadenopathy is present (Paterson and Curzon, 1992). In some teeth, drainage can be established through the root canals, while in others, fluctuant intraoral swellings may be drained using topical analgesia. In these cases the abscess is lanced using a No. 11 scalpel wrapped in one piece of gauze so as to cover the blade. Once the topical gel has been allowed to work for about 1 min the scalpel blade is used to puncture the abscess with one quick stab. Because the blade is disguised in the gauze the child does not see what would appear to him or her to be a very sharp pointed instrument. Relief of pain is almost instantaneous.

As the pulp is non-vital, local analgesia is unnecessary because injection of a local analgesic into inflamed tissues is contraindicated on the grounds that it may spread infection and the inability to achieve analgesia when an acute abscess is present. Sometimes a sharp explorer is sufficient to puncture the swelling and establish drainage. It may be necessary, in severe instances, to resort to extraction under general anaesthesia to establish drainage. This may be most appropriate when a cellulitis is associated with a non-vital maxillary tooth.

Relief of pain from vital inflamed teeth can be achieved by a variety of techniques dependent upon the cause. In some instances, such as a lost restoration with no underlying caries, simply closing the exposed dentine to the oral environment will prevent the pain caused by changes in pH and local temperature. In teeth with deep carious lesions, the superficial necrotic layers of decay can be removed without local analgesia and a temporary restoration placed, usually IRM. In other teeth, the vital, inflamed coronal pulp may have to be removed as in a pulpotomy procedure, when local analgesia will be required.

In most instances, pain relief can be accomplished without extraction; wherever possible this should be done. Extraction signals to the parents that once a toothache occurs, an extraction is necessary. Psychologically this may not be a desirable association to make for either the child or the parents. Furthermore, consideration has to be given to the need for space management. If the toothache has prompted the child to a first visit, it is quite likely that there may be several carious teeth in addition to the one causing the pain. The extraction of the single offending tooth may be performed without consideration of management of the developing occlusion.

Parents may be very demanding in their desire for definitive treatment. The receptionist may frequently be asked, 'Will the tooth be extracted?' 'Telephone' diagnoses cannot be made, and the receptionist should assure the parents that pain will be relieved. However, extraction should not be promised over the telephone. Similarly, if the patient is offered an appointment on the following day, the reason for the delay in scheduling must be tactfully explained.

Indirect pulp treatment (primary teeth)

The technique of pulp capping in primary teeth, either directly or indirectly, is not recommended, although it has its advocates. However, on the basis of many years of experience we now feel that the treatment of choice whenever the pulp of primary tooth is compromised is to perform a vital pulpotomy as soon as possible. As local analgesia will have been used with rubber dam in order to restore a primary tooth, then if the dental caries is found to be deep it is far better to carry out a coronal vital pulpotomy immediately. Because the success rate of vital pulpotomies is well over 90% (Morawa et al., 1975), then this is by far the best approach. Use of an indirect pulp-capping procedure leads to pulp death in many cases and then a non-vital pulpotomy is needed, with a much lower success rate.

Pulpotomy procedures (primary teeth)

Pulpotomy procedures involve removing vital, partially inflamed, coronal pulp tissue, placing a dressing over the amputated pulp stumps and then placing the final restoration. Various medicaments have been recommended for covering the radicular filaments. The initial recommendation of these materials was empirically based. Since then, assessments in animals and humans by clinical, radiographic and microscopical means have allowed us to rank the different pulpotomy procedures using different materials. A brief review of the recommended treatments is relevant.

In primary teeth, the pulpotomy procedure can be performed in a single visit when local analgesia is used. In this instance, the technique is one of vital amputation. Either formocresol, or one of the suggested alternatives such as glutaraldehyde (Ranly, 1984) or ferric sulphate (Fei et al., 1991), are used to cover the amputated radicular pulp stumps.

Single-visit formocresol pulpotomy (vital primary teeth)

Indications

- Carious or mechanical exposures in vital primary teeth

Contraindications

- Cardiac conditions
- Spontaneous pain – pain at night
- Swelling
- Fistula
- Tenderness to percussion
- Pathological mobility
- External root resorption
- Internal root resorption
- Periapical or inter-radicular radiolucency
- Pulp calcifications
- Pathological external root resorption
- Pus or serous exudate at the exposure site
- Uncontrollable haemorrhage from the amputated pulp stumps

Technique (Fig. 18.1)

The procedure is carried out step-by-step in one visit using local analgesia and rubber dam (Duggal and Curzon, 1994). Following the establishment of cavity outline form, all peripheral caries is removed before the pulp is exposed. This important step prevents unnecessary bacterial contamination of the exposed pulp and improves visibility of the exposure site. Following pulp exposure and its evaluation, the roof of the coronal pulp chamber is removed. A high-speed bur, No. 330, with water coolant is used to locate the pulp horns. Bur cuts are made between the horns so that the roof of the chamber is removed. The coronal pulp can be removed either with a sharp excavator or with a large, round bur run at low speed. No attempt should be made to arrest haemorrhage at this stage. The pulp is amputated at the entrance to the root canals. This step is facilitated by knowing the location of the root canals and the depth of the coronal pulp chamber, assisted by the preoperative radiograph. Copious irrigation of the pulp chamber with water will prevent dentine chips from being forced into the radicular pulp, which would occur if air were used.

The whole coronal pulp must be removed, paying special attention to pulp filaments left under ledges of dentine. If these are not removed they would continue to bleed and therefore cloud the diagnosis of the radicular pulp stumps. Care must be exercised not to perforate either the thin pulpal or interproximal wall, or the floor of the pulp chamber, by using excessive force with the round bur (*Fig.* 18.2). A large, round bur (No. 6) run at slow speed with a light touch is recommended or a large, sharp excavator; there is less danger of inadvertently forcing these down the canals as their dimensions would exceed those of the canal entrance in most instances.

Postamputation bleeding is controlled by moistening cotton pellets with a non-irritating solution such as saline or water and placing

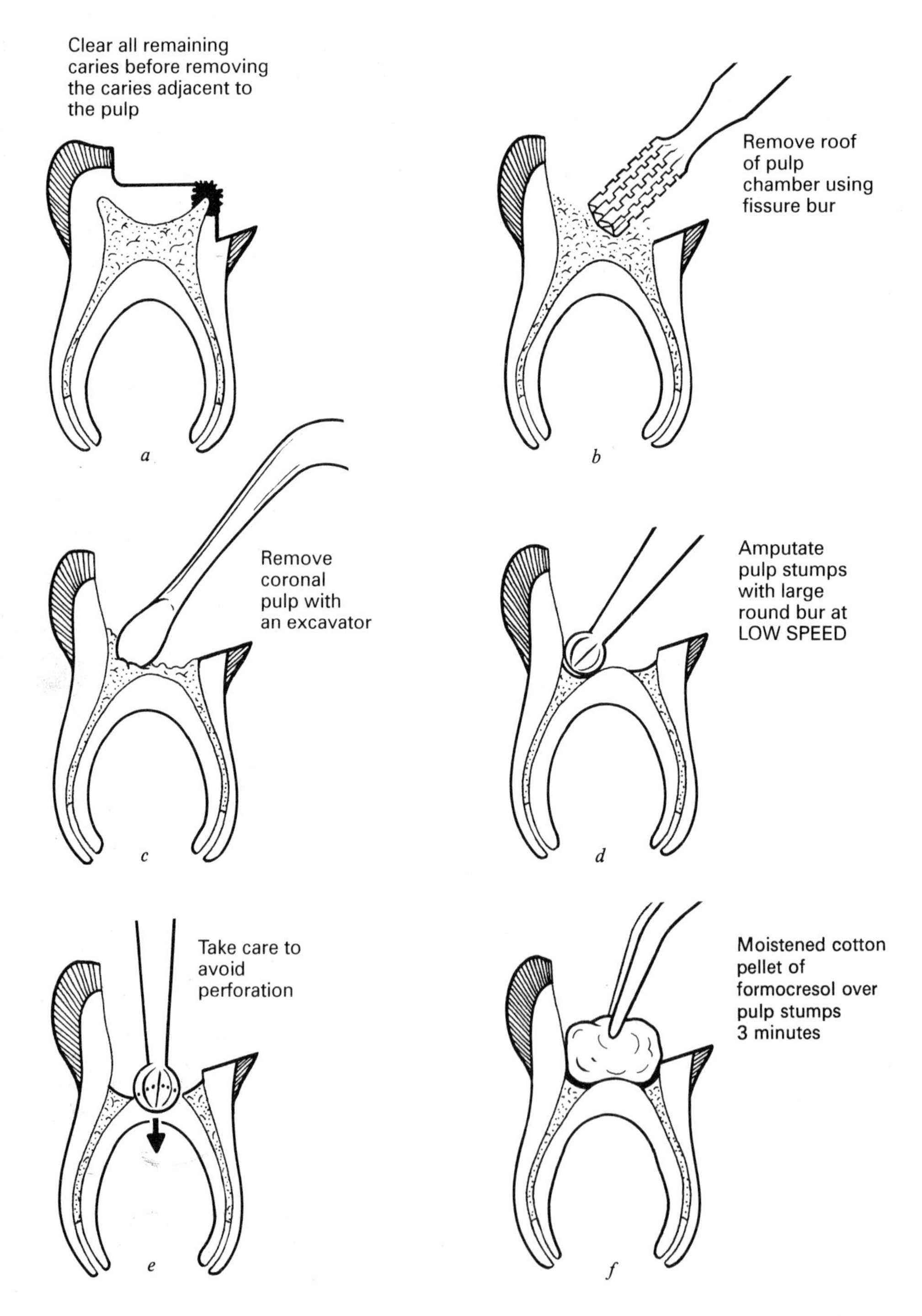
Clear all remaining caries before removing the caries adjacent to the pulp
a
Remove roof of pulp chamber using fissure bur
b
Remove coronal pulp with an excavator
c
Amputate pulp stumps with large round bur at LOW SPEED
d
Take care to avoid perforation
e
Moistened cotton pellet of formocresol over pulp stumps 3 minutes
f

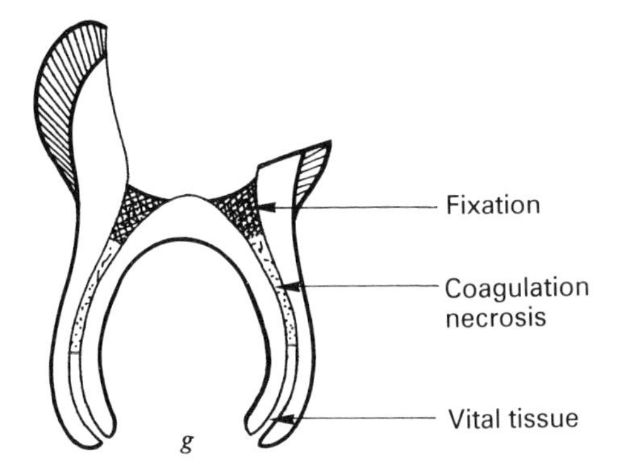

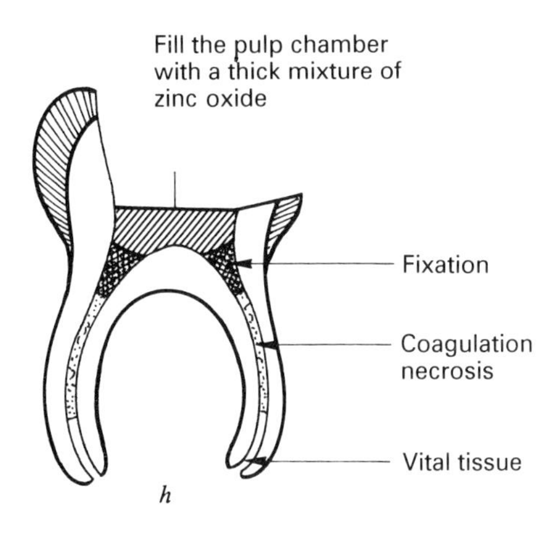

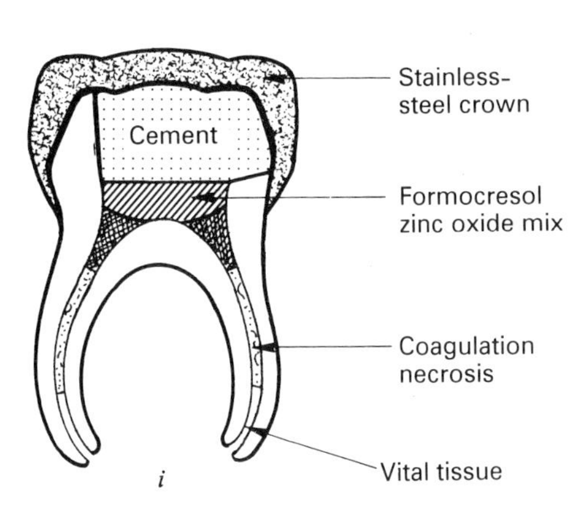

Fig. 18.1 Single-visit formocresol pulpotomy.

them over the amputated stumps for 3 min. The status of the radicular pulp stumps is then assessed. It is important that no material is placed over them that would alter haemostasis, such as a local analgesic with vasoconstrictor. The tooth may be considered suitable for a single-visit formocresol pulpotomy only if bleeding is arrested naturally. The pulp stumps are sensitive to indelicate handling and the clinician must prevent iatrogenic, traumatic haemorrhage when removing the cotton pellet. This problem will be more pronounced in young primary molars with very wide orifices to the root canals. If postamputation haemorrhage persists, a two-visit pulpotomy or pulpectomy should be performed (see Chapter 19).

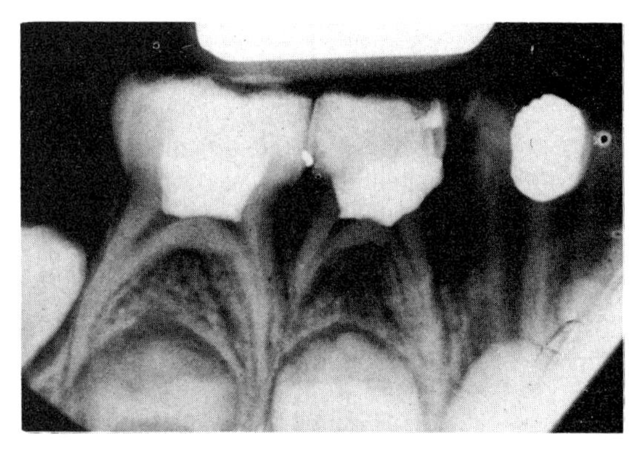

Fig. 18.2. Perforation of the mesial wall in the first primary molar: note the interseptal bone loss. The tooth must be extracted.

The orifices of the root canals are covered for 3 min (Doyle, 1961) with cotton pellets moistened with 1/5th dilution formocresol. The pellets are first saturated with formocresol and later compressed between gauze to remove excess so that they are just moistened with the liquid (*Fig.* 18.3). Excess formocresol is undesirable since it serves no other purpose than to increase the likelihood of a soft-tissue burn should any leakage occur. Buckley's formocresol comprises cresol (35%) and formalin (19%) in aqueous glycerine; it can be made up at the local chemist or pharmacy in small, 10-ml, dark bottles. It has been recommended for some years that a 1/5th dilution be used. It has an indefinite shelf-life, although the screw cap should always be replaced immediately to prevent evaporation of formaldehyde and also to minimize its pungent odour.

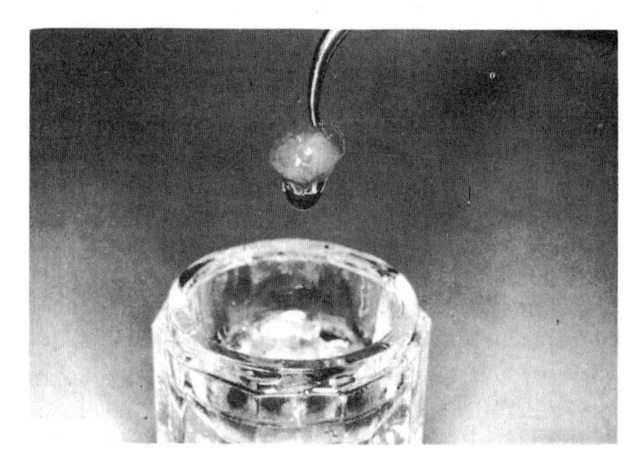

a

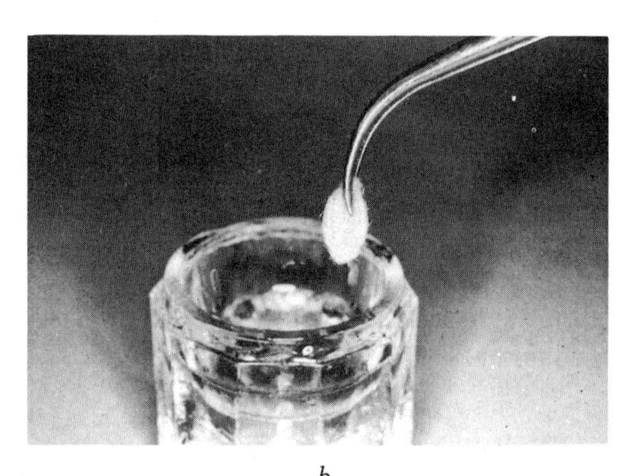

b

Fig. 18.3. *a*, Cotton pellet saturated with formocresol. This should be compressed between gauze to remove excess; saturated pellets should *not* be used. *b*. Dampened formocresol pellet. This is the correct amount of drug for placing in the chamber. Compare to (*a*).

When the formocresol pellet is removed, the radicular pulp stumps should appear dark brown or even black as a result of fixation caused by the drug. If a slight haemorrhage still occurs the procedure should be repeated for 2 more minutes. If after two applications of formocresol the bleeding cannot be arrested, then this indicates irreversible damage of the radicular pulp and a pulpectomy is indicated.

The pulp chamber is filled with a soft mix of a zinc oxide paste (Kalzinol), placed over the pulp stumps and tapped gently into place. If a preformed crown is not placed at the same visit as the pulpotomy, the restoration that is used must prevent the ingress of bacteria and oral fluids that may further irritate the pulp.

Histology

The histological reaction of the radicular pulp to formocresol is represented diagrammatically in *Fig.* 18.1*g–i*. There is universal agreement that pulp fixation occurs after formocresol application. The histochemical study of Loos and Han (1971) confirms that the drug suppresses metabolism, acting as a cytotoxic agent to account for the fixation. Just below the zinc oxide, in the coronal one-third of the canal, is a narrow band of homogeneous, eosinophilic tissue; apical to this is a broader band of pale, eosinophilic tissue which fills the bulk of the canals. The loss of cellular detail accounts for the microscopical interpretation of coagulation necrosis. The apical one-third of the canal contains vital tissue, but opinions differ as to whether this is vital pulp (Doyle, 1961) or ingrowth of connective tissue (Berger, 1965; Hannah and Rowe, 1971). Because these two tissues are histologically similar and because the mechanical disturbance caused by extraction may account for microscopical misinterpretation, no answer can be given. However, the vitality of this apical tissue may be important in the resorption process.

The above description refers to a single-visit (3-min) application of the drug. When formocresol application extends beyond 3 days in the two-visit technique there is an increase in linear, vertical, calcific degeneration (Emmerson et al., 1959). This may narrow the radicular pulp canal and it is speculated that there is an increased potential problem with resorption. Willard (1976) observed this in human primary molars treated by 4-min formocresol application in a single-visit pulpotomy technique. Of 30 treated teeth, 29 demonstrated calcification of the root canal as early as 6 months postoperatively.

Microscopical study of the supporting tissues of teeth treated by single-visit formocresol pulpotomy indicates that there is no untoward effect on the developing permanent tooth (Kennedy et al., 1973). Obviously this research was done in animals so that microscopical evaluation was possible. There have been long-term follow-up studies in children that have shown no effects on the permanent premolars when formocresol pulpotomies have been done on primary molars (Rolling and Poulsen, 1978), although Pruhs et al. (1977) earlier reported a correlation in which the defects on permanent teeth associated with formocresol pulpotomy took the form of mild enamel opacities; these are seldom aesthetically undesirable since they commonly occur on premolars.

Variations in technique

Time of formocresol application

It is of historical interest that the formocresol pulpotomy was first advocated by Sweet (1936) as a multivisit technique. Also, preoperative criteria were less stringent than those previously mentioned and included non-vital teeth. The aim of treatment was to sterilize the pulp chamber by a rotation of drugs (mainly formocresol and beechwood creosote) before filling it with zinc oxide. The multivisit approach was reduced to two visits in vital teeth, a formocresol pellet being left in the chamber in between appointments. The treatment was further reduced from two visits to a single-visit, 5-min application of the drug. Direct comparison of the two- and single-visit formocresol pulpotomy in human primary molars was made by Redig (1968); neither treatment was superior. However, the convenience of the single-visit technique for child and parent, the reduction in the need for further analgesia and isolation, and the opportunity to perform quadrant dentistry make the single-visit (3-min) formocresol pulpotomy superior to a two-visit technique.

Variations in time of formocresol application from days to minutes have been studied (Doyle, 1961; Venham, 1967). Microscopical evaluation indicates that the main action of formocresol occurs within the first 5 min of application (Emmerson et al., 1959). However, since no real attempt is made to monitor the volume of the drug, there seems little sense in accurately timing the application. Indeed, Venham (1967) found identical microscopical appearances in the pulps of monkey teeth exposed to 5 min and to 15 s of formocresol application; however, Venham always incorporated formocresol in the zinc oxide mix that was placed over the pulp stumps. We believe that 3 min is the minimum time required, and that anything beyond will not be detrimental. As the final restoration of choice is the preformed crown, it is clinically convenient to allow the formocresol pellet to remain over the pulp stump during crown contouring and trial fitting. Only rarely does this take less than 5 min.

Dilution of formocresol

Some researchers have been concerned with the cytotoxic damage caused by formocresol and have recommended a 1/5 dilution. Clinical evaluation was made of human primary molars treated by pulpotomy; the amputated stumps were exposed to 1/5 formocresol for 5 min, followed by a zinc oxide–eugenol mix to which 1/5 formocresol was added. Results were equivalent to using full-strength formocresol (Morawa et al., 1975; Fuks and Bimstein, 1981).

Inclusion or omission of formocresol from the sub-base

A further variation in clinical technique is the omission of formocresol from the zinc oxide mix placed over the radicular pulp stumps, after 3 min of direct contact with the wet drug. Microscopical evaluation shows that teeth with only a zinc oxide sub-base and those with formocresol–zinc oxide mixes have identical results (Beaver et al., 1966). Thus this omission is of minimal clinical consequence. Although some authorities still recommend the inclusion of formocresol in the sub-base, current teaching is to omit it.

Concerns about formocresol

Formocresol has recently come under some critical review (Ranly, 1984; Garcia-Godoy, 1986). Three concerns have been raised. Firstly, local toxicity; secondly, the effect of local formaldehyde systemically; and thirdly, mutagenicity and carcinogenicity.

Concerns about the local toxicity of formocresol have been raised because of the histological appearance of tissue fixation. While Ranly (1984) has identified that this does not result in a healing process, the clinical success enjoyed by the technique over several decades appears to have been ignored.

The second concern centres around the potential systemic effect of the formocresol pulpotomy technique (Pashley et al., 1980; Myers et al., 1983). Animal experimentation has demonstrated that full-strength formocresol, when applied to vital pulp tissue, is absorbed systemically and distributed throughout the body. Excretion is via the kidney and lungs; the remaining formocresol is tissue bound to liver, kidney and lungs. The presence, absence and rate of cell recovery from this injury are unknown in experimental animals. The systemic effects of the high numbers of formocresol pulpotomies in the experimental animal needed to produce these changes cannot be equated to a single pulpotomy in a child patient. Ranly (1984) calculated that over 3000 pulpotomies would have to be performed at the same time for formocresol to reach toxic levels systemically.

Ranly's third concern is of mutagenicity and carcinogenicity of formocresol. Since a variety of detoxification steps can occur, he concluded that it is unlikely that the genetic damage reported in cell culture *in vitro* would ever occur *in vivo* following formocresol pulpotomy.

Many of the arguments against formocresol are based upon extrapolation from animal experimentation and laboratory data. Whilst it is appropriate to search for alternatives, it is imperative to re-emphasize the success of formocresol over the past 50 years. Before the clinician should eliminate formocresol from his or her armamentarium, the alternatives need to be shown clinically and histologically to be either as, or more, successful than formocresol. Furthermore, the alternatives have to be as safe as formocresol and proven over the long term.

Glutaraldehyde

Glutaraldehyde has been suggested as an alternative to formocresol in primary tooth pulpotomy. Histological assessment of animal (Davis et al., 1982) and human (Kopel et al., 1980) pulps exposed to a glutaraldehyde pulpotomy technique revealed that a 2% solution results in maintenance of pulp vitality beneath an initial zone of fixation. This initial zone of fixation (as with formocresol) does not proceed apically.

Clinical results (Garcia-Godoy, 1983, 1986) on human primary teeth treated by 2% glutaraldehyde pulpotomy demonstrated 96% success over the first 2 years. Giuliana (1988), using 2% glutaraldehyde, found a 96% success rate at 12 months, while Prakesh et al. (1989) claimed 100% with glutaraldehyde compared with 90% for formocresol. In other studies, Fuks et al. (1990) have shown a failure rate of 18% after 25 months, mainly due to internal resorption.

Other medicaments

Paraformaldehyde devitalizing paste for a two-visit pulpotomy technique has been advocated for many years (Andrew, 1955; Hobson, 1970), although it must be admitted that microscopical evaluation and long-term clinical trials are less well documented than with formocresol. Other commercial products are available but cannot be recommended at present because of the lack of scientific data available from the manufacturers. The medicaments used to devitalize the exposed primary pulp are all similar in that they contain some formalin or paraformaldehyde. All of these compounds suffer from the same fault in that, in our experience, they never work adequately to devitalize the pulp totally. When used, the objective is to place the medicament over an exposed pulp horn and seal it in place for 1–2 weeks. Over this period it is expected that the paraformaldehyde will diffuse through the coronal pulp and devitalize it. In practice this only happens to the part of the coronal pulp adjacent to the paste. When the tooth is opened up to complete the treatment, without local analgesia (because the pulp is now thought to be non-vital!) the child reacts in pain because not all of the pulp tissues have, in fact, been devitalized.

The use of 5% paraformaldehyde as the key constituent in pulpotomies for primary molars has been studied by Hannah and Rowe (1971). Using excellent preoperative criteria, they reported a 98% success over 5 years using 'N_2' as the material placed over the amputated radicular pulp stumps; this was not preceded by wet contact of the amputated stumps with formocresol although the pulpal haemorrhage was controlled by adrenaline-soaked cotton pellets. These results compare very favourably with the success of the single- or two-visit formocresol pulpotomy and they are superior to the two-visit mummifying technique reported by Hobson (1970).

The paraformadehyde technique has been suggested when the time factor or lack of co-operation from the child make it difficult to complete a single-visit pulpotomy, or when an exposure is encountered at the end of a long visit on a young child who is becoming restless. It has been recommended for use when the child does not readily accept local analgesia. However, we vehemently disagree with the concept of exposing unanaesthetized pulps in young children; properly handled local analgesia is less traumatic than a painful vital exposure on a tired child. Correct treatment planning (see Chapter 4) should have included the possibility of pulp therapy and therefore local analgesia should have been provided at the outset. Of course, once local analgesia has been given, there is little justification for not performing a single-visit formocresol pulpotomy.

Beechwood creosote has been recommended and its use is still taught. Its method of application is somewhat similar to paraformaldehyde in that a pledget of cotton wool soaked in the medicament is sealed into a carious cavity, or on an exposed pulp, until the coronal pulp becomes dead. The coronal pulp chamber is then cleaned out and filled with zinc oxide–eugenol. The technique has virtually no research to support its claims and there is no evidence at all as to efficacy and clinical and/or radiographic success. Beechwood creosote is a far more toxic medicament than formocresol and its use has no place in paediatric dentistry.

Ferric sulphate has recently been recommended. The pulpotomy technique is exactly the same as that described but instead of the formocresol a solution of 15.5% ferric sulphate is applied. This chemical causes coagulation of the tissues at the entrances of the root canals, in much the same way as formocresol. A sub-base of zinc oxide–eugenol is placed. Success has been claimed with this technique (Fei et al., 1991) using combined radiographic and clinical assessment after a 1-year follow-up.

Lasers, typically the carbon dioxide laser, have been used experimentally for pulpotomy in dogs (Shoji et al., 1985). It was claimed that the laser caused no pulpal damage but obviously more research is needed, together with clinical trials to determine the effectiveness and the type of laser best suited to pulpotomy techniques.

Cautery (electrosurgery) has been suggested (Ruempling et al., 1983) to fix radicular pulp tissue after amputation of the coronal pulp. Pulpal response was as favourable as that after formocresol. These findings were supported by Shaw et al. (1987). However, further work by Schulman et al. (1987) noted pathological resorption and periapical/furcal pathology. As with lasers, further work on the use of cautery is needed.

Calcium hydroxide has also been recommended for capping the primary radicular pulp stumps. Comparative studies of calcium hydroxide and formocresol in pulpotomies have been performed but the clinical success rate of calcium hydroxide has seldom exceeded 60% (Magnusson, 1970; Schroder, 1978) compared with as high as 98% for formocresol. According to Schroder (1978) the lack of adequate haemostasis before placement of calcium hydroxide adversely affects the treatment outcome. A higher success rate might be achieved by promoting haemostasis of the radicular tissues. Helig et al. (1984) used aluminium chloride on radicular pulp tissue prior to placement of the calcium hydroxide. A more rapid decrease in haemorrhage was noted and after 9 months the aluminium chloride-treated group presented a more favourable result radiographically. There remains at present insufficient evidence to recommend the routine use of calcium hydroxide for pulpotomies in primary teeth.

Conclusion

In conclusion it is worth noting Feigal and Messer's (1990) comments in a critical review of the subject of glutaraldehyde versus formocresol. They concluded that while glutaraldehyde had better fixative properties than formocresol the clinical claims were not yet substantiated. Therefore, any change needs evidence of an improved success and safety. These comments would apply to any new technique or agent. Accordingly formocresol remains, for the present time, the medicament of choice for pulp therapy in primary teeth.

References

Andrew P. (1955) The treatment of infected pulps in deciduous teeth. *Br. Dent. J.* **98**, 122.

Beaver H. A., Kopel H. M. and Saber W. R. (1966) The effect of zinc oxide-eugenol cement on a formocresolized pulp. *J. Dent. Child.* **33**, 381.

Berger J. E. (1965) Pulp tissue reaction to formocresol and zinc oxide-eugenol. *J. Dent. Child.* **32**, 13.

Davis M. J., Myers R. and Switkes M. D. (1982). Glutaraldehyde: an alternative to formocresol for vital pulp therapy. *J. Dent. Child.* **49**, 176.

Doyle W. A. (1961) A comparison of the formocresol pulpotomy technique with the calcium hydroxide pulpotomy technique. Unpublished Thesis, Indiana University.

Duggal M. S. and Curzon M. E. J. (1994) Pulp therapy for

primary teeth. In: *Restorative Techniques in Paediatric Dentistry*. London, Dunitz.

Emmerson C. C. et al. (1959) Pulpal changes following formocresol applications on rat molars and human primary teeth. *J. Calif. Dent. Assoc.* **27**, 309.

Fei A., Udin R. and Johnson R. (1991) A clinical study of ferric sulphate as a pulpotomy agent in ten teeth. *Pediatr. Dent.* **13**, 327.

Feigal R. J. and Messer H. H. (1990) A critical look at glutaraldehyde. *Pediatr. Dent.* **12**, 69.

Fuks A. B. and Bimstein E. (1981) Clinical evaluation of diluted formocresol pulpotomies in primary teeth of school children. *Pediatr. Dent.* **3**, 321.

Fuks A. B. et al. (1990) Assessment of a 2% buffered glutaraldehyde solution in pulpotomies in primary teeth of schoolchildren. *J. Dent. Child.* **57**, 371.

Garcia-Godoy F. (1983) Clinical evaluation of glutaraldehyde pulpotomies in primary teeth. *Acta Odont. Pediatr.* **4**, 41.

Garcia-Godoy F. (1986) A 42-month clinical evaluation of glutaraldehyde pulpotomies in primary teeth. *J. Pedodont.* **10**, 148.

Giuliana G. (1988) Use of glutaraldehyde in the pulpotomy of deciduous teeth. *Stomat. Medit.* **8**, 251.

Hannah D. R. and Rowe A. H. R. (1971) Vital pulpotomy of deciduous molars using N_2 and other materials. *Br. Dent. J.* **130**, 99.

Helig J et al. (1984) Calcium hydroxide pulpotomy for primary teeth. *J. Am. Dent. Assoc.* **108**, 775.

Hobson P. (1970) Pulp treatment of deciduous teeth. *Br. Dent. J.* **128**, 232; 275.

Kennedy D. B. et al. (1973) Formocresol pulpotomy in teeth of dogs with induced pulpal and periapical pathosis. *J. Dent. Child.* **40**, 208.

Kopel H. M. et al. (1980) The effects of glutaraldehyde on primary pulp tissue following coronal amputation: an *in vivo* histologic study. *J. Dent. Child.* **47**, 425.

Loos P. J. and Han S. S. (1971) An enzyme histochemical study of the effect of various concentrations of formocresol on connective tissues. *Oral Surg.* **31**, 571.

Magnusson B. O. (1970) Therapeutic pulpotomy in primary molars – clinical and histologic follow-up. I. Calcium hydroxide paste as a wound dressing. *Odont. Revy* **21**, 415.

Morawa A. P. et al. (1975) Clinical evaluation of pulpotomies using dilute formocresol. *J. Dent. Child.* **42**, 360.

Myers D. R. et al. (1983) Tissue changes induced by absorption of formocresol from pulpotomy sites in dogs. *Pediatr. Dent.* **5**, 6.

Pashley E. L. et al. (1980) Systemic distribution of ^{14}C-formaldehyde from formocresol treated pulpotomy sites. *J. Dent. Res.* **59**, 603.

Paterson S. A. and Curzon M. E. J. (1992) The efficacy of amoxycillin versus penicillin V in the treatment of acutely abscessed primary teeth. *Br. Dent. J.* **174**, 443.

Prakesh C., Chandrah S. and Jaisral J. N. (1989) Formocresol and glutaraldehyde pulpotomies in primary teeth. *J. Pedodont.* **13**, 314.

Pruhs R. I., Olen G. A. and Sharma P. S. (1977) Relationship between formocresol pulpotomy on primary teeth and enamel defects on permanent successors. *J. Am. Dent. Assoc.* **99**, 698.

Ranly D. M. (1984) Formocresol toxicity. Current knowledge. *Acta Odont. Pediatr.* **5**, 93.

Redig D. F. (1968) A comparison and evaluation of two formocresol pulpotomy technics utilizing 'Buckley's' formocresol. *J. Dent. Child.* **35**, 22.

Reumpling D. R., Morten T. H. and Anderson M. (1983) Electrosurgical pulpotomy in primates – a comparison with formocresol pulpotomy. *Pediatr. Dent.* **5**, 14.

Rolling I. and Poulsen S (1978) Formocresol pulpotomy of primary teeth and the occurrence of enamel defects on the permanent successors. *Acta Odont. Scand.* **36**, 243.

Schroder U. (1978) A 2 year follow up of 10 molars pulpotomised with a gentle technique and capped with calcium hydroxide. *Scand. J. Dent. Res.* **86**, 273.

Schulman E. R., McLiver F. T. and Burkes E. (1987) Comparison of electrosurgery and formocresol as pulpotomy techniques in monkey primary teeth. *Pediatr. Dent.* **9**, 189.

Shaw B. W., Sheller B., Barrus B. D. and Morton T. H. (1987) Electrosurgical pulpotomy – a six month study in primates. *J. Endodont.* **13**, 500.

Shoji S., Nakamura, H. and Hariuchi H. (1985) Histopathological changes in dental pulps irradiated with CO_2 laser: a preliminary report on laser pulpotomies. *J. Endodont.* **11**, 379.

Sweet C. A. (1936) Treatment for deciduous teeth with exposed pulps. *Washington Univ. Dent. J.* **3**, 78.

Venham L. L. (1967) Pulpal responses to variation in the formocresol pulpotomy technic: a histological study. Unpublished Thesis, Ohio State University.

Willard R. M. (1976) Radiographic changes following formocresol pulpotomy in primary molars. *J. Dent. Child.* **43**, 414.

Wright G. Z. and Alpern G. D. (1971) Variables influencing children's co-operative behaviour at the first dental visit. *J. Dent. Child.* **38**, 126.

Chapter 19

Pulp therapy techniques – multivisit pulpotomy and pulpectomy

Once the primary pulp has degenerated so that the radicular pulp can no longer be considered healthy, the one-visit pulpotomy is contra-indicated. A two-visit formocresol technique, also known as the non-vital pulpotomy (*Figs* 19.1 and 19.2), has been used in these instances but the success rate is never as good as with the vital pulpotomy. The alternative is to remove as much of the coronal and radicular pulp tissue as possible – a pulpectomy. It should be remembered that the terms 'pulpotomy' and 'pulpectomy' refer to techniques in which the coronal pulp chamber and radicular canals are debrided and later filled, irrespective of pulp status. For simplification of reading, the common terminology, though not strictly accurate, will be used.

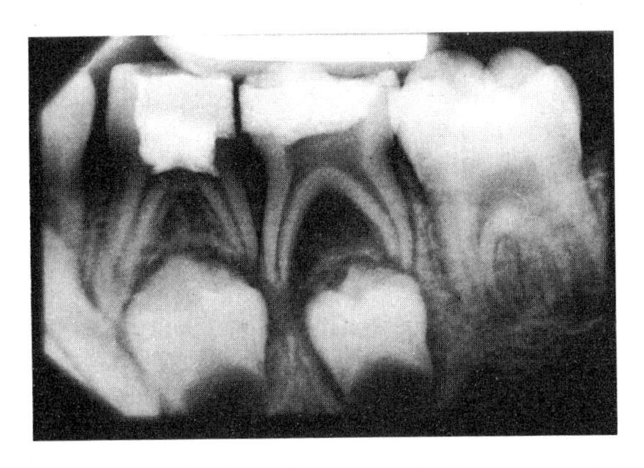

Fig. 19.1. Non-vital mandibular second primary molar with inter-radicular radiolucency. A cotton pellet of formocresol has been sealed in the pulp chamber as an emergency treatment. The tooth was finally treated by a two-visit pulpotomy. A formocresol pulpotomy has been performed on the first primary molar.

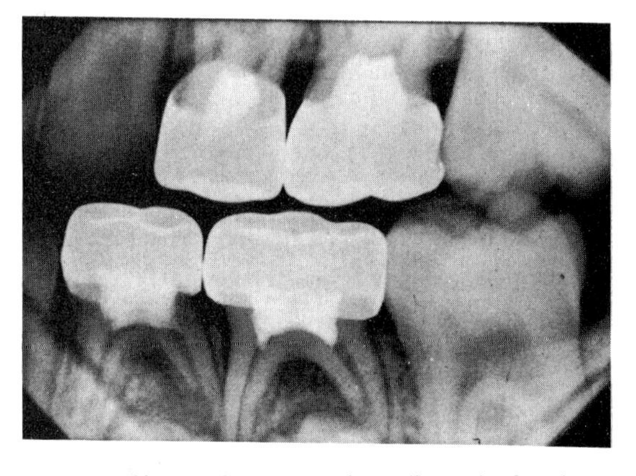

Fig. 19.2. Six-month postoperative radiograph of teeth shown in *Fig.* 19.1 demonstrates bone healing in the bifurcation region.

The success of treating partially vital primary teeth is considerably less than for those with vital, uninflamed pulps. The success is in the order of 50–60% in non-vital primary teeth (Wittich, 1956; Nicholls, 1963). Therefore, the clinician should refer to Chapters 1 and 16 and reconsider the orthodontic implications of extractions. However, the retention of a non-vital, second primary molar in a preschool child is one of the most valuable services that can be provided for the child. The retention of this tooth by heroic pulp therapy during the critical period of first permanent molar eruption can have extensive benefits, if symmetry is maintained by the retention of all other primary teeth (*Figs* 19.1–19.3).

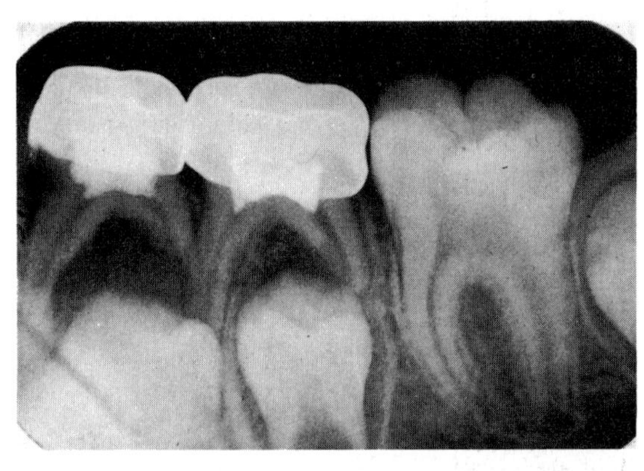

Fig. 19.3. Eighteen-month postoperative radiograph of teeth shown in *Fig.* 19.1 demonstrates good response of supporting tissues to a two-visit pulpotomy on the non-vital second primary molar. Note the resorption on the distal root of the first primary molar: this tooth must be watched carefully.

Two (or more) -visit pulpotomy (partially vital and non-vital primary teeth)

Indications

Historically the indications for a two (or more) -visit pulpotomy procedure in primary teeth are:

(1) inability to arrest haemorrhage from the amputated pulp stumps during a single-visit formocresol pulpotomy;
(2) pus at the exposure site or in the coronal pulp chamber;
(3) presence of an abscess or sinus;
(4) non-vital coronal and/or radicular pulp;
(5) evidence of bone loss in the furcation area.

In our opinion, however, there are really only two indications for performing a two (or more) -visit pulpotomy. These are:

(1) inability to arrest haemorrhage from the amputated pulp stumps during a single-visit formocresol pulpotomy, and
(2) non-vital coronal and/or radicular pulp without the presence of an abscess.

The following preoperative conditions reduce the chances of success (Lawrence, 1966):

(1) internal root resorption,
(2) external pathological root resorption,
(3) gross bone loss at the apex or at the furcation,
(4) pus in the pulp chamber,
(5) pathological mobility,
(6) cellulitis.

Technique

After cleaning out the debris from the pulp chamber (see Single-visit formocresol pulpotomy; Chapter 18) a medicament is sealed on a cotton pellet in the coronal pulp chamber with a temporary cement. This medicament is usually dilute (1/5) formocresol. In the past, other medicaments, such as beechwood creosote or paraform devitalizing paste, have been advocated. However, there have been no research studies to support the use of such medicaments and, indeed, beechwood creosote is considered a very toxic chemical. We only recommend the use of dilute formocresol. Other medicaments, such as glutaraldehyde (Ranly, 1994) can also be used, although the technique is essentially the same. Details of the procedure have been described in Chapter 18. When the pulp is non-vital, devitalization with formocresol or any other paste is obviously redundant; rather, some attempt must be made to control the infection both in the coronal pulp chamber and in the root canals. This can be done either with formocresol or camphorated monochlorophenol. Alternatively, Cresatin, the acetic acid ester of metacresol, is a mild, non-irritating, antibacterial and antifungal agent. It is an effective pulpal anodyne and thus can be used as an intracoronal medicament in primary teeth. It is assumed that the mechanism of action of these drugs in non-vital teeth is by vapour action as well as wet contact. However, the cotton pellet should not be soaked with any drug; instead it should be moist as excess of the drug may irritate the gingiva if it leaks out of the cavity.

At the second visit, 7–10 days later, a non-vital tooth should be symptom-free. The pulp chamber can be filled with a zinc oxide cement in which a drop of dilute formocresol has been mixed. If symptoms persist or an abscess or fistula develops, then a pulpectomy should be performed.

Pulpectomy (partially vital and non-vital primary teeth)

This can be performed as a single- or multivisit procedure for vital and non-vital primary teeth, respectively. The technique is partial or complete according to the penetration of instrumentation. Pulpectomy differs from pulpotomy in that the infected material within the root canals is both pharmacologically and mechanically treated. This is a more biologically sound approach to the treatment of non-vital primary teeth than a two-visit pulpotomy. Flaitz et al (1989) concluded, after an evaluation of multivisit pulpotomy and pulpectomy techniques, that the pulpectomy was superior when the extent of the pulpal changes cannot be determined.

There have been a number of papers describing the technique and claiming success over short and long term (Gould, 1972; Duggal and Curzon, 1989). Recently, a study by Yacobi and Kenny (1991) claimed 76% success for anterior and 84% success for posterior primary teeth over a 12-month follow-up period.

Indications for a pulpectomy

A pulpectomy is ideally indicated instead of a multivisit pulpotomy as described in the previous section. In addition, some further specific indications for a pulpectomy are:

(1) a non-vital tooth associated with an abscess or fistula;
(2) presence of pus at the exposure site or in the pulp chamber;
(3) cellulitis;
(4) extensive furcation pathology.

It is remarkable the degree of repair that is possible with abscessed primary teeth as long as there has not been too much root resorption. Teeth that are mobile, tender to percussion and with considerable cellulitis present can be restored to full function (Paterson and Curzon, 1992) with the use of antibiotics and a pulpectomy.

Single-visit pulpectomy (*Figs* 19.4 and 19.5)

This is applicable to vital teeth where haemorrhage from the amputated radicular stumps is dark red, a slow ooze, and is uncontrollable. Under local analgesia and rubber dam, all accessible radicular pulp tissue is removed with broaches. No attempt should be made to instrument beyond the apex. The canals should be filed with the aim of enlarging them to permit condensation of root-canal filling material. A diagnostic file radiograph is not needed to assess root length but is desirable if practical, as in endodontically treated permanent teeth. Visual comparison of file and root-canal length on the preoperative periapical radiograph will result in sufficient clinical accuracy.

The multiple ramifications of the radicular pulp in a primary molar make complete debridement impossible. Also, the ribbon shape of the root canals, with a narrow mesiodistal width compared to their buccolingual dimension, discourages gross enlargement of the canals. In permanent teeth the object of mechanical preparation is to provide an even, circular, apical one-third of the canal which will be obliterated with an accurately fitting master point. In the primary tooth, attempts to prepare a circular apical one-third mechanically may result in lateral perforation of the canal because of its hour-glass shape. Because of the bizarre anatomy of the root canals the use of barbed broaches as in conventional endodontics may be unsuccessful; at the worst there is increased danger of instrument fracture. Rather, a combined biomechanical preparation of the canals is preferred.

Instruments used in conjunction with irrigating solutions reduce the possibility of fracture, because of the lubricant action of the solution. A 5% solution of sodium hypochlorite has an excellent solvent action and is dilute enough to cause only mild irritation when contacting periapical tissue (Schilder and Amsterdam, 1959). It can be used in a small (15-ml) syringe fitted with a 25-gauge $1\frac{1}{4}$-in (32-mm) needle; provided the needle fits loosely in the canal there is no danger of forcing debris apically. It

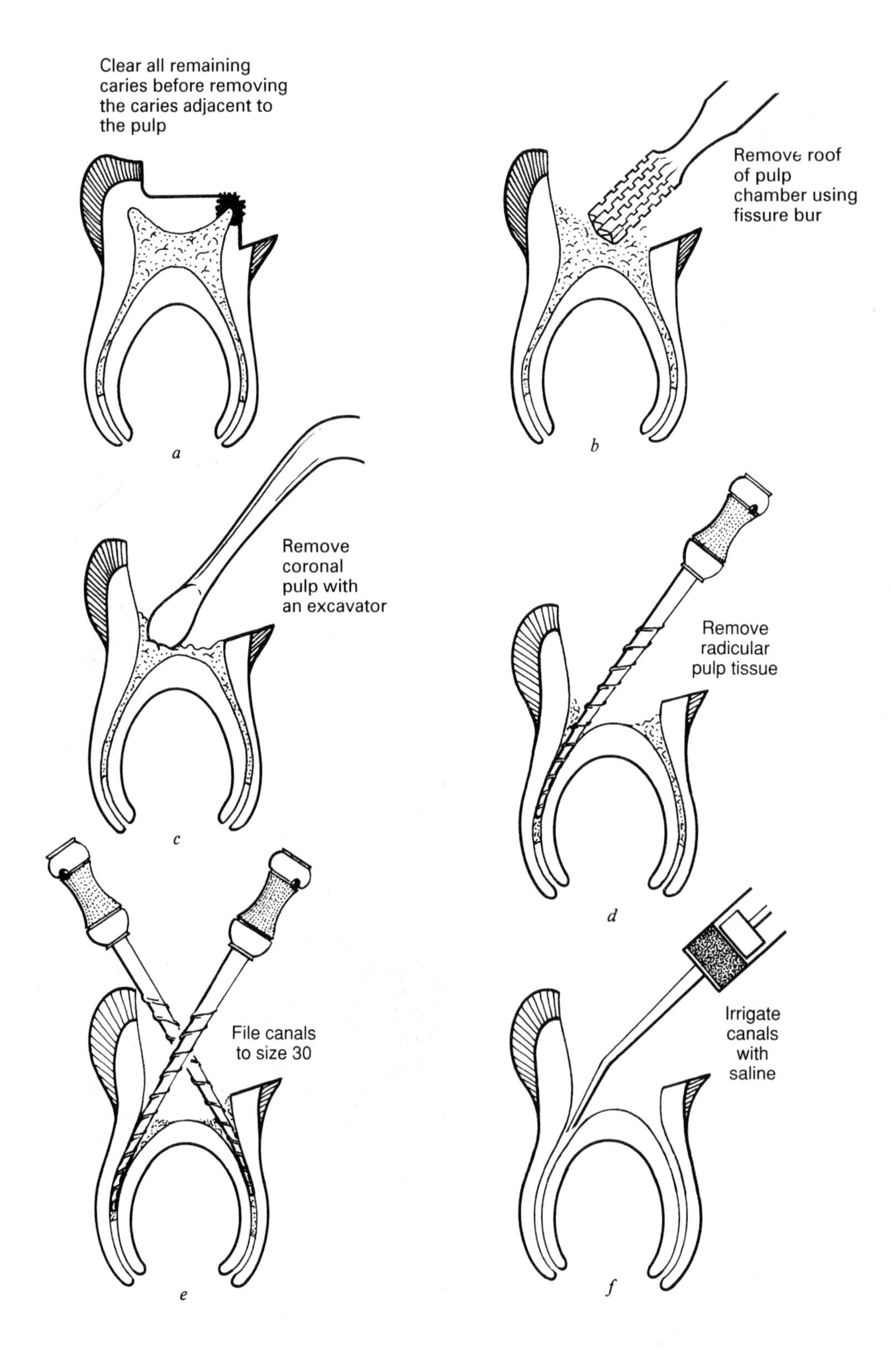
Clear all remaining caries before removing the caries adjacent to the pulp
a
Remove roof of pulp chamber using fissure bur
b
Remove coronal pulp with an excavator
c
Remove radicular pulp tissue
d
File canals to size 30
e
Irrigate canals with saline
f

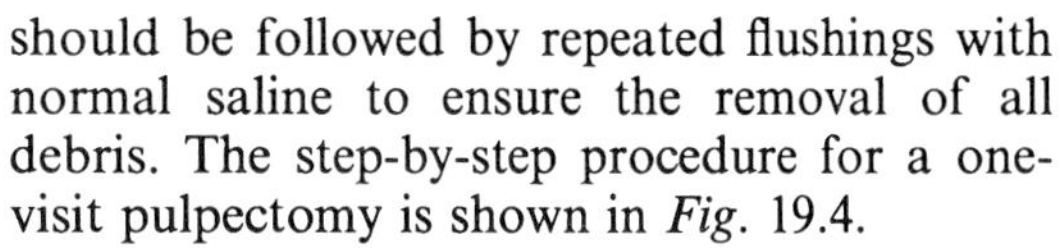

should be followed by repeated flushings with normal saline to ensure the removal of all debris. The step-by-step procedure for a one-visit pulpectomy is shown in *Fig*. 19.4.

Hedstrom files, Nos 15 or 20, are strongly recommended since they remove hard tissue only on withdrawal, which prevents pushing

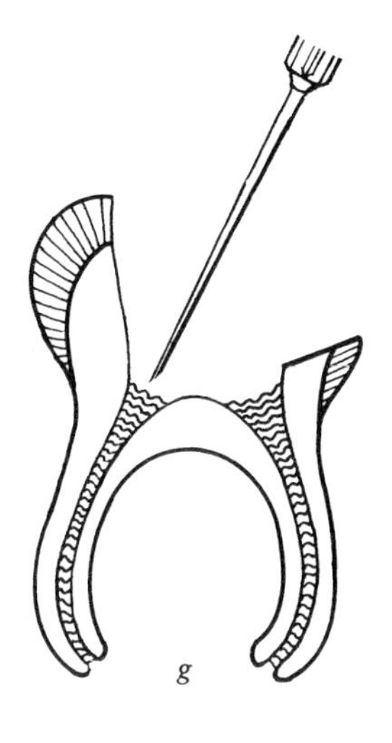

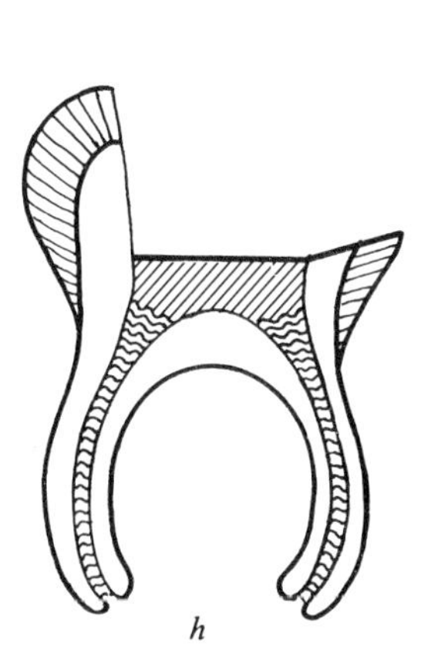

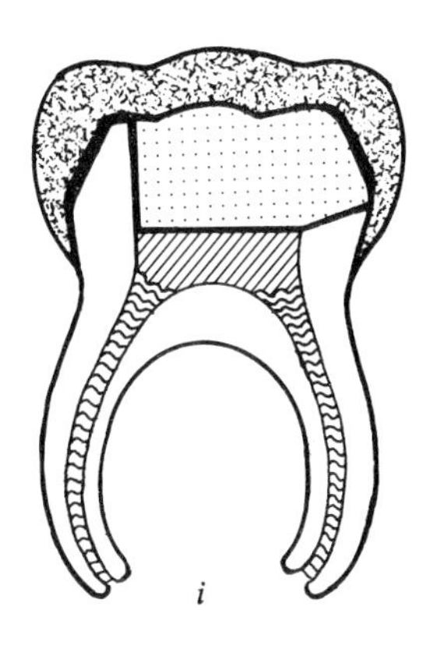

Fig. 19.4. Single-visit pulpectomy procedure.

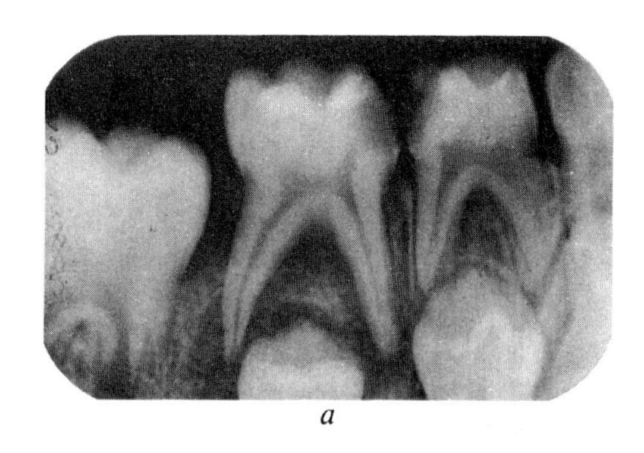

a

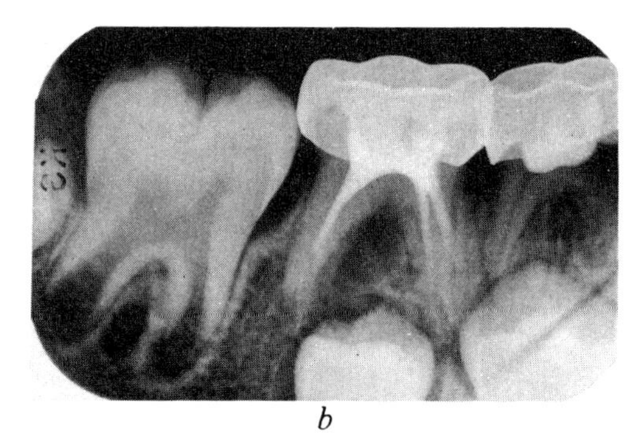

b

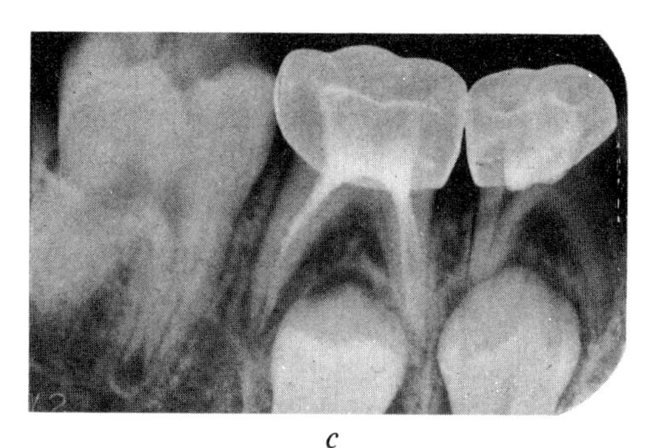

c

Fig. 19.5. Pulpectomy and root-canal filling in non-vital mandibular second primary molar. *a*, Preoperative. Note bone loss and unerupted permanent molar. *b*, 1 year after treatment. Molar erupting. Bone filling in. *c*, 3 years after treatment. Bone healthy. Permanent molar erupted.

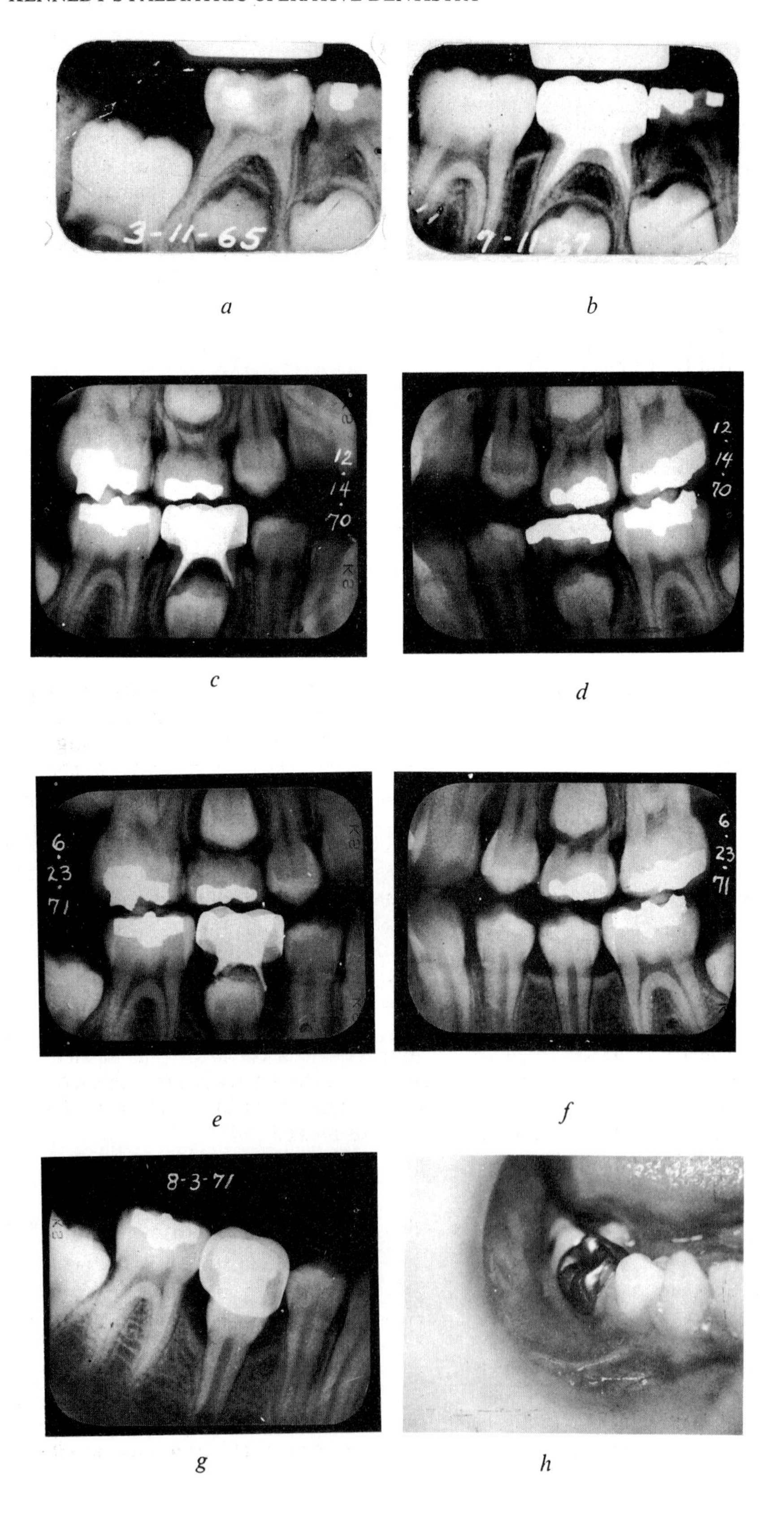

a *b* *c* *d* *e* *f* *g* *h*

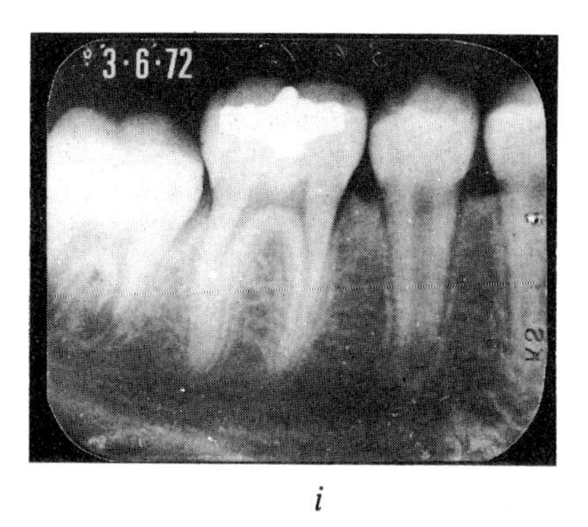

i

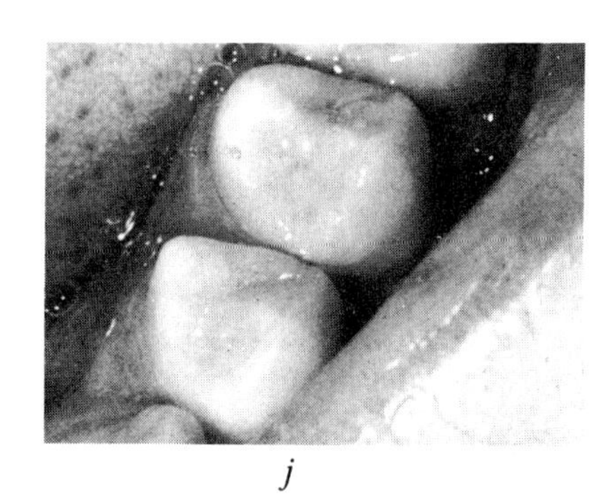

j

Fig. 19.6. Successful pulpectomy and root-canal filling in a mandibular second primary molar. *a*, Preoperative radiograph. *b*, 2 years postoperative. *c*, Slightly delayed resorption compared to untreated antimere in (*d*). *e*, Treated tooth still present. Compare with bitewing radiograph in (*f*). *f*, Antimere to tooth has exfoliated and succedaneous tooth erupted. *g*, Treated tooth deflected buccally. *h*, Deflected, treated tooth. *i*, Erupted premolar. *j*, Photographic evidence of freedom from hypoplasia of succedaneous tooth (mirror image). [Courtesy of Dr Paul Starkey, Indianapolis and *J. Dent. Child.* (1973), **40**, 213.]

infected material through the apices (the maximum size used should be No. 30). For this reason, reamers are definitely not recommended. The limited amount of mouth opening may make access difficult. This can be improved by routinely using a mouth prop and bending the file handles to gain access to the mesial canals of first and second primary molars. The canals should be instrumented to the resistance point; this is evident by tactile sensation and usually corresponds to a curvature in the apical one-third of the root. Each canal should be enlarged three or four instrument sizes greater than the first file capable of working the apex.

After filing, the canals should be irrigated many times (at least 10 flushings are recommended) with saline or chloramine T (Zonite), followed by drying with paper points. A small pledget of cotton wool moist with formocresol is placed in the pulp chamber for 3 min. This is used to 'fix' any remaining pulp tissue in the apical 1–2 mm and any accessory canals that may be present in the floor of the pulp chamber.

The canals are filled when dry with a slurry, the consistency of medium cream, of pure zinc oxide paste. The creamy mix of filling paste can be coated around the walls of the canals with the last-used file or a spiral root-canal filler (Duggal and Curzon, 1994). The spiral root filler should be one size smaller than the last file used and cut with sharp scissors to half its length. This makes it easier to use in a child's mouth but also prevents the filling material being pushed through the apices of the primary tooth. Other techniques are available (Aylard and Johnson, 1987) such as the use of a pressure syringe (Spedding, 1977) or using paper points to carry the paste down into the canals.

Yacobi and Kenny (1991) state that overfilling is not preferrable to underfilling, although experience shows that if small quantities of paste are extruded through the apex then these resorb. For this reason, and that of subsequent exfoliation of the primary tooth, *pure* zinc oxide–eugenol must be used, and not any proprietary brand that may have filler particles present.

Multivisit pulpectomy (*Figs* 19.6 and 19.7)

This procedure is used for non-vital primary teeth and has been studied over the short term (Gould, 1972) and the long term (Starkey, 1973). However, in our experience, most primary teeth can be treated with the single-visit technique. The multivisit pulpectomy is indicated where infection, an abscess or a chronic sinus exist (Paterson and Curzon, 1992).

The clinical technique is similar to that of the single-visit pulpectomy. If the tooth is mobile, if swelling or a fistula is present, or if pus is present in the canals, then only light instrumentation of the canals is recommended at the first visit in order to establish drainage of the pus.

Once the signs and symptoms of swelling and abscess have subsided, usually within 48–72 h, further instrumentation of the canals can be effected (Paterson and Curzon, 1992). Instrumentation can proceed as described previously; local analgesia, to ensure the child suffers no pain, and rubber-dam placement are recommended. This is omitted in cases of swelling and cellulitis. After instrumentation the canals are irrigated as described before.

Between appointments an antibacterial drug, such as dilute formocresol or PMCP, is sealed in the pulp chamber, maintained with a temporary dressing. In instances where the degree of preoperative cellulitis is considerable, drainage will have to be established. A smooth broach should be used to perforate the apices if possible and the tooth left open to drain for no more than 1 day. Leaving the tooth open for longer than 24 h usually results in food packing into the canal. Local measures include warm saline rinses and parental instruction to prevent food packing in the open cavity. Systemic antibiotic therapy is also indicated. The parent should be advised against applying heat externally since this may result in extraoral drainage of the infection. In these acutely abscessed teeth, the coronal pulp chamber can be filled with a formocresol-soaked cotton pellet after 24-h drainage with a dressing.

In these instances, the clinician must realize that swelling may recur after the tooth is closed, so arrangements should be made to see the patient, if necessary, during the weekend or in the evening. However, despite preoperative cellulitis and the need for drainage, pulpectomy in primary molars can be successful and ensure the maintenance of the second primary molar prior to, and during, the active eruption of the permanent first molar (Cartwright and Bevans, 1970).

Appointments are 7–10 days apart. The number of appointments and the timing and extent of instrumentation will be determined by the signs and symptoms at each visit. The canals should not be filled until they are dry and all other signs and symptoms have been eliminated (Lawrence, 1966). The root-canal filling paste is chosen and inserted as in the single-visit pulpectomy.

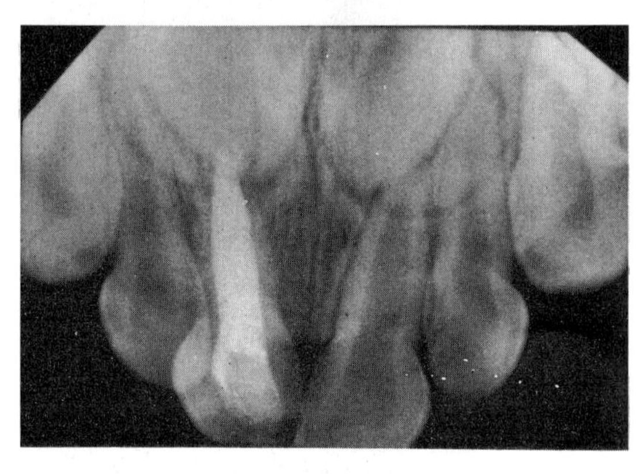

Fig. 19.7. One-year postoperative radiograph of a pulpectomy in a non-vital maxillary primary central incisor. Treatment was performed when the child was 18 months old to maintain space anteriorly in this crowded mouth.

Follow-up of primary teeth with pulpotomy and pulpectomy

Final restoration

For the reasons given in Chapter 14, the ideal restoration for an endodontically treated primary tooth is a preformed (stainless-steel) crown. However, there are instances when it may be acceptable to delay crowning or leave the tooth with an amalgam restoration. For example, extensive occlusal decay in first primary molars due to nursing-bottle mouth syndrome may require a pulpotomy; the short co-operation time of the infant may encourage delay of the crowning unless general anaesthesia is being used. Also the inadvertent or unplanned, traumatic or carious, exposure in a small cavity in a second molar will encourage maintenance with amalgam after formocresol pulpotomy, especially if additional time had not been scheduled to place a crown.

Assessment of success

Rarely does pain occur after pulpotomy and pulpectomy in primary teeth. This may lull the

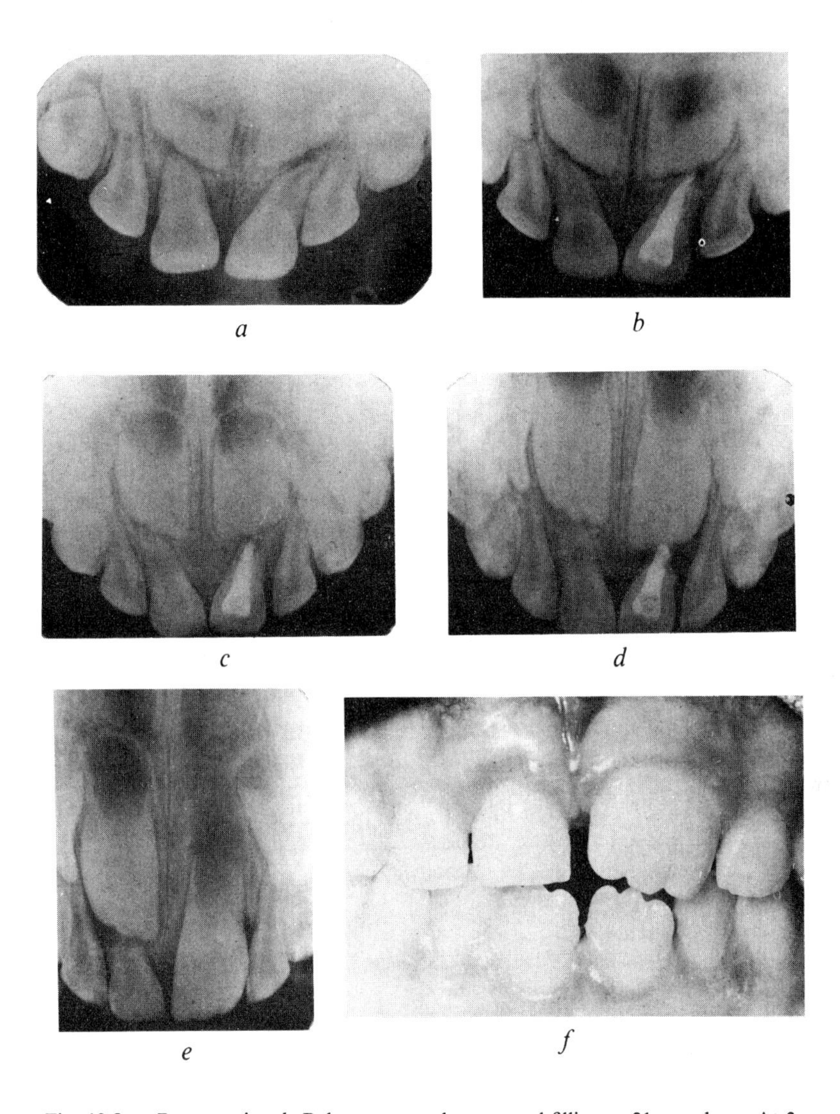

Fig. 19.8. *a*, Preoperative. *b*, Pulpectomy and root-canal filling at 21 months. *c*, At 3 years. *d*, At $4\frac{1}{2}$ years. *e*, At $6\frac{1}{2}$ years. Note premature exfoliation of treated tooth and premature eruption of permanent successor. *f*, Absence of enamel defect on erupted permanent incisor.

clinician into thinking that the treatments are 100% successful. Those who fail to take postoperative radiographs may also claim a low percentage of failures of pulp treatments in primary molars (see *Fig*. 19.7).

Postoperative follow-up at 6-monthly intervals should include an evaluation of signs and symptoms; periapical radiographs should be taken between 12 and 18 months postoperatively. Pathological mobility, the presence of a fistula and, in rare instances, pain (usually to percussion) are clinical evidence of failure. Radiographic evidence of failure is judged by the appearance, or increased size, of a radiolucency, and by external or internal root resorption. Any bone loss is likely to occur at the furcation region and not at the apices (see Chapter 17). The radiographic observation of bone repair is evidence of success, together with absence of signs and symptoms (Barr et al., 1991). Those teeth that show neither an increase nor a decrease in preoperative radiolucency must be considered successfully treated, in the absence of signs and symptoms. However, they must be closely evaluated to observe any changes in size of any radiolucency.

In the study by Yacobi et al. (1991) they reported a higher rate of resorption of the anterior teeth treated with pulpectomy than for posterior teeth. However, as the anterior primary incisors naturally resorb at an early age, and it was only a 12-month study, it would not be surprising for this finding to occur. Delayed resorption of the primary teeth during eruption of the permanent successors post-pulpectomy has not been reported.

Accurate postoperative follow-up requires meticulous maintenance of the patient's records. For example, it is impossible to evaluate a postoperative radiolucency without a preoperative radiograph to serve as a baseline. Preoperative signs and symptoms, such as the type and duration of pain, mobility, and presence of a fistula should be recorded, as well as the medicaments used. With accurate treatment records come pride in one's work and a superior service for the child.

Vital primary teeth treated by pulpotomy that later exhibit fistulae, internal resorption or bone loss should be treated by extraction or by pulpectomy. Most of these teeth have already received a considerable investment of time. Their value in maintaining the integrity of developing occlusion must be reassessed and appropriate treatment performed.

It is a clinical impression that the succedaneous permanent tooth also erupts prematurely (*Fig.* 19.8).

Eruption of the permanent successor

Hobson (1970) reported premature exfoliation of primary teeth treated by two-visit mummification pulpotomy when compared to caries-free antimeres. More rapid external root resorption because of failure to control infection and the inflammatory process accounts for this premature loss. In non-vital teeth treated by pulpotomy and pulpectomy, premature root resorption is more marked.

Any root-filling material placed either in the coronal pulp chamber or in the root canals must be resorbable. Pure zinc oxide fulfils this requirement. However, the material is not of the same texture or hardness as normal tooth or vital pulp. Thus when the erupting permanent successor meets root-filling material, there is a possibility of deflection, but this is most unlikely if pure zinc oxide has been used.

One major disadvantage of pulpectomy compared with pulpotomy in primary teeth is the increased likelihood of resorption problems. However, it has been documented that pulpectomy in a primary molar can be followed by proper eruption of the permanent successor (Starkey, 1973). Most problems associated with resorption arise when the erupting tooth has resorbed the pulpal floor of the primary molar and is contacting the material in the coronal pulp chamber. This is the time when the clinician least suspects trouble. Ankylosis of the primary tooth and deflection of the permanent successor can occur at this critical stage. The improper eruption of permanent successors can negate the benefit of the many previous years of successful pulp therapy.

References

Aylard S. R. and Johnson R. (1987) Assessment of filling techniques for primary teeth. *Pediatr. Dent.* **9**, 195.

Barr E. S., Flaitz C. M. and Hicks M. J. (1991) A retrospective radiographic evaluation of primary molar pulpotomies. *Pediatr. Dent.* **13**, 4

Cartwright H. V. and Bevans G. L. (1970) Management of two abscessed primary molars in a four-year-old child: report of interesting case. *J. Dent. Child.* **37**, 230.

Duggal M. S. and Curzon M. E. J. (1989) Restoration of the broken down primary molar: I. pulpectomy technique. *Dent. Update.* **16**, 26.

Duggal M. S. and Curzon M. E. J. (1994) Pulp therapy for primary teeth. In: *Restorative Techniques in Paediatric Dentistry.* London, Dunitz.

Flaitz C. M. et al. (1989) Radiographic evaluation of pulp therapy for primary anterior teeth. *J. Dent. Child.* **56**, 182.

Gould I. M. (1972) Root canal therapy for infected primary molar teeth – preliminary report. *J. Dent. Child.* **39**, 269.

Hobson P. (1970) Pulp treatment of deciduous teeth. *Br. Dent. J.* **128**, 232, 275.

Lawrence R. P. (1966) A method of root canal therapy for primary teeth. Unpublished Thesis, Emory University School of Dentistry.

Paterson S. A. and Curzon M. E. J. (1992) The effect of amoxycillin versus penicillin V in the treatment of acutely abscessed primary teeth. *Br. Dent. J.* **174**, 443.

Ranly D. M. (1994) Pulpotomy therapy in primary teeth: new modalities for old rationals. *Pediatr. Dent.* **16**, 403.

Schilder H. and Amsterdam M. (1959) The inflammatory potential of root canal medicaments. *Oral Surg.* **12**, 211.

Spedding R. H. (1977) Root canal treatment for primary teeth. *Dent. Clin. North Am.* **17**, 1.

Starkey P. E. (1973) Pulpectomy and root canal filling in a primary molar. Report of a case. *J. Dent. Child.* **40**, 213.

Wittich H. C. (1956) Treatment of pulps of deciduous and young permanent teeth. *J. Can. Dent. Assoc.* **22**, 142.

Yacobi R. and Kenny D. J. (1991) Evolving primary pulp therapy technique. *J. Am. Dent. Assoc.* **122**, 83.

Chapter 20

Pulp therapy techniques – young permanent teeth

General considerations

When young permanent teeth have large carious lesions which are radiographically close to the pulp or involving it, the clinician should evaluate the patient orthodontically. The aesthetic desirability of maintaining anterior permanent teeth should be obvious. Yet heroic, time-consuming and costly pulp treatment to maintain first permanent molars may not be justified when crowding exists. In crowded or potentially crowded mouths, thought should be given to extracting grossly carious first permanent molars, followed where and when necessary by active orthodontic treatment. It is imperative that the child has the benefit of orthodontic consultation before such a drastic step is taken. Orthodontic treatment planning in relation to the first permanent molar has been excellently outlined by Crabb and Rock (1971) and the reader is referred to this article for clinical application.

There are instances when pulpally involved, young permanent teeth must be maintained either permanently or, as is sometimes the case with first permanent molars, temporarily, while awaiting the eruption of other permanent teeth prior to active orthodontic therapy. A complicating factor in treatment is the state of apical development. As a rule, root closure in permanent teeth occurs 3 years after eruption. These teeth often present with large carious lesions involving the pulp prior to normal root closure. This makes conventional endodontic treatment impractical. It will be assumed here that such teeth require maintaining, if only over the short term, after orthodontic evaluation. The retention of the first permanent molar is often required until the bifurcation of the roots of the second permanent molar is seen on a diagnostic radiograph. The formation of the bifurcation indicates the optimum time for extraction of the first permanent molars (Houston et al., 1992). In some children, extensive decay of the first permanent molars may need treatment in order to maintain these teeth for an interim period.

Pulp therapy for the permanent teeth may include the treatment of the permanent incisors. This may be due to dental caries, although these days this is fortunately not common because of the preventive effects of fluoride. Where caries of the permanent incisors has led to a need for pulp therapy the situation is likely to be very serious and careful attention must be paid to the treatment plan needed for the *whole* mouth. More likely these days, pulp therapy for incisors is the result of trauma.

The treatment regimens applicable to young permanent teeth (molars) are:

(1) indirect pulp treatment;
(2) direct pulp capping;
(3) pulpotomy;
(4) pulpectomy – to induce root end repair of the open apex; and
(5) pulpectomy – when the apices are closed.

Indirect pulp treatment

Indirect pulp treatment, while contraindicated in primary teeth, is applicable to vital, young permanent teeth with large carious lesions closely approximating the pulp. The aims of treatment are to remove the bulk of the lesion and to protect the pulp so that it can repair itself by laying down secondary dentine. In this way pulp exposure is avoided.

Indications

- Deep asymptomatic lesions which are radiographically close to, but not involving, the pulp in vital young permanent teeth.
- Signs of neglected mouths, including rampant caries, severe breakdown of the dentition in a young school-age child or pre-teenager.

The first indication follows logically from the material presented in Chapters 16 and 17. The second indication warrants further discussion. When faced with mouths which exemplify problems of this type, the dentist may find that several teeth are possible candidates for some form of pulp therapy. The rate of carious attack is a potential source of frustation to child, parent and practitioner as attempts to tackle the problem tooth by tooth result in permanent treatment to individual teeth while the overall level of disease progresses unhindered. Indeed, several teeth that might have been rescued at the time of initial treatment may be committed to extraction when they finally are treated, the decay having progressed unchecked while other teeth have been cared for. Stabilizing the level of decay in a mouth by indirect pulp treatment in these instances results in the following advantages.

(1) The decay process in each treated tooth is arrested or at least slowed down. This gives the pulp a chance to repair.
(2) The acidogenic bacterial count of the mouth is markedly reduced as the superficial aspects of the carious lesion contain most of the bacteria; by reducing the bacterial flora the oral environment is less conducive to active plaque metabolism.
(3) With lesions closed, time is available to implement a preventive programme and to assess the patient's (parent's) co-operation with this. The use of caries monitoring tests, such as Dentocult® (Ivoclar–Vivadent, Meridian South, Leicester LE3 2WY), is useful here to check on compliance while at the same time carious cavities are brought under control.
(4) The mouth is restored to function and the threat of dental pain reduced or removed.
(5) Pulp exposure is avoided by successful indirect pulp treatment.

Contraindications (individual permanent teeth)

- Spontaneous pain – pain at night
- Swelling
- Fistula
- Tenderness to percussion
- Pathological mobility
- External root resorption
- Internal root resorption
- Periapical or inter-radicular radiolucency
- Pulp calcifications

Technique

Local analgesia is recommended as all the decay except that which would expose the pulp is to be removed. In addition, there are often a number of teeth in a quadrant requiring treatment. Some clinicians doubt the need for local analgesia for this technique as the superficial layers of gross lesions are necrotic. However, as a cavity needs to be rendered caries-free in the coronal aspects, local analgesia is a wise precaution. Failure to anaesthetize a tooth may well lead to pain for the child and compromise future co-operation.

Indirect pulp treatment differs markedly from the simple removal of gross caries, where superficial caries is quickly excavated without analgesia and a dressing placed. This approach is appropriate as an emergency procedure and a cavity preparation is not refined to include the use of rotary instruments. The sequence of treatment and required outcome in specific, indirect pulp treatment is shown in *Fig.* 20.1.

After analgesia and isolation with rubber

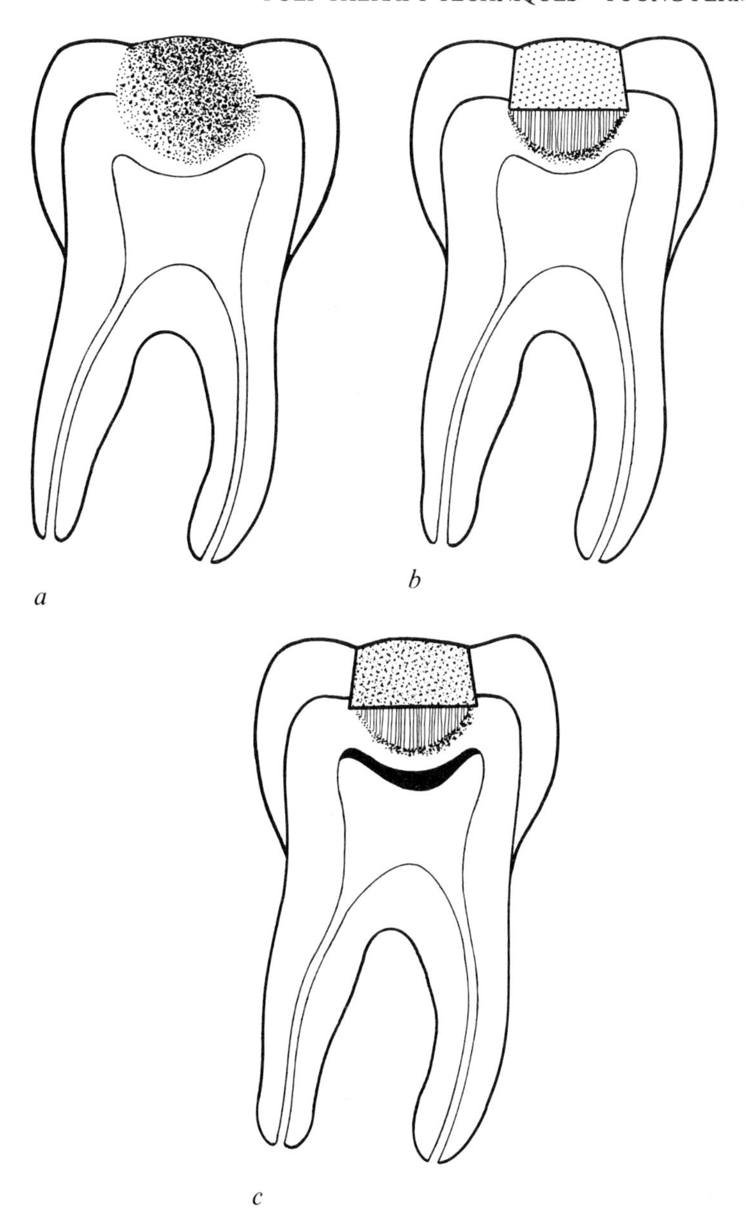

Fig. 20.1. Indirect pulp treatment. *a*, Preoperative appearance of a deep lesion close to the pulp in an asymptomatic vital tooth. *b*, All decay is removed except that which may expose the pulp and a calcium hydroxide base is placed. *c*, The residual decay is arrested and the pulp has repaired by laying down secondary dentine. A final restoration can then be placed.

dam the cavity outline form is made. All margins are left adequately supported and peripheral caries is removed with a large, round bur. The amelodentinal junction must be free from all softened material and stain, even if the stain is firm. All decay, except that which in the operator's experience lies immediately over the pulp, should be removed. The remaining carious material should not be soft, moist or have a leathery texture. Knowledge of pulp-horn morphology, with the use of radiographs and clinical experience, allows the practitioner to estimate at which point the caries removal should stop. The mesiobuccal pulp horns of young first permanent molars are often quite superficially placed and the preoperative radiograph may help to locate them. Should a pulp horn be exposed, then the tooth becomes a candidiate for pulp capping.

A protective base must be placed prior to any temporary restoration; this restoration is intermediate until such time as the continued vitality of the tooth is assured and there is radiographic evidence of pulpal repair. Both zinc oxide–eugenol and calcium hydroxide–methyl cellulose sub-bases stimulate secondary dentine formation (Kerkhove et al., 1967). The clinician should be aware of the possibility of undetected microscopical exposure (Chapter 17) when excavating deep lesions. As zinc oxide induces an inflammatory response in direct pulp capping, so a calcium hydroxide–methyl cellulose sub-base is recommended. It is as effective as zinc oxide–eugenol in indirect pulp capping, and it is the material of choice for direct pulp capping. Although most researchers have used pure calcium hydroxide compounds, the commercially available products are also successful. They have adequate strength to withstand the condensation pressures of amalgam.

The removal of bacteria and substrate, together with an effective seal of restoration (either intermediate or permanent), provides the means whereby the pulp can recover by laying down secondary dentine. When an intermediate restoration is placed, retention and sealing must be assured; accordingly, the use of the reinforced glass-ionomer cements is recommended. Failure of the intermediate restoration will result in unnecessary pulp irritation and an increased risk of pathosis. If necessary the intermediate restoration can be supported by placing an orthodontic band cemented to the tooth.

Parental acceptance of the technique is largely determined by the way that the dentist explains it. The avoidance of direct pulp therapy, particularly in young permanent teeth with incompletely formed apices, is attractive. It is, however, important that the parent realizes the significance of the treatment approach; thus the intermediate restoration should be presented as a 'treatment filling' rather than a 'temporary filling'. As discussed earlier, the term 'temporary filling' should be avoided as it implies that a filling required little effort; this belies the importance of maintaining pulp vitality. Indeed the filling may well be left for many months until a secondary dentine bridge has formed and is certainly therefore not temporary. The term 'treatment filling' implies an active process and it leads logically to the need for further visits to evaluate the success of the indirect pulp capping.

Postoperative evaluation

Successful indirect pulp treatment is evaluated by the absence of signs and symptoms, the radiographic evidence of secondary dentine formation, and the arrest of the lesion judged clinically by the hardness of the floor of the cavity. Before the re-entry visit the signs and symptoms should be checked, as with the preoperative evaluation. In young permanent teeth vitality tests should be performed. Radiographs need not be taken at the next evaluation visit; however, after a 6-month period radiographs will be needed as part of the continuing care of the child. These should include periapicals or bitewings sufficient to show the coronal pulp area of the permanent molar(s) treated indirectly (*Fig.* 20.1*c*). These radiographs will often show a radiopaque area pulpal to the sub-base of the intermediate restoration. This is interpreted as secondary or reparative dentine. However, radiopacities which remain undetected to the eye can still be demonstrated by laboratory techniques (Geller et al., 1971). Thus the clinician should not rely too heavily on the absence of this radiographic finding. Rather the combined evidence of clinical and radiographic findings should be the guide.

The tooth should be re-entered after a minimum of 12 weeks, although some recommend 6–8 weeks (McDonald and Avery, 1994). Traubman (1967) demonstrated that the rate of reparative dentine formation was highest during the first month and then diminished with time. The thinner the pulpal floor, the faster the rate of repair. He also found that reparative dentine continued to form, although at a slower rate, for a period of 9–12 months. Traubman stated that apparent pulp exposures can be avoided by allowing for significant amounts of protective secondary dentine to form before re-entry.

Provided the intermediate restoration is sound and there are no symptoms, clinically or radiographically, no harm is done by leaving the restoration for up to a year. Indeed, if after a year the tooth is entirely symptom-free and a periapical radiograph shows reparative dentine and no furcation or periapical pathology, there is no reason not to leave the tooth well alone and the intermediate restoration is left as a permanent restoration.

In the past, re-entry into the tooth treated by indirect pulp therapy has been recommended (Kennedy, 1986). In this approach, after a period of 6–8 weeks, the treatment filling is removed as well as the sub-base to check on the firmness of the cavity floor. The aim was to confirm that the caries was arrested and hard. Current thinking, and our present view, is that if the tooth has remained entirely symptomless then there is no need to reopen it.

Direct pulp capping

Direct pulp capping in young permanent teeth is applicable to small, mechanical or carious exposures when it is believed that there is no pulp pathology adjacent to the exposure site. The aim is to ensure that the pulp can remain healthy and even repair in response to the capping medicament.

Indications

The technique is indicated in mechanical exposures of less than 1 mm^2 surrounded by clean dentine in vital young permanent teeth. Usually these are teeth with open apices. Direct pulp capping and pulp curettage enjoy a high success rate in young permanent teeth. It is hypothesized that the increased blood supply from the wide open apical foramina of young permanent teeth increases the pulp's ability to respond favourably to direct capping.

Contraindications

The contraindications to direct pulp capping are the same as those for indirect pulp capping (listed above) with the addition of:

- mechanical exposures where an instrument has been pushed inadvertently into the pulp tissue;
- profuse haemorrhage from the exposure site;
- pus or exudate at the exposure site.

The success of the treatment is dependent upon:

- making an accurate preoperative assessment;
- preventing unneccessary bacterial contamination of the exposed pulp;
- avoiding pressure on the exposed pulp (see Technique).

The presence of bacteria has been shown to reduce the chances of successful pulp capping in animal studies (Kakehashi et al., 1965). For this reason, mechanical exposures where a contaminated instrument has been pushed inadvertently into the pulp are a contraindication of pulp capping. The traumatic insult, along with the introduction of bacteria, significantly reduces the chances of success. Similarly, forcing chips of infected carious dentine into the pulp tissue reduces success.

Technique

The rubber dam provides the only means of working in a sterile environment. Thus the anticipated success of pulp capping will be increased when the rubber dam is used, although this remains clinically undocumented. As has been discussed before (Chapter 7) the use of rubber dam should be routine for all restorative work in children; however, should an exposure occur when working under isolation with cotton-wool rolls only, the operator should continue the treatment as quickly as possible and not attempt to place a dam. Bacterial contamination of the exposed pulp would be inevitable during the dam application even if the exposure were to be covered with a cotton pellet. Should contamination occur then the clinician should consider either a partial pulpotomy technique (see below) as described by Mejare and Cvek (1993) or root-canal therapy.

Once an exposure is encountered, further manipulation of the pulp should be avoided. The cavity should be irrigated with saline, chloramine T or distilled water, and the haemorrhage arrested with *light* pressure from sterile cotton pellets. While the pulp-capping material is being placed, pressure, which would force it into the pulp chamber, should be avoided. Calcium hydroxide compounds are recommended for direct pulp capping, although other materials have been suggested (see below). As further pressure is to be avoided, a cement base should be placed prior to any final restoration whenever possible. The marginal

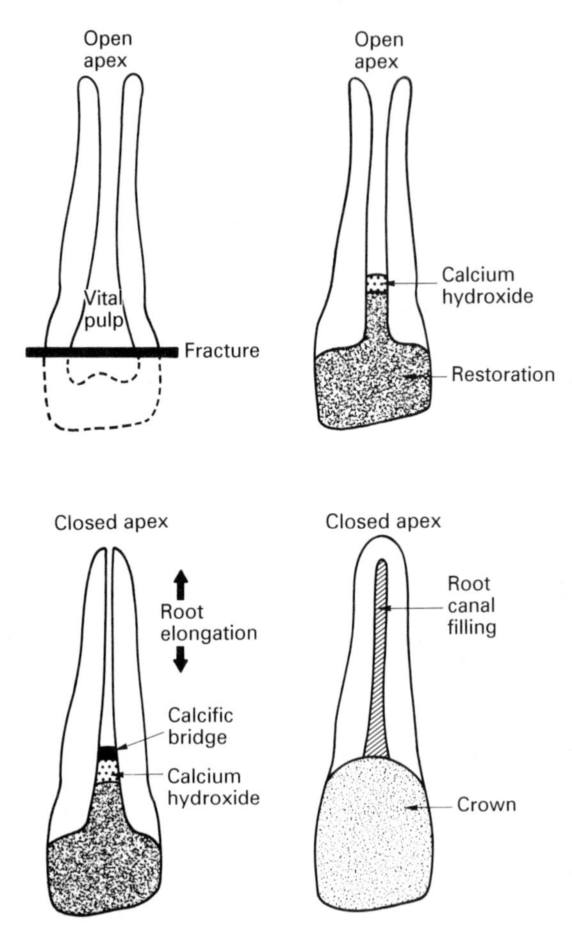

Fig. 20.2. *Top left:* Class 3 fracture, vital pulp; open apex. *Top right:* calcium hydroxide pulpotomy. *Bottom left:* apical closure after calcium hydroxide pulpotomy. *Bottom right:* completed root-canal treatment.

seal of the final restoration must adequately prevent ingress of saliva and bacteria to ensure success.

Choice of direct pulp-capping material

1. Calcium hydroxide

Short-term results (up to 12 months) of pulp capping cariously exposed primary teeth indicate a 75% success (Jepperson, 1971) compared with over 90% for formocresol pulpotomy (Morawa et al., 1975). It is for this reason that the formocresol pulpotomy is preferred for primary teeth. However, for permanent teeth the success rate for pulp capping with calcium hydroxide is much better (McDonald and Avery, 1994) and is to be preferred.

2. Corticosteroid/antibiotic cements

Some clinicians use Ledermix cement for pulp capping. It consists of a powder made up of demethylchlortetracycline hydrochloride and triamcinolone acetonide with zinc oxide and calcium hydroxide, together with a liquid catalyst. Hargreaves (1969) reported its use to be superior to calcium hydroxide in pulp capping primary teeth. However, there have been no other clinical trials of its use in primary teeth. In permanent teeth it also has its advocates.

However, the use of Ledermix can only be as a very temporary measure in an emergency. Rather the clinician should focus on treating the exposure in such a way as to enhance the chances of long-term success. This means the use of pulpotomies or pulpectomies in young permanent teeth.

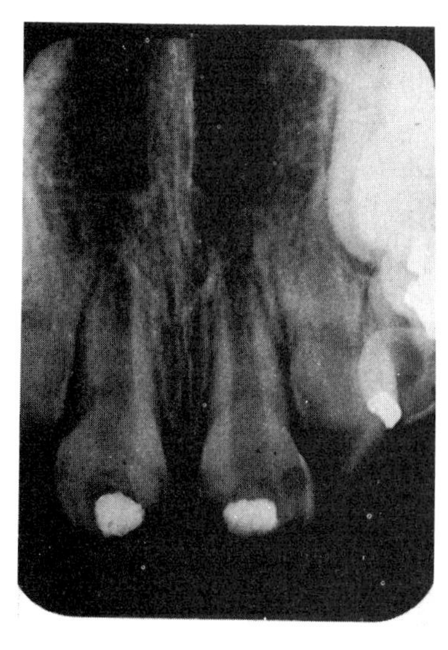

Fig. 20.3. Calcium hydroxide pulpotomies have been performed to treat exposed pulps when the apices are incompletely formed. The child was 7 years old.

Pulpotomy – vital permanent teeth with open apices

Technique

Large, vital exposures in permanent teeth with incompletely formed apices warrant treatment by calcium hydroxide pulpotomy (*Figs* 20.2–20.5). The aim is to remove the infected coronal pulp and place calcium hydroxide over the healthy radicular stumps after the inflamed coronal pulp has been amputated. A calcific barrier should form in response to the calcium hydroxide and the radicular pulp should retain its vitality so that root closure can occur (*Fig.* 20.4). The coronal pulp chamber of the permanent molar is considerably deeper than in primary teeth. In fact, using normal-length burs, there is little chance of perforating the pulpal floor of a permanent molar. Long-shanked burs may be required to remove all coronal pulp. The level of amputation in permanent incisor pulpotomy is at the estimated cementum–enamel junction. Haemorrhage should be arrested with cotton pellets prior to placement of calcium hydroxide–methyl cellulose mixed with water or saline. A final restoration can be placed at the same visit if time permits, or can be placed much later (*Fig.* 20.5).

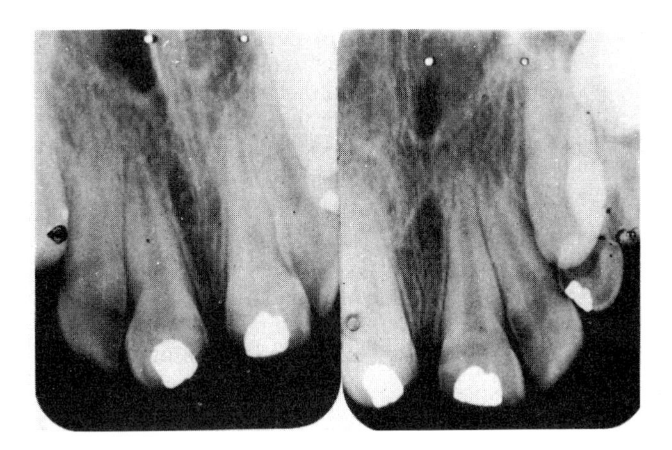

Fig. 20.4. Radiographs $2\frac{1}{2}$ years later than in *Fig.* 20.3 show calcific bridges, continuation of growth in root length and apical closure. Root-canal filling is indicated to prevent further linear calcification of the canal.

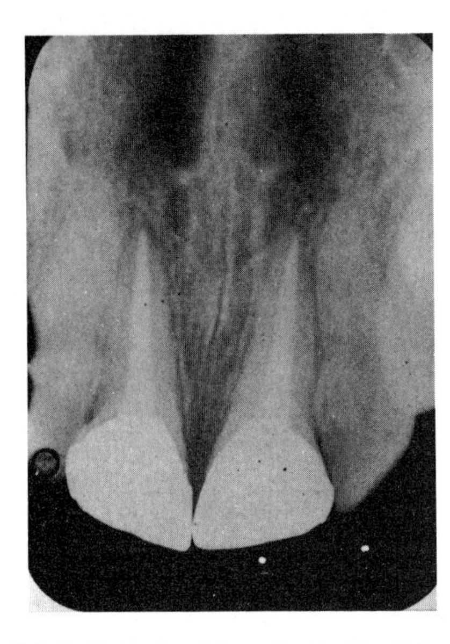

Fig. 20.5. Radiographs of the patient in *Figs* 20.3 and 20.4 taken 1 year after completion of root-canal therapy and crowning. Note well-condensed root fillings and healthy periapical tissues. The child is now 12 years old.

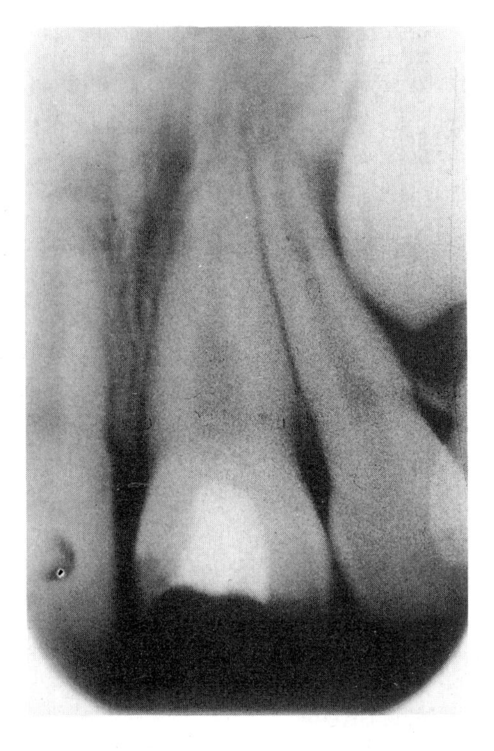

Fig. 20.6. Radiograph showing linear calcification of root canal.

Follow-up

Clinical and radiographical follow-up is identical to that for pulpally treated primary teeth. Apical development is monitored by comparison with the preoperative periapical radiograph and where possible with a normal, untreated antimere. Formation of a calcific bridge, continued apical development, absence of internal resorption and periapical radiolucency are radiographic evidence of success (*Fig*. 20.4). Often there is a linear calcification along the length of the root canal after formation of a calcific bridge (*Fig*. 20.6). This has been labelled calcific metamorphosis and is considered to be a pathological rather than physiological process (Patterson and Mitchell, 1965). It will progress until the canal will appear to be completely calcified radiographically.

Many clinicians are content to call this nature's efforts at root filling. However, microscopical evaluation of such teeth reveals pulp remnants which may slowly become non-vital through self-strangulation. One school of thought favours leaving the tooth well alone and allowing the sclerosis of the root canal to take place. On the other hand, bacteria may migrate within these root-canal spaces, perhaps undetectable on the radiograph, and periapical pathology may result (*Fig*. 20.7). Of course, once the canal has calcified to this extent, it may be impossible to negotiate it with instruments, even with the use of chelating agents such as EDTA (ethylene diaminetetra-acetic acid). This commits the tooth either to extraction or to apical surgery and retrograde root filling.

Calcium hydroxide pulpotomy should thus be considered as the first stage of treatment for vital, cariously or traumatically exposed, permanent teeth with incompletely formed apices, and the aim is to permit normal apical closure (*Figs* 20.2–20.5). The second phase of treatment is conventional root canal filling, once the apices have been closed; in addition to apical closure, the root continues its normal growth to assume normal length and thickening of root canal walls. The state of apical development and the speed of calcific metamorphosis will decide the exact timing of pulpectomy and root-canal therapy. It should be re-emphasized that watchful waiting can result in subsequent inability to instrument a calcified canal.

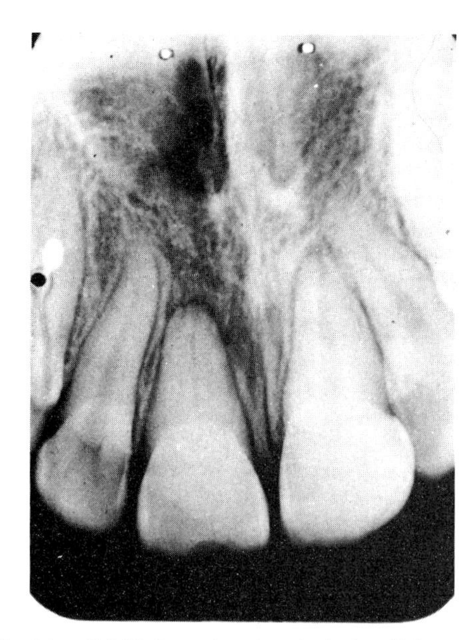

Fig. 20.7. Calcified canal and periapical radiolucency; whenever linear calcification occurs, root-canal therapy must be considered.

Induction of root-end repair – non-vital permanent teeth with open apices

General considerations

The permanent tooth with a vital but degenerating, or a non-vital, pulp and with incompletely formed apices presents a severe problem. The open apex and so-called 'blunderbuss canal' defy attempts at conventional root-canal therapy because the apical dimensions of the canal exceed those at the coronal access area. The treatment alternatives are root-canal therapy followed by apical surgery or induction of root-end repair followed at a later stage by conservative root-canal therapy.

The techniques of root-canal filling and apical surgery are described in texts on endodontics. However, this approach is not recommended as the first choice of treatment for several reasons. First, surgical techniques are to be avoided whenever possible in young children. Second, the thin apical walls of the young permanent tooth make apical surgery even more difficult. If a retrograde filling procedure is necessary to obtain an adequate apical seal, these thin walls do not lend themselves to undercutting to obtain retention or to condensation pressure if amalgam is used. Finally, the root, which is already short because of its incomplete formation, is further reduced by apical surgery. This has potentially far-reaching effects in terms of adequacy of periodontal support. For these reasons, the non-surgical approach of induction of root-end repair is indicated for non-vital permanent teeth with incompletely formed apices. The principles of treatment are to debride and sterilize the canal before filling it with a calcium hydroxide paste; saturating the periapical tissues with calcium ions, together with the elimination of bacteria, stimulates physiological calcific repair at the apex. When repair is complete, conventional root therapy can be performed using lateral and apical condensation against the repaired, calcified apical tissue (*Figs* 20.8 and 20.9). This technique is called apexification.

This treatment is often required in incisors rather than in molars because of the prevalence of untreated Ellis Class II fractures (involving dentine) in 7- and 8-year-olds, whose incisor apices would be incompletely formed. Subsequent pulp death may occur prior to apical closure.

Technique

Preoperative assessment includes clinical evaluation of colour, mobility, tenderness to percussion and swelling. Periapical radiographs may demonstrate the preoperative root length, the extent of apical development, the possibility of root fractures, the integrity of the periodontal membrane and lamina dura, and the existence of periapical radiolucency.

Preoperative swelling warrants drainage through the canal; neither local analgesia nor rubber dam is indicated when opening such a tooth. Drainage, as with primary molar pulpectomy, is supplemented when indicated by antibiotic therapy and local measures, such as warm saline mouthrinses, and should occur for no longer than 24 h. The presence of haemorrhagic exudate should not alarm the student who may interpret this as vital tissue – rather, it is a blood-tinged inflammatory exudate draining from the periapical lesion. When acute signs and symptoms are absent, instrumentation is recommended at the first visit, using local analgesia and rubber-dam isolation. Even though the tooth may be non-vital, there may

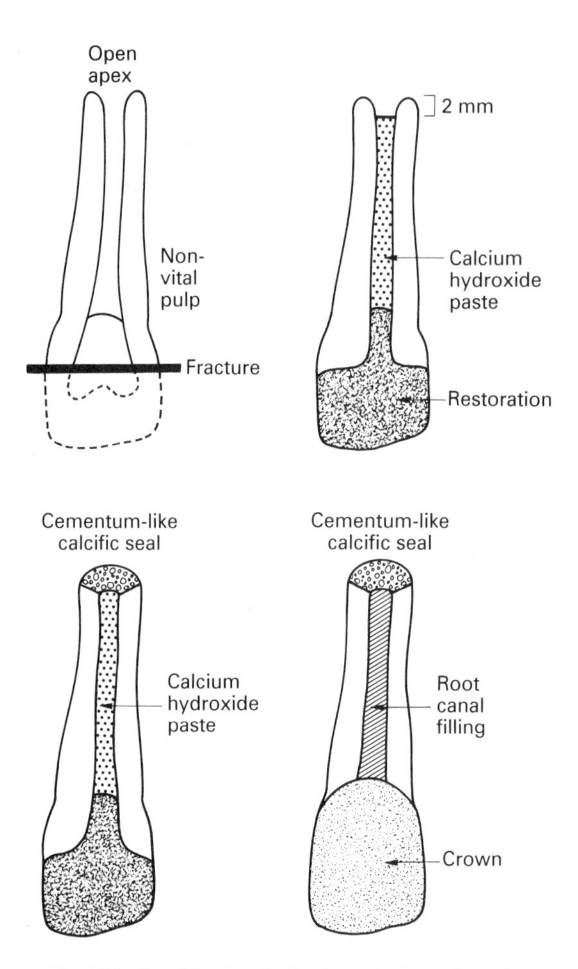

Fig. 20.8. Apexification. Induction of root-end repair.

be tags of vital tissue in the apical parts of the canal. This vital tissue may in fact be ingrowing granulation tissue, which is as sensitive as vital pulp.

Barbed broaches are used to remove debris and necrotic tissue from the canal. A diagnostic radiograph must be taken with an instrument in the canal to assess the correct root length. Care should be exercised to avoid penetration of the apex, since the induction of periapical haemorrhage and the formation of a blood clot do not expedite periapical repair (Ham, 1969). The maxillary central incisor's normal root length is between 22 and 24 mm from incisal edge to apex. Since the root is incompletely formed, the clinician should place the diagnostic instrument appropriately short. After the diagnostic radiograph has been obtained the canal should be debrided to within 2 mm of the radiographic apex. The wide and diverging canal encourages the use of large instruments from the outset. Because of this divergent shape, the file should be worked around the canal at the coronal access to ensure proper mechanical cleansing at the apex. Hedstrom files are used intermittently with copious irrigation by saline to remove infected dentine from the canal walls. The appearance of clean dentine filings should encourage the operator to terminate instrumentation. The canal is irrigated with saline and dried with paper points.

The canal should be filled with calcium hydroxide. The chances of success are greatly improved when the canal is filled in the absence of periapical inflammation (Ham, 1969; Steiner and Van Hassel, 1971). Pure calcium hydroxide is recommended for filling the canal(s) to within 2 mm of the radiographic apex, as its success

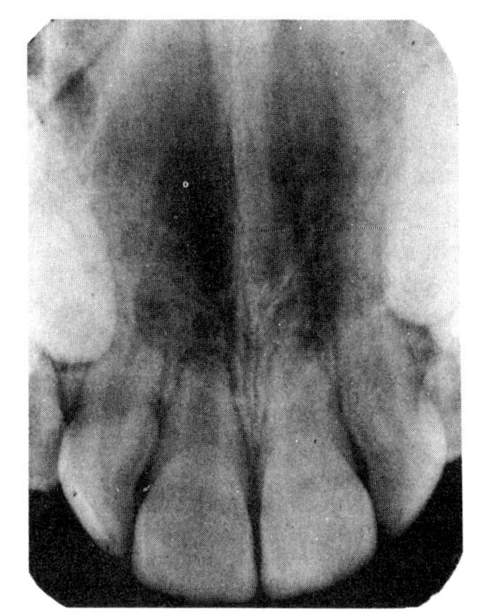

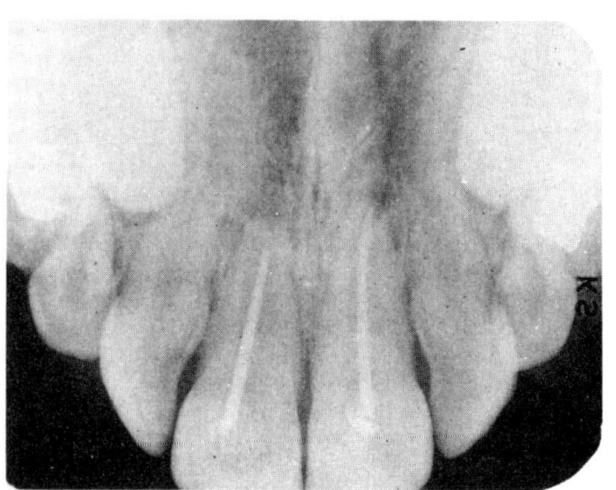

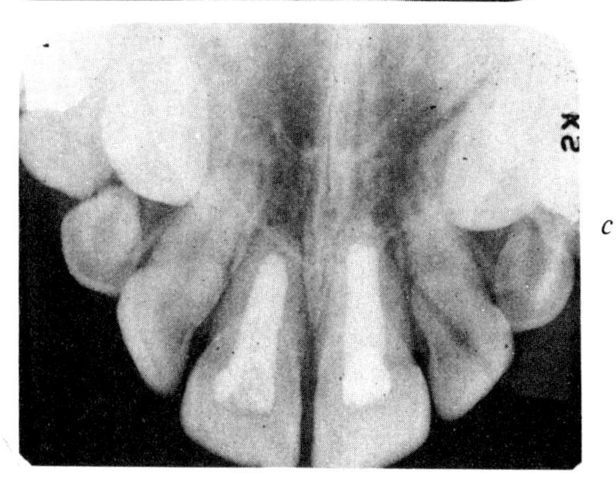

Fig. 20.9. Apexification. *a*, Preoperative, age 8. *b*, Calcium hydroxide paste in canal on loosely fitting gutta-percha point. Apices closing. *c*, Final root-canal fillings.

has been well documented (Frank, 1966; Rule and Winter, 1966); the commercially available products (e.g. Dycal) cannot be recommended because of their short working time. The powder should be mixed with saline to the consistency of a creamy paste. Premixed commercial preparations are also available. The paste can be introduced into the canal to the correct length with a rotary root-canal filler or with a large gutta-percha point. The latter technique lends itself to sealing the point in place at a predetermined distance, which ensures that the calcium hydroxide paste is carried by the tip of the point. Since calcium hydroxide itself is not radiopaque, it should be mixed with barium sulphate powder in equal quantities to facilitate postoperative evaluation, or use a commercial compound such as Hypocal (Ellman International, Inc., Howlett, New York).

Follow-up

The root canal should be re-dressed with calcium hydroxide every 3–4 months because it gradually disappears from the canal. Post-operative follow-up at 6-monthly intervals should include an evaluation of signs and symptoms as well as periapical radiographs. Comparison is made with the preoperative baseline radiograph to see if any change has occurred; the root appearance can also be compared with that of an untreated antimere. Frank (1966) described four types of repair:

(1) The apex is closed with definite though minimum recession of the canal.
(2) The apex is closed with no change in root space.
(3) A radiographically apparent calcific bridge forms just coronal to the apex.
(4) There is no radiographic evidence of apical closure but upon clinical instrumentation there is a definite stop at the apex, indicating some calcific repair.

As this apical calcification most frequently occurs in a horizontal rather than vertical fashion, the term 'apical repair' is preferred to 'apical closure'. However, an increase in the root length seldom occurs, in contrast to the continued root growth after calcium hydroxide pulpotomy in vital, young permanent teeth.

Calcific repair may be complete in 6 months

postoperatively, although it may take as long as 2 or 3 years. In the absence of signs and symptoms, it is imperative that the clinician be patient while awaiting apical repair. Too frequent re-entry into the tooth does not result in increased speed of apical repair, though refilling with calcium hydroxide should be done at 3–6-month intervals. The paste should be removed by further instrumentation and irrigation, the canal dried, and new paste inserted. A further diagnostic file radiograph to assess root length is redundant because accurate records should identify the correct working length of the canal. Once calcific repair has occurred, the calcium hydroxide paste is removed, the canal is irrigated, and the final root filling placed. This can be done at one visit. Because of the wide canal, emphasis must be placed upon lateral condensation to seal the canal adequately. Fortunately the danger of overfilling is eliminated by the apical calcific barrier.

When the calcium hydroxide is replaced, the presence of an apical stop must be checked at that same visit. It is not recommended to use endodontic files to do this as the apical barrier may be fragile in the early stages of its formation and can easily be perforated with sharp files. We recommend the use of gutta-percha points to test this. One point should be placed in the root canal and gently tapped down until an apical barrier is felt.

Histology

As identified from radiographic evaluation, root development is not normal. Rather, calcific material repairs the wide-open apex in a horizontal fashion. Hertwig's root sheath has not been observed in animal histological sections (Ham, 1969; Steiner and Van Hassel, 1971); this may account for the lack of continued apical development in a vertical dimension. The calcified material is similar to cementum and continuous with the cementum on the lateral root surfaces. Despite radiographic evidence of complete bridging, the calcific material has communicating channels between root canal and periapical tissues. This makes permanent root filling mandatory after apexification is complete to ensure a hermetic seal. While it is logical that the success of the completed root-canal treatment following apexification should be as high as conventional with root-canal treatment, this assumption has yet to be clinically documented.

Success

There is abundant clinical evidence of the technique's success over the short term (Frank, 1966; Rule and Winter, 1966). Zelterman et al. (1989) reported a study of partial pulpotomies in 15 permanent molars in children aged 7–17 years, using a calcium hydroxide preparation (Calxyl) placed over the excision sites and covered by zinc oxide, and with the teeth then restored. They showed that in 12 teeth followed-up for 12–99 months, dentinal bridge formation was evident radiographically. However, all these studies lack evidence of continued success after completion of root-canal therapy against the repaired apical tissue. It is hoped that the success will be similar to that of root-canal therapy for teeth with normally closed apices; this awaits long-term documentation. It may therefore be wise to warn the parent that apical surgery may be required at some time. This forewarning is useful should surgery be required later. Also, the parent should understand the need for long-term follow-up when the induction of root-end repair is initiated.

Cvek technique

Recently, a modification of the Cvek technique for permanent incisors has been reported for use on other permanent teeth, premolars and molars (Mejare and Cvek, 1993). The technique requires analgesia and the placement of rubber dam as described before. The carious material in the crown of the permanent tooth is removed with excavators or slow-running, round burs until an exposure occurs. The coronal pulp tissue in the pulp horns is removed using the gentle cutting technique (Granath and Hagman, 1971) to perform a pulpotomy involving the infected pulp horns. After arrest of the haemorrhage, pure calcium hydroxide is applied to the exposed pulp surfaces, ensuring that there is no blood clot involved. The cavity is then filled with a temporary or semipermanent restorative material and followed clinically and radiographically. The tooth should remain symptom-free at recall and radiographs should show formation of a secondary dentine bridge (*Fig.* 20.10).

Out of 31 teeth treated with this technique only two failures were reported over an average

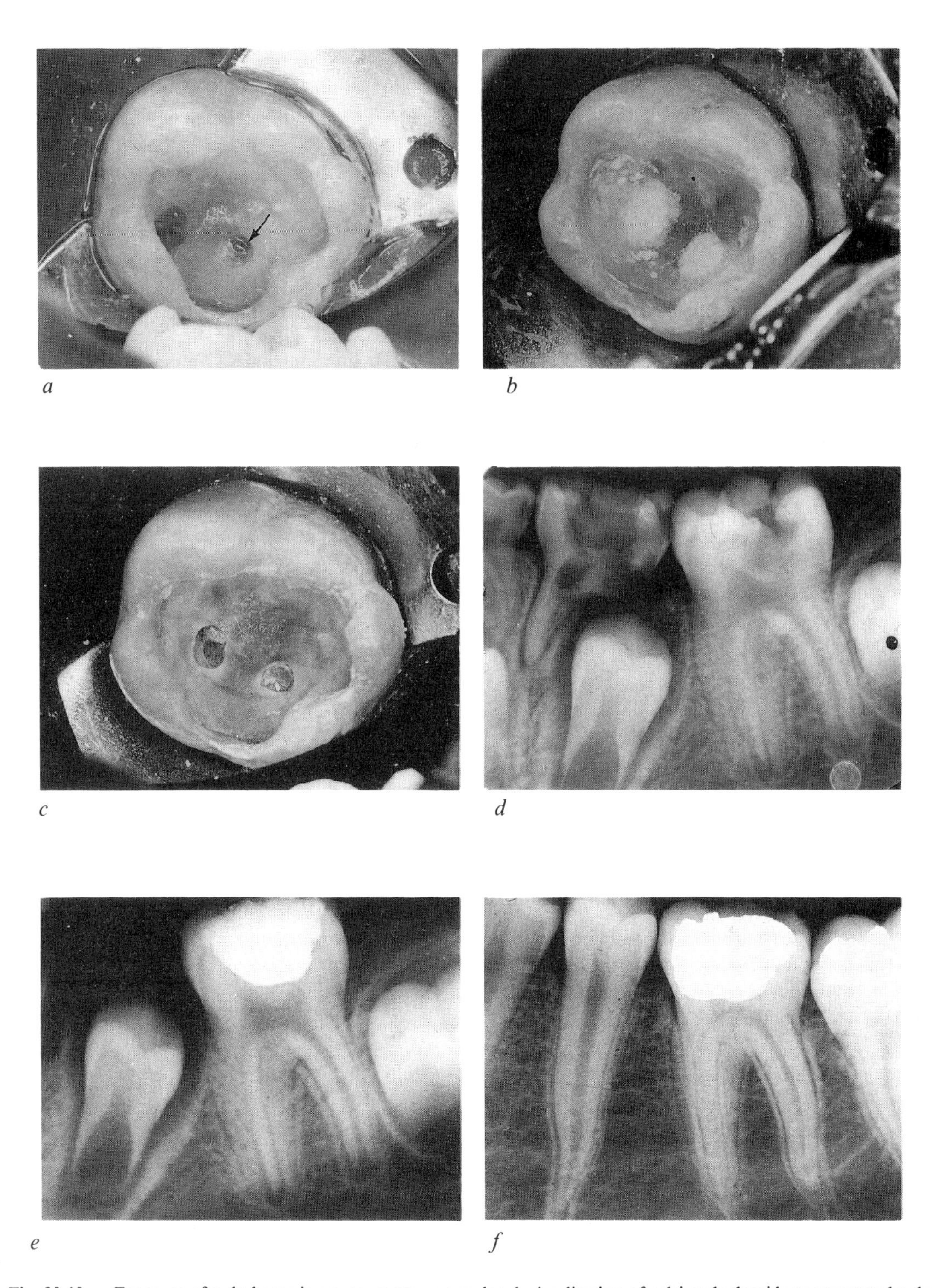

Fig. 20.10. *a*, Exposure of pulp horns in young permanent molar. *b*, Application of calcium hydroxide to amputated pulp horns. *c*, Appearance of hard tissue barriers 3 months after treatment. *d*, Radiograph showing carious exposure. *e*, Radiograph taken 6 months later showing evidence of pulpal repair. *f*, Radiograph 2 years later showing secondary dentine bridge. (Courtesy of Drs I. Mejare and M. Cvek.)

treatment time of 56 months. A variation of the technique does not require the removal of all carious or leathery dentine in one go. A step-wise technique, first advocated by Magnusson and Sundell (1977), is used, spread over two to three visits with approximately 2 weeks between visits. However, as in the report by Mejare and Cvek (1993), there did not appear to be any better rate of success for the single versus the multivisit technique. Therefore there seems to be no reason to prolong the treatment but to carry it out in one visit and restore the permanent tooth at the same time. It has recently been demonstrated that the frequency of pulp exposures is lower when the step-wise approach is used (Mejare, 1995).

Modified formocresol pulpotomy

Permanent molars only

This approach is now some years old and, while it has its advocates, we feel that the Mejare–Cvek technique is more appropriate, even for short-term treatment of permanent molars. However, a partially vital or non-vital permanent molar with open or closed apices must occasionally be maintained over the short term awaiting active orthodontic treatment. Conventional endodontics may be contraindicated if investment of time is to be minimal. Success has been reported using a modification of the formocresol pulpotomy in these teeth (Trask, 1972). The technique is identical to that described for primary teeth, except that the formocresol pellet is sealed permanently in the tooth. Postoperative sensitivity, for 24 h and controlled by an analgesic, has been observed in vital treated teeth. According to Trask, no deleterious effect has been reported from leaving the formocresol pellet in place for an extended time. On the other hand, a two-visit formocresol pulpotomy can be performed (*Figs* 20.11–20.13). The procedure is suggested as an alternative to extraction, and though it is no substitute for conventional root-canal therapy, it is an economic alternative in the short term. Its use can be encouraged in selected cases, prior to active orthodontic care, in the knowledge that the tooth can always be extracted if the treatment fails.

Recently, Housseni (1992) reported on 120 cases of formocresol pulpotomies in permanent molars, although the age of the patients was 16–25 years. After 10 years the success rate for teeth originally diagnosed as having acute pulpitis was 92.3% compared with 84% for those with chronic pulpitis. As noted above, the technique may have its uses when it is necessary to maintain permanent molars for a number of months.

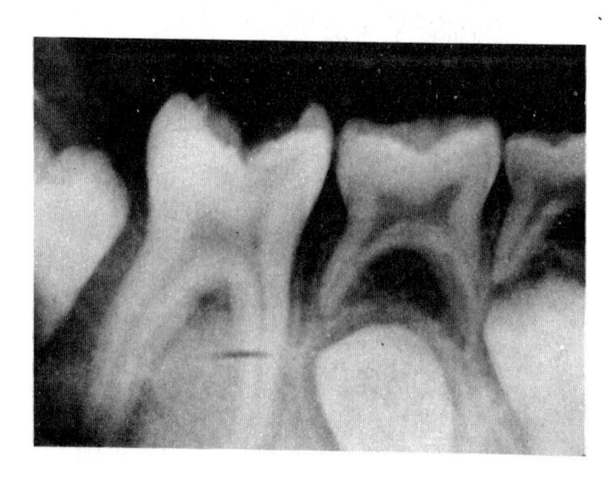

Fig. 20.11. Preoperative radiograph of non-vital first permanent molar. The poor quality film just shows a radiolucency around the incompletely formed distal apex. For economic reasons a two-visit formocresol pulpotomy was performed in this uncrowded mouth, see *Figs* 20.12 and 20.13.

Pulpectomy – closed apices – permanent teeth

Once the apices have been closed and the pulp is non-vital, root-canal therapy should be instituted (see texts on endodontics). It is also indicated in vital permanent teeth with exposures too large for pulp capping. Non-vital permanent teeth with periapical bone loss should always be treated conservatively before resorting to apical surgery. Such lesions will often repair in response to elimination of infection and effective sealing of the canal (*Figs* 20.14 and 20.15).

Very recently, bone morphogenic proteins have attracted interest in dentistry as a means of inducing the pulp tissue to regenerate dentine and hence heal the pulp faster after surgical removal of infected material (Ranly, 1994). A number of materials have been proposed and

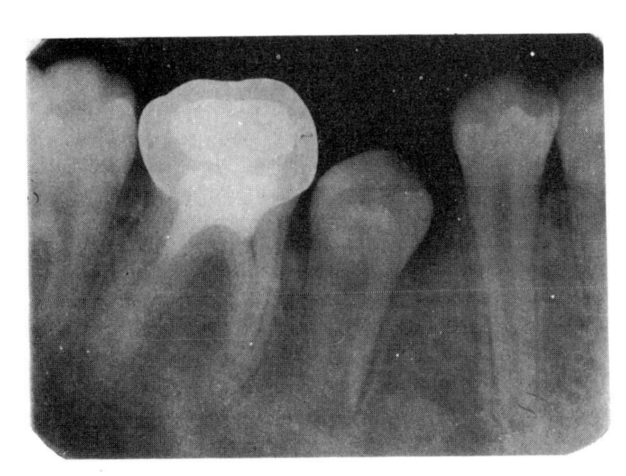

Fig. 20.12. One year after a two-visit formocresol pulpotomy the radiolucency (*Fig.* 20.11) has disappeared and the distal apex has closed.

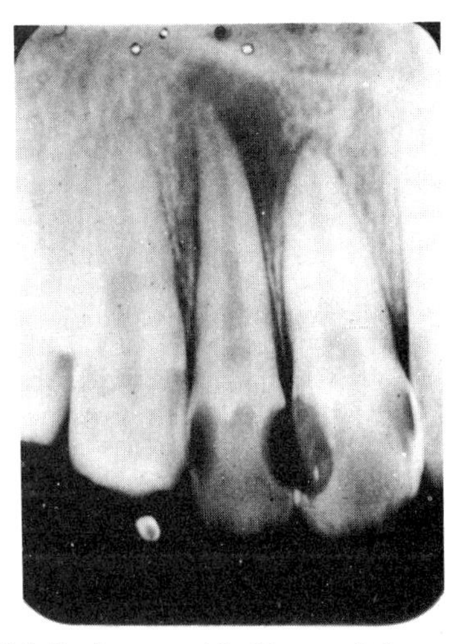

Fig. 20.14. Twelve-year-old with non-vital permanent central and lateral incisors. Note size of preoperative radiolucency.

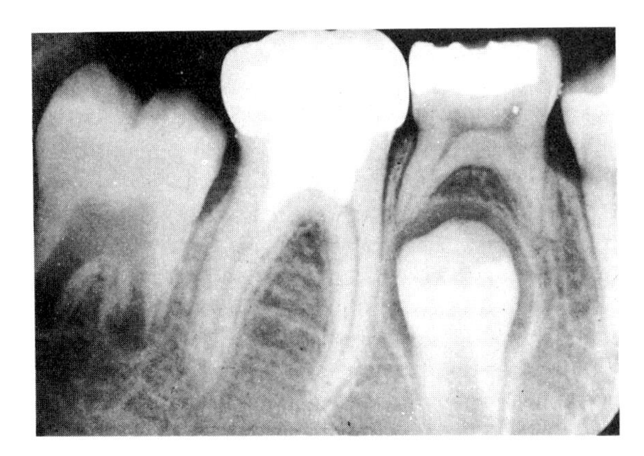

Fig. 20.13. The case illustrated in *Figs* 20.11 and 20.12, 3 years later. Periapical tissues are normal. Linear calcification has occurred in the root canals

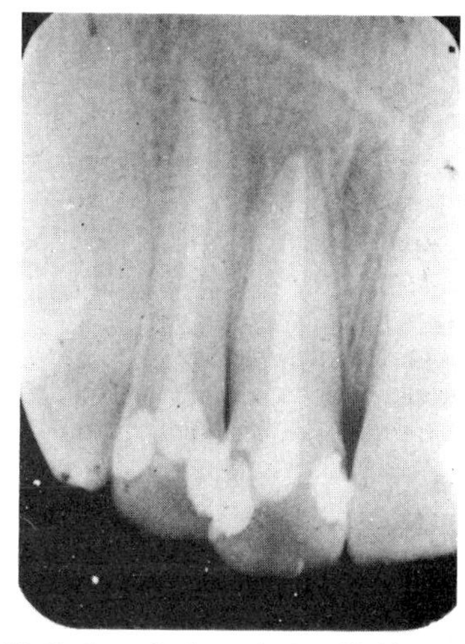

Fig. 20.15. Both teeth shown in *Fig.* 20.14 were treated by pulpectomy and root canal filling. Six-month postoperative radiograph demonstrates periapical bone repair.

tested but none as yet has reached the stage of clinical use, neither have any been used for clinical trials over long periods of time. However, studies have shown that reparative dentine can be induced biologically (Rutherford et al., 1993) and it is only a matter of time before they become available.

References

Crabb J. J. and Rock, W. P. (1971) Treatment planning in relation to the first permanent molar. *Br. Dent. J.* **131**, 396.

Frank A. L. (1966) Therapy for the divergent pulpless tooth by continued apical formation. *J. Am. Dent. Assoc.* **72**, 87.

Geller J. S., Klein A. I. and McDonald R. E. (1971) Association between dentinal sclerosis and pulpal floor thickness: television radiographic evaluation. *J. Am. Dent. Assoc.* **83**, 118.

Granath L. E. and Hagman G. (1971) Experimental pulpotomy in human bicuspids with reference to cutting technique. *Acta Odontol. Scand.* **29**, 153.

Ham I. W. (1969) A study of induced apical closure in pulpless teeth with open apices. Unpublished thesis, Indiana University.

Hargreaves J. A. (1969) Proceedings, Second International Symposium of Dentistry for Children, Sienna.

Housseni A. A. (1992) A clinical evaluation of root resorption by formocresol treatment in 120 cases of pulpotomy in permanent molars. *J. Clin. Pediatr. Dent.* **17**, 11.

Houston W. J. B., Stephen C. D. and Tulley W. J. (1992) *A Textbook of Orthodontics*. 2nd edn. London, Wright.

Jepperson K. (1971) Direct pulp capping in primary teeth – a long term investigation. *J. Int. Assoc. Dent. Child.* **2**, 10.

Kakehashi S., Stanley H. R. and Fitzgerald R. J. (1965) The effects of surgical exposures of dental pulps in germ-free and conventional laboratory rats. *Oral Surg.* **20**, 340.

Kennedy D. B. (1986) *Paediatric Operative Dentistry*. 3rd edn Ch. 17. Butterworth-Heinemann.

Kerkhove B. C., Herman S. C., Klein A. I. and McDonald R. E. (1967) A clinical and television densitometric evaluation of the indirect pulp capping technique. *J. Dent. Child.* **34**, 192

McDonald R. E. and Avery D. R. (1994) Treatment of deep caries, vital pulp exposure, and pulpless teeth. In: *Dentistry for the Child and Adolescent*. 6th edn. St Louis, Mosby.

Magnusson B. O. and Sundell S. O. (1977) Stepwise excavation of deep carious lesions in primary molars. *J. Int. Assoc. Dent. Child.* **8**, 36.

Mejare I. (1995) Comparison of step-wise and partial pulpotomy technique in permanent molars (personal communication).

Mejare I. and Cvek M. (1993) Partial pulpotomy in young permanent teeth with deep carious lesions. *Endodont. Dent. Traumat.* **9**, 238.

Morawa A. P. et al. (1975) Clinical evaluation of pulpotomies using dilute formocresol. *J. Dent. Child.* **42**, 360.

Patterson S. S. and Mitchell D. F. (1965) Calcific metamorphosis of the dental pulp. *Oral Surg.* **20**, 94

Ranly D. M. (1994) Pulpotomy therapy in primary teeth: new modalities for old rationales. *Pediatr. Dent.* **16**, 403.

Rule D. C. and Winter G. B. (1966) Root growth and apical repair subsequent to pulpal necrosis in children. *Br. Dent. J.* **120**, 586.

Rutherford R. B. et al. (1993) Induction of reparative dentine formation in monkeys by recombinant human osteogenic protein-1. *Archs Oral Biol.* **38**, 571.

Steiner J. C. and Van Hassel M. J. (1971) Experimental root apexification in primates. *Oral Surg.* **31**, 409.

Trask P. A. (1972) Formocresol pulpotomy on (young) permanent teeth. *J. Am. Dent. Assoc.* **85**, 1316.

Traubman L. (1967) A critical and television radiographic evaluation of indirect pulp capping. Unpublished thesis, Ohio State University.

Zeltermann U., Eliyahu M. and Sarnat H. (1989) Partial pulpotomy in carious permanent molars. *Am. J. Dent.* **2**, 147.

Index